Organ Transplantation

A Manual for Nurses

Barbara A. Williams, RN, BSN, is presently a staff nurse in the cardiovascular intensive care unit at Stanford University Hospital, Stanford, California. She was an assistant clinical nursing coordinator for 7 years in the cardiovascular intensive care unit at Stanford University Hospital. She has over 17 years' experience in intensive care nursing and has written guidelines, instructions, and flowsheets for nursing protocols.

Ms. Williams received her BSN degree with distinction from San Jose State University, San Jose, California. Her certificate as a Nurse Anesthetist is from Westend University Hospital, Berlin, West Germany. She presents lectures on transplant issues nationally and internationally. Ms. Williams is a member of the International Society for Heart Transplantation, the American Association of Critical Care Nurses, and the American Heart Association.

Kathleen L. Grady, RN, MS, is the clinical nurse specialist for heart and heart–lung transplantation at Loyola University Medical Center and clinical assistant professor at the Marcella Niehoff School of Nursing, Loyola University, Chicago. She has over 18 years of experience in intensive care nursing, and for 14 of those years she has had experience with heart transplantation.

Mrs. Grady participated in the development of the heart/heart–lung transplantation program at Loyola. She has published numerous articles on heart transplantation, and she lectures locally, regionally, and nationally on transplantation. She is co-investigator on a $1.2 million National Institutes of Health grant for "Predictors of Quality of Life after Transplantation." Mrs. Grady received her BSN from Mercy College of Detroit, graduating summa cum laude, and her MS from the University of California, San Francisco, graduating magna cum laude. She is enrolled in doctoral education at Loyola University and is seeking her PhD in Nursing. Mrs. Grady is a member of many professional organizations, including the International Society for Heart Transplantation, American Heart Association, American Association of Critical Care Nurses, and the Midwest Nursing Research Society.

Doris M. Sandiford-Guttenbeil, RN, BSN, is a staff nurse in the Cardiovascular Intensive Care Unit at Stanford University Hospital, Stanford, California. Her professional career encompasses over 20 years of nursing experience. She has presented lectures on the left ventricular assist device, published an article on heart transplantation, and written various nursing guidelines.

Mrs. Sandiford-Guttenbeil received her RN diploma from Chicago Wesley Memorial Hospital School of Nursing and her Bachelor of Science and Nursing degree from Northwestern University. She is certified in intra-aortic balloon pump (IABP) and left ventricular assist device system (LVAS) and serves on the Adult Critical Care Transport Team. Mrs. Sandiford-Guttenbeil also serves as a preceptor and presents various inservices.

Organ Transplantation

A Manual for Nurses

Barbara A. Helene Williams, RN, BSN

Kathleen L. Grady, RN, MS

Doris M. Sandiford-Guttenbeil, RN, BSN

Editors

Springer Publishing Company
New York

Springer Publishing Company, Inc.
536 Broadway
New York, NY 10012

91 92 93 94 95 / 5 4 3 2 1

Library of Congress Cataloging in Publication Data
Organ transplantation : a manual for nurses / Barbara A. Williams,
    Kathleen L. Grady, Doris Sandiford-Guttenbeil, editors.
        p. cm.
    Includes index.
    ISBN 0-8261-7230-X : $48.95
    1. Transplantation of organs, tissues, etc.—Nursing.
I. Williams, Barbara A. II. Grady, Kathleen L. III. Sandiford-
Guttenbeil, Doris.
    [DNLM: 1. Organ Transplantation—nursing.   WY 161 068]
RD129.8.074   1991
610.73'677—dc20
DNLM/DLC
for Library of Congress   91–4720
                                                              CIP

Printed in the United States of America

Any medical or therapeutic agent or procedure described in this book
should be applied by the practitioner under appropriate supervision in
accordance with professional standards of care and the unique
circumstances of each situation. Medically qualified readers are advised to
consult the instructions and information included in package inserts of
each drug or therapeutic agent before administration, particularly when
using new or infrequently used drugs.

This book is dedicated to all organ donors, recipients, and health care providers.

For the things we have to learn before we can do them, we learn by doing them.

—Aristotle

CONTENTS

Part III Special Issues in Transplantation

FOREWORD

This volume is extremely important for the entire current and future field of transplantation. Nursing care of the patient before and after transplantation is the focus of this book, and probably nowhere in medicine is the importance of nursing so clearly defined as in the care of the transplant recipient.

The authors provide significant and pertinent information for nurses just beginning their activities in transplantation as well as for those experienced in the field. Whereas the transplant physicians and surgeons, the social workers, and various others are important in the transplantation project, the nursing staff is still the most important component of the total picture.

This book is strongly recommended, even for the families of transplant recipients, who must carry forward into the months and years after the transplant work begun by an expert nursing staff.

All in all, the information contained in this book has a very special pertinence to all aspects of care for the transplant recipient, whether it be kidney, heart, heart–lung, lung, liver, or bone marrow.

NORMAN E. SHUMWAY, MD
Professor and Chairman
of Cardiovascular Surgery,
Stanford University School
of Medicine
Stanford, California

FOREWORD

Organ transplantation has come a long way from pure research, speculation, and science fiction fantasy to accepted medical therapy, life extension, and a chance for continued life for thousands of dying patients.

The technology and research that has made organ transplantation possible has changed the options of many critically ill patients. This technology has also increased and broadened the opportunities in which to explore and deliver nursing care. New skills and theory are now required of the nurse expected to deliver total care for the patient undergoing organ transplantation.

It has added a tremendously exciting area of specialty in both medicine and nursing. To become expert in this area is a challenge to nursing. This book can assist those who have not had the expanded experiences in organ transplantation.

It is written by clinical experts in each area of organ transplantation. These clinicians have each performed a role in "a bridge to life" for many. Their personal and professional experiences, combined with their vigorous study of organ transplantation makes the information in the book extremely accurate and of great value. Every area of transplant nursing is thoroughly explored and explained.

Having been involved in cardiac transplantation as a staff nurse, head nurse, and presently a nurse administrator, I am proud and excited to introduce these authors to all who are interested in promoting or delivering expert care to the transplant patient. The book's authors have presented a thorough, expert clinical approach to nursing care, enabling nurses to take a major role in building the "bridge to life,"—transplantation.

LAUREL GUNDERSON, RN, MPA
Assistant Director of Nursing
Critical Care Region
Stanford University Medical Center
Stanford, California

PREFACE

As medical teams from hospitals across the country perform increasing numbers of organ transplantations and as new centers emerge, a nursing book focusing on transplantation is needed. We designed this book for health care professionals, especially nurses, who care for transplant patients and their families.

Organ Transplantation: A Manual for Nurses addresses the nurse's role and responsibilities regarding the transplant candidate's acceptance into the program, pre- and postoperative care, discharge planning, and rehabilitation.

We discuss nursing diagnoses, interventions, and patient outcomes for various transplanted organs, including kidney, heart, heart–lung, lung, liver, and bone marrow. Immunological aspects of transplantation, infection control, and donor procurement are discussed in separate chapters. Neonatal/infant heart transplantation and pediatric organ transplantation chapters have been included and add uniqueness to our book with their special nursing care considerations. A chapter on the application of mechanical assist devices as a bridge to transplantation describes new approaches to patient management and nursing care. Other important chapters focus on psychosocial issues and quality of life after transplantation. We enthusiastically share our experiences in this new frontier with our nursing colleagues.

Our book provides a foundation of nursing care for the novice transplant nurse and sharpens nursing management skills for the experienced transplant nurse. Better-educated nurses make better nurses! Nurses are the transplant patients' advocates and are accountable for their care delivery. Without knowledgeable and experienced nursing care, there would not be organ transplantation. Nursing is a vital link in this dynamic area of health care. Nurses need to actively continue to stimulate new concepts and nursing–care techniques.

ACKNOWLEDGMENTS

This book came together with the contributions from many people. I am grateful to all. The cooperation given by Kathleen L. Grady and Doris M. Sandiford-Guttenbeil has been memorable. Their speedy and continued labor is appreciated. I thank you.

Dr. Shumway is a strong advocate for nurses. His interest and participation were important for the conception of this book. I thank you.

Laurel Gunderson along with the North-ICU nursing staff helped to foster an attitude that lead toward the basic idea of this book. They have provided an environment for my continued education and growth. I thank you all.

The devotion, intense efforts, and expertise of the contributing authors made possible the first hand, in-depth presentation of the subject matter. I thank you all.

Donna Dowdney deserves a special "thank you" for her editorial assistance, inspiration, and sage counsel.

Lois Manning and Margaret Fisher provided great assistance and patience in preparation of the manuscript. I thank you.

Springer Publishing Company editors Philip Rappaport and Pamela Lankas calmed waters from the contract negotiation to the printing. I thank you both.

Terry C. Williams for his unequivocal support throughout the process of this book. I thank you.

Norman H. Lehrer for his strong encouragement to write this book. I thank you.

BARBARA A. H. WILLLIAMS

I deeply appreciate all the help and support given over the past three years that enabled this book to be published. Namely, I wish to thank the publishers, the contributors, my co-workers and friends, and John and Luisa, my husband and daughter.

DORIS M. SANDIFORD-GUTTENBEIL

I would like to thank Roque Pifarre, MD, Professor and Chairman, Department of Thoracic and Cardiovascular Surgery, Surgical Director, Heart Transplantation, and Maria Rosa Costanzo-Nordin, MD, Associate Professor, Department of Medicine, and Medical Director, Heart Transplantation, Loyola University of Chicago, for their support and encouragement in the writing of our book.

I would also like to thank Barbara Williams and Doris Sandiford-Guttenbeil, my editor colleagues from California, with whom I have worked closely as our book has developed and grown. The editors from Springer Publishing Co. have encouraged and facilitated our efforts.

All of the authors have been generous in giving of themselves to this worthy undertaking. A very special thank you to the Loyola University of Chicago, Hines Veteran's Administration, and University of Illinois authors who shared their time and expertise in bringing this book to fruition: Janet L. Cohan, Eileen G. Collins, Bonnie B. Grusk, Elizabeth Hubbell, Pamela K. Jacobsson, Anne Jalowiec, Rosanne Perez-Woods, and Kathleen M. Siebold.

Finally, I would also like to dedicate this book to my family (Patrick, my husband, and Sean and Erin, our children) for whom I have undertaken this endeavor.

KATHLEEN L. GRADY

CONTRIBUTORS

Marguerite E. Brown, RN, BSN, received a bachelor of science degree in nursing from Columbia University in 1972. She began working at Stanford University Medical Center in 1973. Her positions have included assistant clinical nursing coordinator for the cardiovascular intensive care unit, and for the past 6 years she has been the donor coordinator for the heart, heart–lung and lung transplant program.

Catherine M. Cebulski, RN, BSN, was graduated from Salve Regina College in Newport, Rhode Island, with a bachelor of science degree in nursing. Ms. Cebulski has been working at the University of California in San Francisco for the past 6 years on the adult hematology/oncology/bone marrow transplant unit. She has been the head nurse of this unit for the past 2 years.

Janet L. Cohan, RN, BSN, MS, is presently a clinical specialist in the Kidney Transplant Clinic at the University of Illinois Hospital in Chicago. She graduated from Ohio State University at Columbus and received her master of science degree in medical surgical nursing from Rush University in Chicago.

Bernice Coleman, RN, MSN, CCRN, is a clinical nurse specialist in cardiovascular surgery at Cedars-Sinai Medical Center in Los Angeles, working with the lung transplant team. She received her undergraduate degree in nursing from the University of Bridgeport in Connecticut, in 1979 and her master's degree, with a clinical concentration in cardiovascular surgery, from Yale University School of Nursing in 1983.

Eileen G. Collins, RN, MSN, is a clinical nurse specialist for the heart transplant program at Hines Veterans Administration Hospital, Hines, Illinois. She received her BSN and MSN degree from Loyola University of Chicago.

Elizabeth Ann (Betsy) Collins, RN, is a care review coordinator and infection control nurse at Stanford University Medical Center in Stanford, California. She was graduated from DePaul Hospital School of Nursing in St. Louis, and received certification in infection control after studies at the University of California, San Diego.

Vicki L. Fioravante, RN, is a transplant coordinator at Pacific Presbyterian Medical Center, San Francisco, specializing in liver transplantation. She has published articles and has delivered numerous presentations in that area of nursing. She received her nursing diploma from Robert Packer Hospital School of Nursing In Sayer, Pennsylvania.

Bonnie B. Grusk, RN, MSN, is a nurse clinician with the cardiac transplant program at Loyola University Medical Center in Maywood, Illinois, and has over 5 years experience in caring for heart transplant candidates and recipients. She received her BSN degree from Illinois Wesleyan University, and her MSN degree at Loyola University of Chicago.

Eleanor Anne Hedenkamp, RN, MS, is a pediatric cardiovascular clinical nurse specialist at Stanford University Hospital, Stanford, California. She received her bachelor of science degree from Stanford University School of Nursing, and her master of science degree in maternal child health was completed at the University of California, San Francisco.

Elizabeth A. Hubbell, RN, has been the coordinator of therapeutic apheresis at Loyola University Medical Center since 1982. She has served a term as president of the Chicago-based Apheresis Forum and remains on the board of directors for the Forum.

Pamela K. Jacobsson, RN, BSN, MS, is a clinical specialist in the Division of Transplantation at the University of Illinois Health Science Center in Chicago. She was graduated from the University of Wisconsin at Madison with a bachelor of science and nursing degree and later received her master of science degree at Depaul University in Chicago.

Anne Jalowiec, RN, Ph D, is an associate professor in community health nursing at the Niehoff School of Nursing, Loyola University of Chicago. She received her master of science and nursing degree as a family practitioner and her doctorate in nursing science from the University of Illinois.

Joyce Johnston, RN, BSN, was graduated from Loma Linda University, Loma Linda, California, with a bachelor of science in nursing. She has been involved in the development of the pediatric cardiac transplant program at Loma Linda University Medical Center since November 1986 in the capacity of nurse clinician.

Nancy D. Meister, MSW, has been the transplant team social worker at the University of Arizona Medical Center, Tucson, Arizona, from 1983 to 1989. She is currently a clinical social worker at the Cancer Center at the University of Arizona. She received a master's degree in social work from the University of California, Berkeley, in 1968. She is an ACSW and board-certified diplomate in clinical social work.

Danielle Newman, RN, is the pediatric kidney transplant coordinator at the Medical Center at the University of California, San Francisco. She was graduated from the College of the Desert in 1983 with an AA degree in nursing.

Johanna Salamandra, RN, CCTC, CPTC, is the clinical lung transplant coordinator for the Lung Transplant Program at Cedars- Sinai Medical Center in Los Angeles,

California. She received her nursing diploma from the Hospital of the University of Pennsylvania School of Nursing in Philadelphia in 1976 and has 11 years of critical care experience.

Kathleen M. Siebold, RN, BSN, CPTC, is the senior procurement coordinator at Loyola University Medical Center in Maywood, Illinois. She received her BSN from Marcella Niehoff School of Nursing at Loyola University, and she is currently pursuing a master's degree in nursing.

Kimberly Stephens, RN, BSN, MSN, received her bachelor's degree from Mount St. Mary's College in Los Angeles and her master's degree in nephrology nursing from the University of California, San Francisco. She has worked as a renal transplant clinical nurse specialist at Stanford University Hospital, and is actively involved in the American Nephrology Nurses Association.

Karen Ulfig, RN, BSN, MSN, received her bachelor's degree from the University of Michigan and her master's degree from the University of California, San Francisco. Formerly, she was a pediatric BMT clinical nurse specialist at the University of California, Los Angeles.

Carol S. Viele, RN, MS, has her bachelor of science degree and master of science degree from the University of Michigan. Her current title is clinical nurse specialist, hematology-oncology- bone marrow transplant, at the Medical Center of the University of California, San Francisco, where she has worked since 1981 in her role.

Rosanne H. Perez-Woods, Ed D, RN, CPNP, is the Niehoff Chair and professor of maternal child nursing at Loyola University of Chicago. Dr. Woods received her BS from St. Xavier College. Her MSN is from Indiana University in Indianapolis, and her certificate as a pediatric nurse practitioner is from Methodist Hospital and Indiana University. Her doctorate, with a double major in education and nursing, is from Indiana University in Bloomington.

PART I

Fundamentals of Organ Transplantation

CHAPTER 1

ORGAN PROCUREMENT

Kathleen M. Siebold
Marguerite E. Brown
Vicki L. Fioravante

Over the past 10 years, the public and health care professionals have found themselves immersed in the drama of transplantation through newspaper, magazine, and television accounts. The media's efforts have made people aware of the successes of transplant operations and the critical shortage of donor organs. Table 1.1 illustrates the rapid growth in transplants performed in the United States.

Factors limiting the availablity of donor organs can be addressed through education of the public and health care professionals. Health care professionals can identify potential donors and initiate the organ donation process in a timely manner. Critical care nurses are the vital link for potential donors and their families in relation to this process.

This chapter is an overview of the organ and tissue donation process. Details of U.S. legislation, brain death declaration, clinical management of the organ donor, and specific information on surgical techniques in procurement will be addressed. It is hoped that knowledge gained from this chapter will allow the nurse to participate in the organ donation process and continue to help advance the science and art of transplantation nursing.

LEGISLATIVE ISSUES

The Uniform Anatomical Gift Act (UAGA), adopted in 1972 by all 50 states, was the first legislation to have a major impact on organ and tissue donation. This law allowed an individual over the age of 18 to donate all or any part of

TABLE 1.1 Organ Transplantations Performed in the United States

Organ	Year				
	1984	1985	1986	1987	1988
Kidney	6968	7695	8976	8967	9123
Heart	346	731	1368	1438	1647
Heart–Lung	22	30	45	41	74
Liver	308	605	924	1199	1680
Lung	N/A	N/A	N/A	9	31

Source: 1984 through 1987 information from Department of Health and Human Services. The 1988 statistics are from the UNOS Scientific Registry, reprinted with permission.

his/her body for the advancement of medical or dental science, therapy, or transplantation. In the absence of a previously signed consent or directive from the deceased, the law stipulated the order of persons who could grant permission for the donation.

This legislation described the use of a donor card, which notes what an individual would like to donate and requires the signature of the donor and two witnesses. Despite the fact that the donor card serves as a legal document, in some states, the Organ Procurement Organization (OPO) or hospital will request written consent from the next of kin before any recovery of organs and/or tissues can begin. Some states are recommending an amendment to their UAGA that would recognize the written wishes of the deceased over those of the family.

Subsequent transplant legislation included Public Law 92-603, adopted in 1972, which created the End Stage Renal Disease (ESRD) program. This legislation provided, for the first time, federal responsibility for financing care for all persons with irreversible kidney failure and for reimbursing most of the costs associated with kidney dialysis and transplantation services.

Legislative efforts were again activated by the rapid growth in organ transplantation in the 1980s, when the Food and Drug Administration approved use of the immunosuppressive drug cyclosporine A. Use of this drug improved extrarenal organ morbidity and mortality rates. Hence, during this time there was rapid growth in the development of new transplant programs. Subsequently, Congress established a federal task force on organ transplantation in October 1984 in response to growing public concern about the shortage of donor organs and the efficiency of organ procurement. This task force wrote a report in 1986 that addressed many complex issues relating to the field of organ transplantation. The task force made recommendations on the following topics:

1. Organ donation and procurement.
2. Organ sharing within the United States.
3. Access by patients to donor organs and transplant procedures.
4. Diffusion and adoption of organ transplant technology.
5. Future directions and research issues (Task Force on Organ Transplantation, 1986).

The task force also concluded that many opportunities for organ donation were being lost because families were not aware of their potential to donate or were too distraught at the time of a family member's death to think of that option. Therefore, it was recommended that routine-inquiry policies be adopted by all hospitals, reflecting a trend that had already begun in many states.

Congress then incorporated task force recommendations into the Omnibus Reconciliation Act (OBRA) of 1986. This law provides that hospitals participating in Medicare and Medicaid develop written protocols to identify and refer potential organ and tissue donors and to

1. Assure that families of potential donors are made aware of their option to donate organs and tissues or their option to decline to donate.
2. Encourage discretion and sensitivity with respect to the circumstances, views and beliefs of such families.
3. Require that an organ procurement organization designated by the Secretary of Health and Human Services be notified of potential organ donors (AHA, AMA, UNOS, 1988).

This condition of participation by the hospitals coincides with the routine-inquiry approach. OBRA became effective November 21, 1987. Individual states have also adopted versions of routine-inquiry laws, and compliance with federal law does not exempt hospitals from the requirements that may be applicable within their state law.

BRAIN DEATH

Because confusion still exists in understanding the difference between severely brain-injured patients who are in a comatose state and those who have sustained cessation of their entire brain function, a clear understanding of the definition of brain death along with its clinical findings is essential. Nurses are the vital link with all organ donor families for questions and special concerns they may have during this tragic time.

With the advent of ventilators and new drugs, heartbeat, blood pressure, and respiration can continue following the loss of all brain functions. Despite all efforts to maintain the donor's circulation, irreversible cardiac arrest usually occurs within 48 to 72 hours in adults and up to 10 days in children (Soifer & Gelb, 1989).

In the late 1960s, physicians were faced with the ethical dilemma of removing patients from life support without strong medical clarity on the definition of brain death. In the United States, a definition of irreversible coma was proposed in 1968 by the Ad Hoc Committee of the Harvard Medical School. The clinical characteristics described by this group include the following:

1. Unreceptivity and unresponsivity, even under the most intensely painful stimuli.
2. No movement or breathing.
3. No reflexes.
4. Flat electroencephalogram (EEG)—not necessary but of confirmatory value; repeated at least 24 hours later with no change.

The validity of such data depends on the exclusion of two conditions: (a) hypothermia (temperature below [32.2°C]) and (b) removal of central nervous system depressants, such as barbiturates (Ad Hoc Committee, 1984).

The conclusions of this committee had a major impact on physicians, theologians, and ethicists; and the concept known conversationally as "brain death" emerged (Bernat, 1987).

More recently, in 1981, the President's Commission for the Study of Ethical Problems in Medicine and Biomedical and Behavior Research published guidelines for the determination of death. This group reaffirmed the clinical criteria for the determination of brain death, once again asserting that laboratory confirmation such as EEG and cerebral angiography are desirable when objective documentation is needed to substantiate the clinical findings. This commission stipulated that the following model statute be adopted in every jurisdiction:

Uniform Determination of Death Act

An individual who has sustained either irreversible cessation of circulatory and respiratory functions or irreversible cessation of all functions of the entire brain, including the brain stem, is dead.

The determination of death must be made in accordance with accepted medical standards (President's Commission, 1981).

This definition has been endorsed by many professional organizations and has even been adopted as part of many state laws on brain death. For use as accepted medical standards and for compliance with state laws, many physicians consider the clinical criteria in evaluating if a patient is brain dead.

Clinical Criteria

The following clinical criteria apply to all patients: (a) coma and absent cerebral function, (b) absent brain stem reflexes, and (c) apnea testing.

Coma and Absent Cerebral Function. The cause of coma must be established and be sufficient to account for the loss of brain function. In addition, the patient must exhibit complete loss of consciousness, vocalization, and spontaneous movement, with the exception of purely spinal reflex withdrawal. Deep tendon reflexes may be maintained because they are integrated at a purely spinal level (Bernat, 1987). Patients without brain function have no response to even the most painful stimuli.

Absent Brain Stem Reflexes. Absence of brain stem function requires a perceptive and experienced physician using adequate stimuli (President's Commission, 1981). Brain stem functions that should be tested include the following:

Test	Response in Brain Dead Patients
Pupillary light	Lack of constriction with light, fully dilated pupils
Corneal	No blink or absence of spontaneous eye movement
	Absence of doll's-eyes response (eyes don't move with respect to the head position)
Oculovestibular and oculocephalic	Absence of spontaneous eye movement and negative reflexes
Oropharyngeal	Absence of pharyngeal movement (no gag or swallow)
Respiratory	Absence of respiratory effort when removed from the ventilator

For these brain stem reflexes to be tested,

1. The patient must not be significantly hypothermic.
2. Should not have significant levels of central nervous system depressants circulating in the body.
3. Patients with severe shock should be treated with vasopressors and or fluids to achieve a minimal systolic blood pressure of 90 mmHg (Bernat, 1987).

Apnea Testing. Cessation of brain stem function should include the absence of respiratory reflexes. An accepted method of apnea testing involves ventilation with pure oxygen or an oxygen and carbon dioxide mixture for 10 minutes prior to withdrawal of the ventilator. This is then followed by a passive flow of oxygen via the endotracheal tube. This procedure allows $PaCO_2$ to rise without hazardous hypoxia. Hypercapnia adequately stimulates respiratory effort within 30 seconds when $PaCO_2$ is greater than 60 mmHg (President's Commission, 1981). Testing of arterial blood can help to confirm this level. Apnea is said to be present if there are no respiratory efforts, gasping, sighing, or hiccuping during this time.

Exclusions

The brains of infants and children have increased resistance to damage and may recover substantial function even after exhibiting unresponsiveness on neurological examination for longer periods compared with adults (President's Commission, 1981). Therefore, it remains controversial to apply brain-death tests to patients under 5 years of age. However, it has been concluded that adult tests probably are valid in the child over 12 months of age. In younger children and neonates, it is highly desirable to perform confirmatory tests along with extending the interval between exams (President's Commission, 1981).

Observation

The time interval between serial examinations is important in proving that whole brain dysfunction is irreversible. It is recommended that the length of the interval depends on the clinical situation and age of the patient. For example:

Children 7 days to 2 months
Two examinations and EEGs separated by at least 48 hours.
Children 2 months to 1 year
Two examinations and EEGs separated by at least 24 hours.
Children over 1 year–adults
1. If cause of coma is known, 12 hours, and in the presence of a positive confirmatory test, time can be decreased to 6 hours.
2. In the instance of a diffuse hypoxic-ischemic insult after cardiopulmonary arrest, the interval should be *24* hours (Special Task Force, 1987).

Confirmatory Tests

Confirmatory tests are used as aids in the diagnosis of brain death and are not required to confirm the diagnosis of brain death if the clinical criteria are fulfilled.

Intracranial Blood Flow. Intracranial blood flow ceases in brain death, and the demonstration of absent intracranial blood flow is an excellent confirmatory test (Bernat, 1987). Intracranial blood flow can be shown to be absent using contrast angiography, radionuclide angiography, and xenon computed tomography (CT). Contrast angiography has the major disadvantage of requiring an invasive and potentially high-risk procedure, whereas radionuclide angiography with portable gamma camera is the most sensitive, easiest, safest, and most widely available confirmatory blood flow test (Bernat, 1987).

Electroencephalograms. The EEG is not an ideal confirmatory test because it produces too many false-positive and false-negative results (Bernat, 1987). Electrocerebral silence may be seen in conditions other than brain death. These false-positive results may occur when there is a reversible metabolic or toxic disorder and when there is a bilateral hemispheric infarction sparing the brain stem (Bernat, 1987). False-negative determinations can also occur when the electroencephalographer cannot distinguish between the actual brain waves and the many types of artifacts resulting from intensive care unit (ICU) machines (Bernat, 1987).

ORGAN PROCUREMENT IN WESTERN EUROPE

Europe is unique in the area of organ procurement. Since there are a multitude of countries, it would seem almost impossible to foresee the development of one network for the distribution of organs. However, Western Europe has several networks that work together.

The organ-matching service located in the Netherlands is called the European Transplant Service (ETS). For registration of kidney patients and allocation of donor kidneys, this service is utilized by the Netherlands, Belgium, Luxembourg, Germany, and Austria. The United Kingdom Transplant Service (UKTS) serves the United Kingdom and Ireland. France Transplant and the Rhone-Mediteranée serve France, and Scandia Transplant Service provides services for Norway, Sweden, and Denmark. Northern Italy is covered by Italy Transplant. Spain does not yet have a national organ-matching system, although the Catalonian region is well organized. Each organization serves its respective area; however, if there is no suitable recipient within that area, the organ will be offered to another transplant service. This provides for a large amount of international exchange to Eastern Europe or even further. The above organ-matching services encourage kidney sharing.

Extrarenal organ sharing is managed differently. Each heart, heart–lung, and liver recipient is registered within its own organ-matching system. If the patient's condition becomes critical, the organ-matching system, on request, registers the patient with other European services. As with kidneys, each service retains the right to treat its own population first. If there is not a suitable match, the organ can be offered to another country or system in the hope of benefiting the recipient listed as urgent.

In Western Europe there are only a small number of extrarenal transplant centers, so patients who need a heart, heart–lung, or liver transplant may travel to another country, where the treatment is available. Under the European Economic Community (EEC) agreements, patients are entitled to treatment in another member country free of charge to the patient, and reimbursement is made at the government level. As more programs are established, fewer patients will need to travel to another country for end-stage organ failure.

Western Europe is also faced with gaps between supply and demand for donor organs. Some countries have adopted policies of opting in. Under an opting-in system, organs are retrieved in two specific situations. First, the prior consent of the deceased is binding, and second, authority to remove organs from the deceased person who did not give approval or disapproval is granted to a close relative. In contrast, Austria and Belgium have adopted an opting-out system, in which it is assumed that the patient would have wished to be a donor unless he/she had stated otherwise during his/her lifetime. Little improvement in donor supply has been seen using these methods of request. European programs are currently interested in required request referral systems, as practiced in the United States, but little progress has been made toward that end.

Coordinators within the United States have assisted European coordinators with compilation of educational material for public and professional use. It is believed that the development of educational programs will help reduce the potential for disruption and confusion within ICUs and therefore increase the number of multiple organ donors (Wight, 1988). While disruption may be decreased with education in the ICUs, the potential for confusion still exists within the operating room.

The operating rooms in Western Europe have the potential for accommodating four surgical teams who speak different languages. A unique program pioneered in Cambridge, England, provide's one single team that is trained to remove and preserve all organs and tissues for transplantation. It has met with much success and it is hoped that more teams will be trained throughout Europe to provide such services.

Western Europe is making strides in the right direction, toward organization of their transplant networks. The problem of language is unique to Western Europe, and one program has instituted an effective solution. However, like the United States, problems concerning the supply of donor organs persist; and like the United States, the Western Europeans have instituted educational programs.

ORGAN PROCUREMENT ORGANIZATIONS AND THE UNITED NETWORK FOR ORGAN SHARING

The organ donation system in the United States is organized through Organ Procurement Organizations (OPOs). The primary purpose of OPOs is to procure donated organs and distribute them to the appropriate recipients. OPOs have four basic functions that they are required to perform: recovery, preservation, and transportation of donated kidneys and the maintenance of a system to locate prospective recipients for all recovered organs. To accomplish these goals, OPOs provide a variety of services to the hospitals within their area, as follows:

1. Developing a relationship with the hospital's administration in order to discuss legal, financial, and ethical issues and formal agreements.
2. Providing professional education for medical and nursing personnel with respect to the hospital's needs.
3. Assessing potential donors and coordinating the clinical management of organ and tissue donors.
4. Discussing organ and tissue donation with families and obtaining consent with respect to the hospital's policy.
5. Assisting with quality assurance for the donation program by providing feedback to the administration and staff on every organ and tissue donor. Also conducting death record audits as outlined by the particular hospital (AHA, AMA, UNOS, 1988).

All organs are distributed centrally through the United Network for Organ Sharing (UNOS). UNOS is the federally appointed organ procurement and transplant network (OPTN) for the United States. All organ allocation criteria are defined through the UNOS organ-matching system.

The UNOS system is a computerized network that lists all potential organ recipients in the United States. Its policies are to ensure equitable organ allocation among transplant centers and among patients medically qualified for organ transplant. UNOS is also charged with operating a scientific registry, and as such it collects, reports, and analyzes data on all human organ transplants in the United States. UNOS has also adopted minimum procurement standards for OPOs with respect to identification and evaluation of potential donors. (See Table 1.2.)

DONOR IDENTIFICATION

The types of organs and tissues that may be donated are dependent on the circumstances of the patient's death. Patients may suffer brain death or cardiopulmonary death.

Brain Death. A patient suffering total irreversible loss of brain function is pronounced brain dead, after which the patient's cardiopulmonary system is maintained artificially by use of a ventilator and supportive care to adequately perfuse the vital organs with oxygen- enriched blood. This type of patient may donate vital organs (kidneys, heart, lungs, liver, pancreas, and small bowel) and tissues (corneas, bone, and skin).

Cardiopulmonary Death. A patient who has suffered irreversible cessation of circulation because of inadequate perfusion to the organs; therefore, this patient may donate only tissues (corneas, bone, and skin).

**TABLE 1.2 UNOS Minimum Standards for Donor Testing by
Organ Procurement Organizations (OPO)**

With respect to donor identification, the OPO must identify potential donors by:
  Verifying that the death has been pronounced in accordance with state law.
  Determining any contraindications for donor acceptance including
    Malignant tumors (primary brain tumors are acceptable unless cerebral venous
      shunts or cerebral peritoneal shunts have been put in place)
    Current sepsis
    Repeated human immunodeficiency virus (HIV) antibody seropositive results
OPO evaluation for potential donors must include the following:
  History and physical
  Chart review
  Hands-on physical examination
  Vital signs
  Pertinent testing to include:
    For all donors
      CBC
      Electrolytes
      ABO typing
      Hepatitis screen
      VDRL or RPR
      FDA licensed HIV-Ab screen
      Blood and urine cultures if hospitalized 72 hr
    Renal-specific
      Urinalysis
      Creatinine
      BUN
    Liver-specific
      Liver enzymes
      Total bilirubin
      Direct bilirubin
      PT
    Heart specific
      12-lead EKG
      Cardiology consult
      Chest x-ray
      Blood gases
      PTT
    Systems review

Source: From *UNOS Articles of Incorporation, By-Laws, Policies* (pp. 2–3) by United Network of
Organ Sharing, 1988. Richmond, VA: Author. Reprinted with permission.

TISSUE DONATION

Tissue can be donated following brain death with or without circulatory arrest. Corneas are usually recovered within 6 hours after death. Bone and skin may be recovered within 24 hours after death. Other tissues that may be recovered include heart valves, saphenous veins, middle ear bones, and bone marrow (see Table 1.3). A history of sepsis, hepatitis B, syphilis, or human immunodeficiency virus (HIV) infection will preclude donation of tissues. Any questions should be conveyed to the local OPO or tissue bank in the area. Tissues can be recovered in hospital operating rooms (sterile bone procurement), morgues, and coroner's offices.

As in organ procurement, proper clinical techniques and respect for the deceased are practiced. For example, when the eye is enucleated, prosthetic orbits are placed in the eye socket, and when bone is removed, rods are used to replace the long bones.

The demand for tissue far outweighs its supply. Eye injuries in children that require corneal or scleral tissue for repair occur 160,000 times annually. Many other types of surgical repairs can be accomplished through tissue donation (see Table 1.3).

TABLE 1.3 Age Restrictions and Use of Donated Tissues

Tissue	Donor age	Use
Bone	15–60 yr	Neurosurgical repairs and spinal fusions
Cartilage	2–30 yr	Facial reconstruction and otologic repairs
Dura mater	2–70 yr	Surgical repairs of head injuries and reconstruction of the middle ear
Eye	1–75 yr	Corneal transplants and sclera repairs
Fascia lata	6–70 yr	Neurosurgical repairs and otologic surgery
Heart valves	0–55 yr	Mostly utilized in pediatric surgery to repair congenital defects
Pituitary	0–no limit	Extraction of growth hormone to treat children with dwarfism
Saphenous Vein	12–60 yr	Source of vascular tissue for coronary or peripheral bypass grafts
Skin	15–75 yr	Dressings for patients with extensive third-degree burns
Temporal bones	0–75 yr	Repair of hearing loss caused by disease of the middle ear

ORGAN DONATION

Organ donation can occur when patients meet brain-death criteria. Common diagnoses of organ donors are listed in Table 1.4. Generally, organ donors may range in age from newborn to 65 years. Certain medical conditions will preclude organ donation; therefore, obtaining a history from family members is critical, especially when the donor is unknown to the physicians caring for him/her. The following conditions preclude organ donation:

1. Malignant tumors, except primary brain tumors.
2. Current sepsis.
3. Repeated seropositive HIV results (National Organ Procurement and Transplant Network, 1988). OPOs encourage hospitals to call with specific questions.

In addition to general criteria for organ donation, there are also organ-specific criteria (see Table 1.5). Each organ has donor age restrictions, and specific laboratory and diagnostic tests are required to assess organ function.

The clinical course of the donor is also evaluated, from the time of admission to the hospital, and includes hemodynamic stability, drugs used to maintain stability, and invasive procedures required during hospitalization. A decision as to which organs are suitable for transplant is made by the respective organ recovery team involved. One organ recovery team may decline to recover an organ, but another team may have a desperate need for that organ.

Clinical Management of an Organ Donor

Maintenance of optimal perfusion and function of organs is the primary focus in the care of an organ donor. Severe neurological injuries produce physiologic abnormalities that must be managed during preoperative and in-

TABLE 1.4 Common Diagnoses of Organ Donors

Diagnosis	Cause
Acute head trauma	Gunshot wounds, automobile or motorcycle accidents, homicide, or child abuse
Anoxic encephalopathy	Aspiration, drug overdose, drowning, prolonged cardiopulmonary resuscitation (CPR), apnea, or birth asphyxia
Intracerebral bleed	Cerebral vascular accident (CVA), craniotomy surgery, ruptured cerebral aneurysm, or subdural hematoma
Primary lesion brain	Glioblastoma or astrocytoma
Other	Sudden infant death syndrome or central nervous system defects

TABLE 1.5 Organ-Specific Donor Criteria

Organ	Criteria

Kidney	• Newborn to 65 years
	  No history of renal disease
	  Normal or acceptable BUN and creatinine

Liver	• Newborn to 50 years (donors over 50 may be considered
	  by some transplant centers)
	  No history of hepatic disease
	  No evidence of hepatic trauma
	  Normal or acceptable liver function tests

Heart	• Newborn to 45 years (donors over 45 years may be
	  considered for possible heart donation depending
	  on local or national needs)
	  No history of heart disease or previous cardiac surgery
	  No evidence of severe cardiothoracic trauma
	  No prolonged cardiac resuscitation

Heart–Lung	• Newborn to 45 years
	  Same criteria as heart donor, plus following pulmonary
	  criteria:
	  No history of pulmonary disease
	  No evidence of pulmonary infection, pulmonary
	    trauma, or pulmonary edema
	  Clear lung fields on chest film
	  Able to maintain PaO_2 of greater than 150 mmHg
	    on FIO_2 of 40% with 5 cm PEEP

Lung	• Newborn to 45 years
	  No history of pulmonary disease
	  No evidence of pulmonary infection, pulmonary
	    trauma, or pulmonary edema
	  Clear lung fields on chest film
	  Able to maintain PaO_2 of greater than 150 mmHg on
	    FiO_2 of 40% with 5 cm PEEP

ative care of the organ donor. Maintenance of circulatory blood volume is of utmost importance in regulating the cardiovascular stability of brain-dead patients. Injuries that cause hemorrhage, hypoxia, acidosis, or decreased pulmonary compliance or drugs like mannitol and furosemide (used to lower intracranial pressure) further deplete circulating volume. Those situations predispose the patient to hypotension, which can be remedied by liberal administration of electrolyte solutions and blood transfusions when necessary. The nursing care plan summarizes the major nursing diagnoses associated with care of the organ donor and the necessary interventions required to maintain a relative state of homeostasis until the organs can be recovered by the respective procurement teams. (See Nursing Care Plan at the end of this chapter.)

Consent Process

The consent process in organ donation occurs during an emotional and traumatic time for the family. In some instances, several days may have passed between the injury and the pronouncement of death; other situations may give the family considerably less time to adjust to the loss and accept the death of their family member. In either instance, the first step in helping the family is to provide an adequate explanation of brain death. Discussion usually occurs when the attending physician informs the family of the terminal condition that the injury has produced. Families will often need to have further discussions if brain death and its finality have not been clearly understood. It is helpful to explain how the use of machines and medications enable heartbeat, blood pressure, and breathing to continue after death has occurred.

Initiation of consent for organ donation should be authorized by the patient's attending physician. The option of organ donation should be presented only after the family has been informed of their relative's death and has been given the time to assimilate that information. A family may be approached by a physician, nurse, procurement coordinator, social worker, patient representative, chaplin, or anyone else designated by the hospital administrator. Generally, a procurement coordinator may be in the best position to provide a full explanation to the family concerning organ donation. Discussions concerning organ and tissue donation should occur in a quiet, private setting. Sometimes, there may be reluctance on the part of hospital personnel to inquire about donation for fear of burdening the family with an additional emotional trauma. This assumption deprives the family of making a decision which may, in fact, give them comfort, by relieving feelings of senselessness associated with the death. It is the family's right to have the choice to donate, and by virtue of state and federal legislation, it is the responsibility of hospital personnel to inform them sensitively of this option.

The following list of questions and answers cover typical areas that are discussed when speaking to families about organ and tissue donation.

Q. How will people benefit from the donation?

A. Corneal donation will enable two people to see. Facial reconstructions, brain surgeries, and back surgeries are possible from tissue donation. A burn patient utilizes donated skin as a temporary dressing which promotes healing of the burned area. Two people will be able to lead normal lives without dependence on a machine through kidney transplantation. A child or an adult may live because of heart or liver transplantation.

Q. Is there any cost incurred through the donations?

A. No, all costs related to recovery of organs and tissues are borne by the organ procurement organization and ultimately, the transplant programs. There is also no payment for donation.

Q. Will the decision to donate affect funeral arrangements?

A. No, the removal of organs and tissues will not interfere with customary funeral or burial arrangements. The appearance of the body is not altered. Funeral and burial expenses remain the responsibility of the family.

Q. Will anyone know I have donated, and what will I learn about the recipients?

A. The decision to donate is a confidential one. You may tell others only if you wish. Names and information about donors and recipients are kept confidential. Generally, donor families are informed about the sex and age of the recipient and the initial outcome of the surgery.

Q. How long will it take to accomplish the donation, and how will it be done?

A. If multiple organs are being recovered, time will be needed to assemble the various transplant teams. This may take 8 - 12 hours. The removal of organs will take place in a sterile environment (an operating room); every effort is made to expedite the recovery process.

Q. Who will receive the vital organs?

A. The vital organs will be transplanted into those individuals who need them most urgently. Recipient selection is based on medical criteria such as blood type, the results of tissue-typing procedures, and body size. Social and financial status is never a factor in selecting recipients.

Another area of consent is the donor card. According to the Uniform Anatomical Gift Act, any person can donate all or part of his/her body after death, for medical research, education, or therapy. Even though a signed donor card exists, in practice, consent is always sought from the next of kin. Consent is pursued to avoid conflict that might arise should the next of kin disagree with the decedent's decision to donate organs and tissues. Unless there has been prior notice of opposition by the decedent, any of the family members (in order of priority) may give consent for organ/tissue donation: spouse, adult son or daughter, either parent, adult brother or sister, grandparent, guardian of the decedent at the time of death.

The consent form must be signed and witnessed. In accordance with UNOS policy, consent by the next of kin and the medically/legally responsible person (e.g., medical examiner) must be documented by the OPO.

Should the circumstances of the decedent's death require the county coroner or medical examiner's (ME) permission for removal of organs and tissues, permission must be documented in the decedent's medical record, in compliance with the hospital's policy. The majority of organ donors will be under the jurisdiction of the coroner/ME. Those cases include but are not limited to the following:

1. Deaths from homicide or suspicion of homicide.
2. Deaths from suicide or suspicion of suicide.
3. Deaths due to accidental or traumatic injury.
4. All deaths from poisoning or suspected poisoning.
5. All deaths resulting from abortion.
6. Deaths during or following diagnostic, therapeutic, surgical, or anesthetic procedures.

Despite having permission from the next of kin, coroners or ME's ultimately decide whether organs and tissues can be removed. After permission is granted, it is important to allow the family adequate time alone with their family member to express their good-byes. In most instances, the family will leave the hospital after this has occurred. The family should be informed about any major delay in the organ/tissue recovery process and also told of the completion of the procedure, if they so desire.

Donor Referrals

The majority of potential organ donors die in the critical-care unit. Therefore, critical care nurses are the major caregivers to potential donors, recipients, and their families. Again, nurses are the vital link to the organ and tissue donation and the transplantation process. Management of the brain-dead organ donor is a challenging role for the critical-care nurse. Active communication of clinical information to transplant coordinators is also a vital service that nurses perform. Although emotionally and physically draining, the effort put forth to support the organ-donation process will often result in several lifesaving operations. The important role that nurses play in these positive outcomes cannot be overstated.

When a potential organ donor is identified, the local OPO and tissue bank should be notified. Any person may refer a potential donor to the OPO. In all cases, it is advisable that the permission of the attending physician be given prior to contacting the OPO. The OPO has procurement specialists on call 24 hours a day to assist with all aspects of organ and tissue recovery. They work collaboratively with donor hospital personnel to facilitate the donation process.

Initial evaluation of donor suitability occurs with the first phone call. Pertinent donor information will be asked for at this time and includes the following:

1. Name.
2. Age, sex, race.
3. Height, weight.
4. Blood type.
5. Date and time of admission.
6. Diagnosis, cause of death, and any other injuries that have occurred.
7. Past medical/social history.
8. Clinical status (hemodynamics during hospitalization).
9. Brain death declaration.

Organ Recovery

Once the referral has been made to the OPO, a procurement coordinator will often be sent to help with family consent, assist in donor management, and begin the process of placing organs. Except for the kidneys, most recovery teams prefer to remove the particular organ they specialize in.

In general, the on-site coordinator, after completing the evaluation of the donor, will call in the specific donor information to the UNOS computer for compatible donor-recipient matches. (Each organ-specific match will be discussed under its respective heading). Obtaining a list of potential recipients begins the time-consuming task of organ placement.

In general, patient match will be established on the basis of urgency of need. Patients whose needs are most urgent will be at the top of the list, and their respective centers will be called first. The on-site coordinator must inform the prospective transplant centers of vital information about the donor.

After accepting an organ, the respective teams will confer about an acceptable operating room time. The time for the donor surgery must be mutually acceptable to all of the teams involved, including the host operating room team. Procurement team transportation arrangements are usually made by their own coordinators. However, if procurement teams are flying from another state or a distant center, the on-site procurement coordinator will be asked to assist those teams with local ground transport (between the airport and the hospital).

Kidney

Kidney Donor Assessment

Acceptable criteria for kidney donors include the following:

Age	0–65 years
History	No history of significant hypertension, arterio- or atherosclerotic vascular or renal disease
Evaluation of the abdomen	Close attention to any adominal trauma

More specific tests include those minimally required by UNOS plus urine culture and sensitivity tests.

Kidney Donor/Recipient Matching

Kidney matching relies strictly on identical blood-type and histocompatibility testing. All retrieved cadaver donor kidneys are tissue-typed to achieve the best possible result, which is a well-functioning and perpetually functioning allograft.

Kidney Donor Surgery

The procurement surgery for kidneys can take $\frac{1}{2}$ to $1\frac{1}{2}$ hours. A midabdominal incision is made, and the colon is deflected left or right. The ureters are identified and ligated with hemoclips or ties. The aorta is dissected free and ligated at both internal iliac vessels and proximally to the heart. The kidneys are flushed with Eurocollins solution via the aorta with the insertion of a Foley catheter while the vena cava is drained (see Figure 1.1). After flushing, the kidneys are removed en bloc and put in a sterile basin of iced saline. The kidneys are then inspected and further dissected—carefully split right from left. The kidneys are then placed in appropriate sterile containers and put in a container of ice. This is simple cold storage, similar to that used for many other organs.

There have been significant improvements in kidney preservation techniques that have contributed to higher graft success rates. Cold storage can maintain the kidneys from 24 to 48 hours. Another popular method for kidney preservation is hypothermic pulsatile perfusion, which can maintain the kidneys for up to 72 hours.

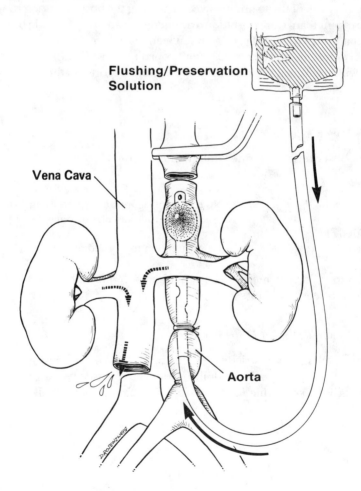

Flushing/Preservation Solution

Vena Cava

Aorta

FIGURE 1.1 Cadaver donor nephrectomy.

Hypothermic pulsatile perfusion preservation uses a perfusate of albumin or colloid solution. Once the kidneys are flushed during removal, the renal arteries are then cannulated so that the kidneys can be placed on the preservation device (see Figure 1.2). The kidneys are maintained on the preservation device until the time of transplantation. It has been shown that a specialized approach to the management of the cadaver donor, coupled with the use of hypothermic pulsatile perfusion—even for extended periods—achieves excellent graft survival and quality of function for kidneys (Feduska, 1987).

Heart

Heart Donor Assessment

The potential heart donor undergoes close evaluation prior to acceptance of the organ. In addition to UNOS required tests mentioned earlier, other information that may be asked includes the following:

Age	0–45 years (criteria may differ for each center)
Weight	Accuracy important
Cardiac arrest	Specific information on duration and drugs used during the arrest
History	Specific heart history and any history of drug use
Evaluation of chest/abdomen	Inspection and notation of areas of traumatic injury
Hypotension	During hospitalization, noting duration
Vasopressor use	During hospitalization, noting dosages and duration

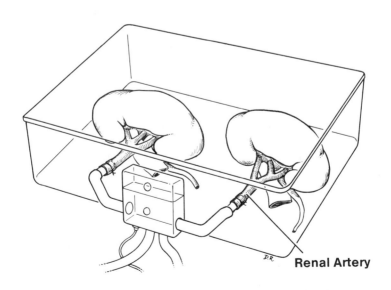

Renal Artery

FIGURE 1.2 Kidney preservation device.

Additional tests:
Echocardiogram, angiogram if   Very important if any of the above data are
donor over 40 yrs. CPK and   questionable
isoenzymes.

Heart Donor/Recipient Matching

The most important considerations in matching a donor and recipient are compatible blood type and body size. The actual height and weight of the donor must be precisely determined. It has been demonstrated that, during the first 20 years of life, cardiac dimensions increase progressively with age and correlate well with body size. Also, male hearts are usually larger than female hearts (Scholz, Kitzman, Hagen, Ilstrup, & Edwards, 1988).

Donor Operation

The success of all organ transplants depends on a well-removed and properly preserved organ. For heart transplantation, the donor cardiectomy is performed through a median sternotomy. Once the pericardium is opened, the heart is examined for evidence of contusion, coronary artery disease, valvular disease, or congenital abnormalities. The ascending aorta, superior vena cava, and inferior vena cava are then dissected free. A line for infusion of cardioplegia solution is carefully flushed to eliminate air bubbles and is connected to a short infusion catheter or needle which is then inserted into the anterior surface of the ascending aorta. (See Figure 1.3.) The superior vena cava is ligated, and the inferior vena cava is cross-clamped at the level of the diaphragm. The distal aorta is also cross-clamped, while the left and right inferior pulmonary veins and the inferior vena cava are immediately divided. Simultaneously, an infusion of 500–1000 ml of cold cardioplegia solution (to lower metabolic requirements of the heart) via the catheter in the aorta is started. Electromechanical arrest of the heart is accomplished. Once the cardioplegia solution has been infused, the infusion line is removed, and the heart is removed from the chest.

The heart is then repeatedly rinsed in basins containing a cold saline solution. For transport, the heart will be placed in a suitable sterile container with iced saline and totally submerged. The heart is kept cold by surrounding the container with ice in a suitable box for transport. Hearts for transplantation are preserved for up to 4 hours, which dictates travel from the transplant center of up to 1,500 miles.

Heart–Lung

Heart–Lung Donor Assessment

The difficulty of finding suitable donors is currently the limiting factor in cardiopulmonary transplantation (Jamieson & Ogunnaike, 1986). Brain death

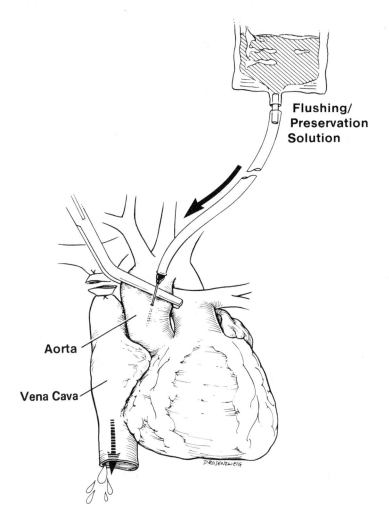

**Flushing/
Preservation
Solution**

Aorta

Vena Cava

D. ROSENZWEIG

FIGURE 1.3 Cadaver donor cardiectomy.

is accompanied by rapid decline in pulmonary status as a result of pulmonary edema, aspiration, or infection from prolonged intubation. Hypothermic pulmonary preservation is also unreliable, and the transfer of a brain-dead donor to a recipient hospital is often unacceptable to the family. Therefore, only 20% of donors with acceptable hearts for transplantation will also have acceptable lungs (Finch & Jamieson, 1987). These factors have severely limited the pool of donors for heart–lung transplantation.

Assessment is crucial in the evaluation of a potential heart–lung donor. Although some of the criteria and tests will be the same as for a cardiac donor, careful observation of pulmonary status is essential.

Although each center's criteria may differ slightly, generally the following additional information will be necessary:

Factor	Data
Age	0–45 years (criteria may differ for each center)
Evaluation of chest	Inspection for chest injury
Prolonged periods of hypoxia	Noting acid–base shifts and their duration
History	Smoking; family history of lung diseases, previous chest surgeries, or occupational exposure to chemicals

Additional lab tests: donor $PaO_2 > 150$ mmHg on FiO_2 40%; Gram's stain of bronchial secretions; chest x-ray (CXR), anterior/posterior (AP). The patient must be free of atelectasis, infiltrates, edema, and contusions.

To exhibit adequate oxygenation, the donor PaO_2 must be greater than 150 mmHg on 40% FiO_2, with matching peak inspiratory pressures of less than 30 mmH_2O for normal tidal volumes. Additional requirements are a close chest size match because efficient pulmonary function requires that the lungs fit well within the recipient's chest cage.

Heart–Lung Donor/Recipient Matching

The matching of a donor and recipient is based on compatible blood type, body size (height and weight), and lymphocyte compatibility. To assess size matching for the lungs, the donor center may be asked for specific thoracic measurements from the CXR (taken on full inspiration). These may include the following (see Figure 1.4):

1. Left and right bronchial diameter (in millimeters).
2. Transverse chest measurements from AP, CXR (in centimeters).
3. Vertical chest measurement from AP CXR, including both right and left side (in centimeters).
4. Circumference (outer chest circumference at nipple level)

Heart–Lung Donor Operation

The procedure is done through a median sternotomy followed by a complete anterior pericardiectomy, to include both phrenic nerves and the remnants of the thymus gland. The ascending aorta, innominate artery, superior vena cava, and inferior vena cava are dissected free, and the azygos vein is ligated and divided. The trachea is encircled with umbilical tape at a level as high as possible so as not to disturb the vasculature of the trachea. The donor is systemically heparinized to prevent microthrombosis. Asystole is induced with cardioplegia solution infused directly into the heart. The lungs are flushed with modified iced (4°C) Collins' solution via an infusion catheter

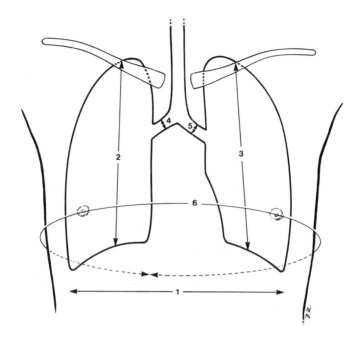

FIGURE 1.4 Thoracic dimensions required for heart–lung and lung donor–recipient matching. 1, Transverse chest measurement from anterior–posterior (AP), chest x-ray (CXR) (cm); 2, right vertical chest measurement from AP, CXR (cm); 3, left vertical chest measurement from AP, CXR (cm); 4, right bronchial diameter (mm); 5, left bronchial diameter (mm); 6, circumference of outer chest at nipple level.

inserted into the main pulmonary artery (see Figure 1.5). Ventilation is continued during this period to distribute the perfusion throughout the lungs. Six to 10 L of topical cold solution are allowed to flow into the chest cavity. The trachea is cross-clamped above the level of the carina while the lungs remain inflated. The donor heart and lungs are excised and placed in a sterile basin of cold solution.

The removal of the heart–lungs must be carefully coordinated with the recipient operation to decrease the ischemic time of the graft (Finch & Jamieson, 1987). The heart and lungs are placed in a suitable container filled with ice-cold solution and are kept cold while being quickly transported to the recipient location.

Another method of heart–lung preservation is the use of cardiopulmonary bypass and deep hypothermia to cool the donor organs without flush perfusion before immediate explantation. Still another method that some transplant centers use simulates the organ's physiologic state by autoperfusion and

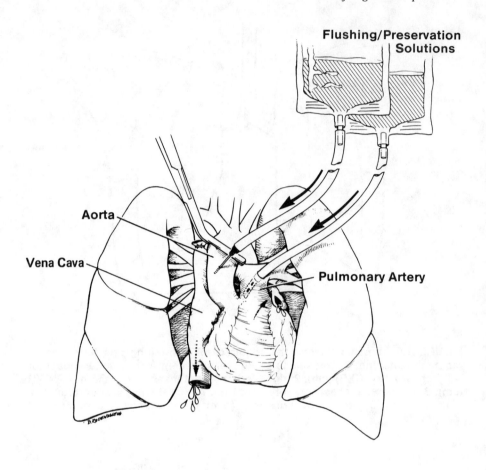

FIGURE 1.5 Cadaver donor heart–lung recovery.

ventilation. Preservation accomplished by this method maintains the heart–lung block in a dynamic state that provides a means of transport for these donor organs over long distances (Kontos et al., 1988). This autoperfused working heart–lung block may provide successful cardiopulmonary preservation for up to 6 hours before transplantation (Kontos et al., 1988). The more traditional, cold-storage preparation allows ischemic times of up to 4 hours. The future development of lung preservation techniques for distant procurement will increase the number of available donors. Today some transplant centers still require that heart–lung donors be transported to the recipient transplant center. For special considerations in donor procurement of single and double lung transplantion see Chapter 6.

Liver

Liver Donor Assessment

Most multiple-organ donors are also considered as potential liver donors. The upper age limit for liver donors is generally 50 years; but in extremely urgent situations, wherein the recipient will die within 24 hours without a transplant, a liver from a donor of any age will be considered. Two children may benefit from a single adult liver donor, the liver being split and shared between the two recipients. In addition, segmented liver donation from a living related donor (often parent to child) is being practiced today. These surgical techniques may assist with donor shortages and be widely practiced in the future.

The potential donor undergoes close evaluation prior to acceptance of the organ. The potential donor should have no history of malignancy (other than primary brain tumor), liver disease, alcohol or IV drug abuse, or any other systemic disease that may affect the liver.

The following laboratory studies will be needed in addition to the basic requirements established by UNOS:

Gamma GTP
Hepatitis screen: hepatitis A, hepatitis B surface antigen, hepatitis B surface
    antibody, hepatitis B core antibody
Viral studies: CMV

Cardiopulmonary function of the donor must be maintained until the liver is flushed with its preservation fluid.

Liver Donor/Recipient Matching

The most important consideration in matching liver donor and recipient is blood-type compatibility and body size. Therefore, accurate height and weight of the potential donor must be determined.

Previous studies have found that the liver is not as immunologically active as other organs; unlike the kidney, no relationship has been found between tissue matching and rejection (Tzakis et al., 1987). HLA typing and donor/recipient cross-matching is performed retrospectively for informational purposes.

Liver Donor Operation

Successful liver transplantation depends on a well-preserved and functioning liver. The organ donor is transported to the operating room and prepped from the neck to groin. A complete midline incision is made from the suprasternal notch to the pubis. There are two methods of hepatic recovery: the standard technique and the rapid technique (Starzl, Miller, Broznick, & Makowka,

1987). The standard technique requires 2 to 3 hours of meticulous dissection prior to flushing the liver.

With the increasing frequency of multiorgan donors, the rapid-flush technique is being utilized by many surgeons. The rapid-flush technique requires no preliminary dissection, with the exception of locating the proximal aorta and cannulating the portal vein and distal aorta. Once the other procurement teams are ready, the aorta is cross-clamped, and an infusion of cold lactated Ringer's solution is infused via both cannulae (see Figure 1.6). The liver is also cooled topically with sterile iced saline. Following perfusion with Lactated

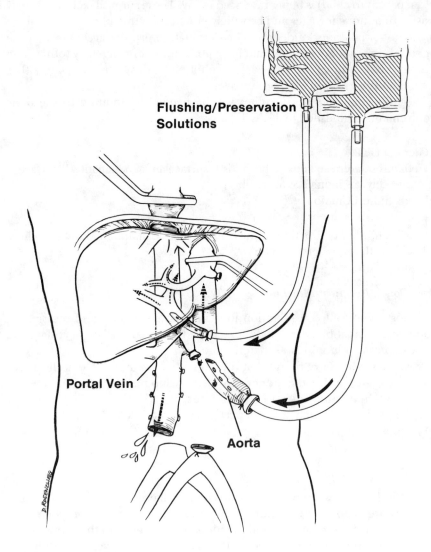

FIGURE 1.6 Cadaver donor hepatectomy.

Ringer's, the liver is perfused with a cold preservative solution. The solution currently used was developed at the University of Wisconsin and has extended the cold ischemia time to as long as 24 hours. Once the liver is completely flushed and cooled, the hilar dissection is then completed in an entirely bloodless field.

Liver preservation is achieved with simple cold storage. Once the liver is removed, it is placed in an appropriate container, packed in ice, and transported to the transplanting center.

FOLLOW-UP

Preservation of organs and tissues is the final step in procurement prior to transplantation. Once the organs and tissues are transplanted, the results are communicated by the OPO to everyone involved.

A letter is written to the donor family noting the outcome of all organs and tissues procured. The recipient's name is kept confidential in all correspondence. Letters are also sent to nurses, physicians, social workers, clergy, and ancillary persons involved. The follow-up letter serves to promote the positive aspect of the donation process: knowing that some good resulted from a tragic event. In some instances, it assists the family as they progress through the stages of grief.

Confidentiality is also maintained with respect to the donor's name in communicating information to the recipient. Most of the donor information is communicated by the physician. The amount of donor information told to the recipient is left up to the discretion of the physician; recipients are usually told the sex and age of their donor.

CONCLUSION

Advances in medical science and immunology will forever contribute to success in transplantation. However, the short supply of donor organs may still persist long into our future. Therefore, it is imperative that nurses, who provide expert clinical care to donors and their families, be knowledgeable about the organ and tissue donation process. They are the professionals, with an understanding of the transplant system, who identify potential donors early in their hospitalizations and maintain adequate physiologic stability of organ perfusion. In this way, nurses contribute in a meaningful way to saving the lives of patients suffering from end-stage organ failure.

NURSING CARE PLAN OF THE ORGAN DONOR

Organ Donor Management

Nursing diagnosis	Expected outcome	Nursing interventions
1. **CIRCULATION,** alterations in vascular fluid volume deficit related to Failure of autonomic nervous system (ANS) → ↓ vasomotor tone → arterial vasodilation → pooling of intravascular volume → ↓ central central venous pressure (CVP) → ↓ preload → hypotension (Levison & Copeland, 1987) Decreased posterior pituitary function and no excretion of antidiuretic hormone (ADH) → diuresis Hyperosmolor agents used during the acute phase of the patient's injury Trauma/hemorrhage	Patient will exhibit adequate hydration as evidenced by CVP: 4–10 cm H_2O PAW: 4–12 mmHg Urine output 1–2 cc/kg/hr Normal vital signs (see p. 35)* Serum electrolytes within normal limits Hematocrit above 30%	1. Measure intake and output hourly. 2. Monitor vital signs—heart rate, blood pressure, CVP or pulmonary artery pressure (PAP). 3. Administer IV replacement fluid therapy as ordered. 4. Monitor urine and serum electrolytes Q4°, especially if patient is having diuresis. 5. Administer inotropes and synthetic ADH replacement drugs as ordered; monitor medications to prevent further loss, and evaluate. 6. Provide eye care to prevent injury to eyes from dryness, especially if patient is going to be a cornea donor.

*   *   *

Nursing diagnosis	Expected outcome	Nursing interventions
2. **BODY TEMPERATURE,** alterations in effective thermoregulation related to Injury with loss of hypothalamic function Loss of thyroid hormone secretion from the pituitary No efferent neurologic supply from the ANS	Patient will maintain body temperature at normal level or above 37°C to prevent development of spontaneous ventricular arrhythmias.	1. Assess temperature by use of an indwelling temperature probe, either rectal or esophageal to obtain temperature Q1°. 2. Maintain temperature (36°C–38°C): Use a warming blanket or warming lamps Use heated mist in the ventilator system 3. Maintain environmental temperature at a comfortable setting. 4. Monitor temperature of all fluids, colloids, crystalloids.

*   *   *

(continued)

Organ Donor Management (continued)

Nursing diagnosis	Expected outcome	Nursing interventions
3. **RESPIRATORY FUNCTION,** alterations in impaired gas exchange related to Loss of brain stem function Loss of respiratory drive Mechanical ventilation with endotracheal or tracheal intubation Neurogenic pulmonary edema Aspiration pneumonia related to trauma	Patient will exhibit adequate gas exchange by Maintaining PaO_2 within normal range Clear breath sounds bilaterally	1. Assess pulmonary status Q1°: Auscultate breath sounds Note CVP/PAW pressures Monitor V/S Q1° Monitor ABGs Q4° and 20–30 min after ventilator changes 2. Maintain airway patency using sterile suctioning technique to remove tracheobronchial secretions: document characteristics of secretions Obtain sputum specimens as ordered. 3. Assist with chest x-rays. 4. Observe for signs of dehydration and overload. 5. Note response to drug therapies.
	* * *	
4. **ELIMINATION PROCESS,** altered: diuresis related to destruction of the hypothalamic–pituitary axis resulting in a decrease in circulating ADH and central diabetes insipidus (DI)	Patient will exhibit adequate urinary output as evidenced by Urine output of at least 100 cc/h or 1–2 cc/kg/h Patient will maintain adequate hydration as evidenced by Normal vital signs for age of patient, Normal CVP or PA pressures	1. Assess fluid balance of patient: Monitor intake/output Q1° Check V/S, monitor for hypotension Check CVP/PA pressures 2. Administer IV replacement therapy, crystolloids, colloids, or blood products as ordered and monitor results. 3. Administer and monitor vasoactive drugs. 4. Monitor urine and serum electrolytes, Q4°. Check for hypernatremia, hypokalemia, hyperglycemia, or hypomagnesemia. Administer fluids or drugs that may correct above scenarios as ordered.

(continued)

Organ Donor Management (continued)

Nursing diagnosis	Expected outcome	Nursing interventions
	* * *	5. Obtain urine/serum osmolality as ordered.
5. **GRIEVING,** related to the acute loss of a family member; defining characteristics: Hopelessness Fear of unknown Abandonment Helplessness	Short-term: Family will be able to express their feelings about the death of their family member. Family exercises control by making decisions about the care of the deceased and may consider organ/tissue donation. Long-term: Family begins making plans for the future.	1. Assess the family's perception of the loss. Plan time to listen to the family Encourage the family to express their feelings about the loss of their family member Give ample opportunity to ask questions 2. Assist the family to understand the grieving process and to accept their feelings as normal, under the circumstances. 3. Encourage the family to make simple decisions related to care issues. 4. Encourage use of support persons, i.e., clergy, social work, or organ procurement personnel. 5. Assist the family to begin to formulate goals for the future.
	* * *	
6. **CARDIAC OUTPUT,** alteration in: decreased related to Failure of ANS and loss of vasomotor tone → ↓ CVP, and ↓ preload Hypovolemia	Patient will exhibit hemodynamic stability as exhibited by Adequate cardiac output (CO) and BP Adequate peripheral perfusion Urine output 1–2 cc/ kg/hr Absence of pulmonary edema Normal hematocrit and hemoglobin	1. Monitor heart rate and blood pressure hourly and PRN. 2. Monitor CVP or pulmonary artery pressures hourly; if no central lines, auscultate breath sounds. 3. Monitor intake and output hourly. 4. Administer IV fluids as ordered. 5. Monitor electrolyte values and replace as ordered. 6. Administer vasoactive drugs, pitressin, and/or desmopressin and observe their results.
	* * *	

(continued)

Organ Donor Management (continued)

Nursing diagnosis	Expected outcome	Nursing interventions
7. **PHYSICAL REGULATION** alteration in immune system and potential for infection related to Immobility Invasive monitors Indwelling tubes and catheters	Patient will demonstrate absence of infection as evidenced by Normal temperature Absence of purulent secretions Cultures without pathogens Clear urine, odorless, without sediment Clean wound incisions, without purulent drainage IV sites without inflammation	1. Assess patient's risk for development of infection by Obtaining a good medical/surgical history both past and present Close observation and documentation of all invasive and indwelling lines and catheters, using aseptic technique in the care of all lines Chart any deviations from normal in consistency and color of secretions 2. Minimize the patient's risk by Using good handwashing before and after care Wearing gloves to prevent sepsis Repositioning the patient to prevent pneumonia 3. Monitor vital signs, noting elevations in temperature. 4. Monitor lab values, especially complete blood count with differential. 5. Send sputum, urine and blood or any other peculiar wound drainage for cultures as ordered. 6. Administer antibiotics as ordered.
	* * *	
8. **CIRCULATION ALTERATIONS** in vascular tissue perfusion related to Hypovolemia	Patient will exhibit hemodynamic stability as evidenced by Normal vital signs Normal arterial	1. Assess: Heart rate Rhythm Blood pressure Temperature

(continued)

Organ Donor Management (continued)

Nursing diagnosis	Expected outcome	Nursing interventions

Central nervous system (CNS) dysfunction
Traumatic injury (multisystem)
	blood gases (ABG)
	Fluid balance maintained; input = output
	Normal Hgb/Hct/WBC, and coagulation studies
	Patient will exhibit good skin integrity as evidenced by
	Good peripheral pulses
	Absence of cyanosis
		CVP/PAP
		2. Administer vasopressor/inotropic support as needed—no more than 10µg/kg/min.
		3. Monitor skin color and temperature.
		4. Monitor ABGs Q4°.
		5. Measure and record I/O Q1°, record and report changes.
		6. Assess causative factors of hypovolemia and treat causes.
		7. Administer fluids/blood products as ordered, noting outcomes.
		8. Initiate measures to improve perfusion:
		  Keep patient warm
		  Elevate lower extremities
		9. Perform pulmonary toilet as ordered.
		10. Monitor lab values, especially electrolytes, Hgb/Hct/WBC; frequency of labs will depend on severity of the patient's condition.

	* * *	

9. **PHYSICAL INTEGRITY,** alteration in:
Potential impairment of skin integrity related to immobility
	Patient will exhibit absence of skin impairment, as evidenced by clean and dry skin without redness or breakdown so that patient may be a skin donor.	1. Assess skin Q/shift and prn:
		  Document any skin condition change
		  Monitor and report progress of reddened areas.
		2. Keep skin clean and dry.
		3. Reposition patient Q 2 hr if appropriate.
		4. Maintain adequate hydration to ensure good skin turgor.
		5. Use preventive skin care devices:
		  Egg crate mattress
		  Water mattress

(continued)

Organ Donor Management (continued)

Nursing diagnosis	Expected outcome	Nursing interventions
		Pillows as padding Air beds 6. Keep linen clean and free of wrinkles. 7. Use lotions to lubricate dry skin.
	* * *	
10. **PHYSIOLOGIC PROCESS** altered: not otherwise specified; potential for coagulopathy related to Necrotic brain releasing large amounts of fibrinolytic agents (plasminogen activator), which is released into the systemic circulation (Levinson & Copeland, 1987).	Patient will not exhibit coagulopathy, as evidenced by normal lab values for prothrombin time (PT) and partial thromboplastin time (PTT).	1. Assess the patient's risk of developing a coagulopathy: Monitor trauma sites for active bleeding, especially those patients with direct injuries to the brain Monitor lab values for deviations from normal PT/PTT and bleeding times. 2. Administer appropriate replacement factors as ordered and monitor their results—*do not* give Episolin aminocaproic acid because it may induce microvascular thrombosis which may cause donor graft failure.
	* * *	
11. **MUCOUS MEMBRANES:** alteration in, related to brain death.	Patient will exhibit absence of corneal abrasions, so the patient can be a cornea donor.	1. Administer natural tears Q2°—do not use Lacrilube® ointment. 2. Cover and close eye with sterile gauze pads. 3. Inspect eyes Q2° describe and document condition and report changes.

*Heart rate normals:		*Blood pressure (BP) normals:	
0–1 mo.	120–160/min	0–1 yr	60/40– 90/60 mmHg
1 mo. –1 yr.	100–120/min	1–2 yrs	65/50– 95/70 mmHg
1–8 yrs	80–100/min	2–6 yrs	75/55–100/75 mmHg
		6–10 yrs	80/60‹110/80 mmHg
		10–14 yrs	85/65–120/85 mmHg
		14 yrs +	90/70–140/90 mmHg

REFERENCES

Ad Hoc Committee of the Harvard Medical School. (1984). A definition of irreversible coma. *Journal of the American Medical Association, 252*(5), 677–680.

American Hospital Association, American Medical Association, United Network for Organ Sharing (UNOS). (1988). *Required request legislation: A guide for hospitals on organ and tissue donation.* Richmond, VA: UNOS.

Bernat, J. L. (1987). Ethical and legal aspects of the emergency management of brain death and organ retrieval. In G. Henry (Ed.), *Emergency medicine clinics of North America* (pp. 659–676). Philadelphia: W. B. Saunders.

Feduska, N. J. (1987). *The recovery and preservation of organs for transplantation.* F. O. Belzer (Ed.), Pro/Com.

Finch, E. L., & Jamieson, S. W. (1987). Anesthesia for combined heart and lung transplantation. In B. R. Brown & J. G. Copeland (Eds.), *Anesthesia and transplantation surgery* (pp. 109–131). Philadelphia: F. A. Davis.

Jamieson, S. W., & Ogunnaike, H. O. (1986). Cardiopulmonary transplantation. *Surgical Clinics of North America, 66*(3), 491–501.

Kontos, G. J., Borkon, A. M., Baumgartner, W. A., Fonger, J. D., Hutchins, G. M., Adachi, H., Galloway, E., & Reitz, B. A. (1988). Improved myocardial and pulmonary preservation by metabolic substrate enhancement in the autoperfused working heart-lung preparation. *The Journal of Heart Transplantation, 7*(2), 140–144.

Levinson, M. M., & Copeland, J. G. (1987). The organ donor: Physiology, maintenance, and procurement considerations. In B. R. Brown & J. G. Copeland (Eds.), *Anesthesia and transplantation surgery* (pp. 31–45). Philadelphia: F. A. Davis.

National Organ Procurement and Transplant Network. (1988). *UNOS articles of incorporation, by-laws, policies.* Richmond, VA: Author.

President's Commission for the Study of Ethical Problems in Medicine and Biomedical and Behavioral Research. (1981). Guidelines for the determination of death. *Journal of the American Medical Association, 246*(19), 2184–2186.

Special Task Force. (1987). Guidelines for the determination of brain death in children. *Pediatrics, 80*(2), 298–300.

Task Force on Organ Transplantation. (1986). *Organ transplantation: Issues and recommendations* (DHHS Publication # HEZ0.9002: OR 3/2). Washington, DC: U.S. Government Printing Office.

Scholz, D. G., Kitzman, D. W., Hagen, P. T., Ilstrup, D. M., & Edwards, W. D. (1988). Age-related changes in normal human hearts during the first 10 decades of life. *Mayo Clinic Procedures, 63*, 126–136.

Soifer, B. E., & Gelb, A. W. (1989). The multiple organ donor: Identification and management. *Annals of Internal Medicine, 110*, 814–822.

Starzl, T. E., Miller, C., Broznick, B., & Makowka, L. (1987). An improved technique for multiple organ harvesting. *Surgical Gynecology/Obstetrics, 165*, 343–348.

Tzakis, A. G., Gordon, R. D., Makowka, L., Esquivel, C. O., Toto, S., Iwatsuki, S., & Starzl, T. E. (1987). Clinical considerations in orthotopic liver transplantation. *Radiological Clinics of North America, 25*(2), 289–297.

Wight, C. (1988). Organ procurement in Western Europe. *Transplantation Proceedings, 20*(1), 1003–1006.

CHAPTER **2**

IMMUNOLOGICAL ASPECTS OF ORGAN TRANSPLANTATION

Eileen G. Collins
Elizabeth A. Hubbell

A normally functioning immune system is vital to human health but has disastrous implications for the transplant recipient. The immune system is a diverse network of organs, cells, and complex signaling systems for inter-communication. It identifies and eliminates all foreign invaders or, more simply, anything that is non-self (Lafferty, 1988). A transplanted organ, unless donated from an identical twin, is considered foreign or non-self to a normal host recipient.

In order for a transplanted organ to survive in recipients, researchers have developed a combination of therapies to deceive the normal immune responses. These alterations include masquerading the transplanted organ as self, partially or selectively blinding the immune system so that it does not recognize the transplanted organ as foreign and suppressing the immune response that results from recognizing non-self.

The transplant nurse is in a key position to make important observations for detecting potential complications of these therapies. This chapter dis-cusses the immune response, the rejection process, immunosuppressive the-rapies, and the care of the patient in rejection.

THE IMMUNE RESPONSE

The immune response hinges on the body's ability to recognize foreign matter, which may be bacteria, viruses, fungi, parasites, or transplanted organs. Such recognition is known as differentiating self from non-self and is controlled by an individual's genetic inheritance. Understanding the immune responses requires explanations of their three major components: major histocompatibility complex (MHC), effector cells, and soluble mediators.

Major Histocompatibility Complex

The major histocompatibility complex (MHC) is a group of genes located on chromosome 6 in humans. The MHC was formerly known as the human leukocyte antigen (HLA) system. The MHC defines self for the immune system by directing placement of certain unique protein markers on selected cell surfaces, called histocompatibility antigens, which can be detected in the laboratory. Testing defines a portion of a person's genetic makeup, compares that individual's similarity or lack thereof to a potential donor organ, and predicts the quality of responses to antigens or future susceptibility to autoimmune diseases.

The MHC has two regions. The Class I region of genes has three major loci called A, B, and C. These three loci direct the production of cell surface markers or antigens, consisting of two chains: a single heavy chain expressing specificity unique to the individual and a smaller chain that is common to all Class I molecules. There are numerous Class I antigens. At least 70 loci are now defined on the A and B regions alone. These known loci are numbered A1, A2, B1, etc.

The Class II region was initially assigned to a single locus, D, but now has been subdivided into DR, DQ, and DP regions. The DR subregion marks all antigen-presenting cells (APCs). Circulating monocytes may ultimately function as APCs and have rich displays of Class II gene products on their surfaces. These circulating monocytes become macrophages after entering the spleen, lymph nodes, liver (Kuppfer cells), lung, skin (Langerhans cells), nervous tissue (microglial cells), and peritoneal fluid. These gene products determine when and how vigorously antigens will be presented to the rest of the immune system.

The DR region is of primary importance in defining self-specificity and preventing auto-directed harmful responses. Recipients with donor-matched D regions tolerate allografts much better than do those with mismatched D regions. This has been proven in the setting of renal, bone marrow, and, retrospectively, cardiac transplantation. Current methods for complete MHC typing are time-consuming and sometimes the typing is not performed before transplantation.

Effector Cells of the Immune System

Effector cells of the immune system are macrophages and lymphocytes. Lymphocytes are generally divided into two major subsets: thymic-derived lymphocytes and bone marrow derived lymphocytes.

Macrophages

Macrophages are mononuclear cells originating from the bone marrow that have MHC Class II surface markers and are multifunctional (Johnston, 1988). They play key roles in almost all facets of the immune response. Macrophages are found in the thymus, where they are essential to the maturation of lymphocytic cells; more important, they delete potential cells that may develop reactivity toward the host. Researchers have recognized circulating and interstitial macrophages for their phagocytic and scavenging abilities. Recent research has uncovered their central role as APCs. These cells internalize antigens, process them, and redisplay them on their surfaces. The entire process occurs in close physical association with MHC Class II surface products, which determines whether the processed antigen will attract or be ignored by other immune cells. Thus, the individual's immune system determines each antigen's destiny, whether or how the host will deal with it. APCs, especially macrophages, are proficient producers of many immunologic cytokines, especially interleukin 1 (IL-1), which can activate the rest of the immune system.

Lymphocytes

Lymphocytes, which are also mononuclear white blood cells, arise from the same stem cell that is the precursor of all leukocytes. They can mature either in the thymus, where they are called T lymphocytes or T cells, or in the bone marrow, where they are called B lymphocytes or B cells (Stobo, 1987). Laboratory testing separates lymphocytes into these major subsets by analysis of their surface markers and functions.

Thymic-Derived lymphocytes. Cells that are destined to become T cells migrate into the thymus early in fetal life. Only 5% of these cells leave the thymus as mature T lymphocytes (T-Ly, thymocytes, or T cells). Researchers presume that the 95% that do not survive had reactivities directed against the host and were deleted for self-protective reasons.

T cells differentiate into subsets that function as helper cells, cytotoxic (or killer) cells, or suppressor cells. Monoclonal antibodies that have been developed to be highly specific against single T-Ly surface markers, receptors, and enzymes can distinguish these subsets in tissue and biological fluids. Current terminology refers to these surface markers as clusters of differentiation (CD) with a specific numerical designation (see Table 2.1.) For instance, CD3 is the code for T cells that display a surface marker composed of three particular polypeptide chains, formerly called the T3 receptor. The CD3 marker is in close physical association with a T cell's antigen-specific receptor and is considered the standard marker for a mature T-Ly. The total number of T cells present in clinical samples is determined by quantification of the CD3-bearing cells. These cells were previously known as T3, and the monoclonal antibody to detect CD3 cells is still often referred to as anti-T3. Table 2.1 contains a list of known CD and terms that have been used synonymously.

CD3 cells can then be further differentiated into subsets with differing and key functions by using additional monoclonal antibodies to detect other surface markers. Helper T cells not only have CD3 markers but they also are distinguished by a CD4 determinant. They are CD3,4, or helper T-Ly. These cells are the predominant lymphocyte circulating in peripheral blood and can be viewed as cells constantly in search of an antigenic encounter. Upon contact with an APC or allograft that is presenting an antigen in the appropriate fashion, T-helper cells orchestrate the ensuing immune response. Simultaneously, once specific antigenic recognition occurs, the APC provides IL-1, which primes the CD3,4 helper cell to produce its own interleukins, 2, 3, and 4. Interleukin 2 (IL-2) is the prime growth and differentiation factor that rapidly expands the population of antigen-specific CD3 T-Ly into CD3,8 cytotoxic cells that will attack any cell displaying the antigen, for example, viral-infected cells and allografts. To prevent promiscuous destruction of cells and tissue, there is simultaneous expansion of a subset of cells that have the

TABLE 2.1 T Lymphocyte Terminology

Cluster of differentiation	Description/synonyms
CD2	Cells displaying sheep red blood cell receptor (SRBC+) present on all T cells OKT11 Thymocytes
CD3	Mature T lymphocytes T-Ly, OKT3, T cells
CD3,4	T Helper cells OKT4
CD3,8	T killer cells OKT8, cytotoxic T cells
CD3,9	T-Ly displaying a transferrin receptor OKT9

ability to modulate or suppress ongoing immune responses. These are called suppressor cells and can be either macrophages, which act relatively non-specifically, or antigen-specific CD3,8 Ly. Eventually, the suppressor system will dominate and dampen most ongoing responses, especially as the amount of inciting antigen that is activating helper T-Ly is removed or destroyed.

Nature Killer Cells (NK). Another name for this subset of lymphocytes is large granular lymphocytes. These larger cells can spontaneously attack certain viral-infected or tumor cells without prior exposure to them and without T cell help. The role of NK cells in the destruction of allografts is unknown, but they have been detected in some early rejection responses.

Bone Marrow-Derived Lymphocytes. Commonly called B cells, these cells are characterized by the presence of a highly specific immunoglobulin (sIg) and dense display of Class II determinants on their surfaces. The latter enables the B cell to act as an antigen-presenting cell. Once a specific antigen combines with its sIg, it can be internalized, processed, and presented to an appropriate helper T cell, which, in turn, activates the process of B cell growth and differentiation by secreting B cell interleukins such as IL-3, IL-4 and IL-6. B cells can also activate this process on their own if multiple sIg sites are bound with specific antigen. Regardless of which activating process is occurring, B cells rapidly internalize their sIg and differentiate to highly efficient protein-producing plasma cells that secrete antibodies specifically targeted at the antigen. These antibodies can coat their target cells and then mediate their destruction by attracting and binding killer monocytes and lymphocytes to them. Antibodies coated on bacteria or other specific targets markedly enhance the efficiency of phagocytosis by neutrophils and monocytes. Antibodies can rapidly mediate cell destruction by binding to a target, by activating the complement system. This complex series of destructive enzymes and corresponding inhibitors effects osmotic lysis of cells that are under attack and can rapidly cause organ destruction because it may inhibit blood supply.

Soluble Mediators of the Immune Response

Immune cells "talk" to one another through a very complex communication network of soluble, low-molecular-weight peptides called cytokines or interleukins, which can activate or suppress various lymphocyte subsets (Dinarello & Mier, 1987). The most notable interleukin is IL-2, the growth factor for T cells after they have been activated by some specific antigen. Resting T cells have few receptors for IL-2 on their surfaces. After antigen activation of the cell and IL-1 exposure, new, highly avid IL-2 receptors are rapidly synthesized and appear on the T cell surface to promote maximal cellular proliferation. A positive feedback system is set in motion as more and more cells and IL-2 become available during continuing antigen exposure. Other interleukins are produced during this time by both B and T cells to enhance B cell growth and differentiation to plasma cells in a similar fashion. Researchers are just beginning to comprehend the full spectrum of interleukin effects on diverse cells and tissue. Advances in understanding the action of interleukin will provide major new avenues for manipulating immune responses in humans.

THE REJECTION PROCESS

Once an allograft (or its passenger leukocytes) is recognized as non-self, it may be assaulted or rejected in two ways, through *cellular* or *humoral* rejection. The efficiency of the immune system is admirable. During any ongoing immune response, the inciting antigen causes a parallel expansion of both B and T memory cells specific for these antigens. When these antigens are subsequently encountered, an even more rapid reaction occurs. Memory cell expansion after antigen encounter is the principle that underlies the efficacy of immunization.

Cellular Rejection

The cycle initiated by helper T cells that have been sensitized by allograft antigens culminates in the production of allograft-specific killer T cells and is known as cellular rejection. Stated simply, cellular rejection occurs when Class II allograft antigens, displayed either on donor endothelium or on donor "passenger" leukocytes in the graft, incite antiallograft T helper cells to promote the expansion of a donor-specific population of cytotoxic T cells and simultaneously recruit macrophages into the area of the allograft by releasing various cytokines. Macrophages, in turn, release IL-1, which further fuels the reaction by enhancing T cell production of IL-2. The cytotoxic T cells then attack allograft antigens, especially those with Class I determinants, and damage the organ. The net result of a cell-mediated rejection is an allograft infiltrated with a rich mixture of CD3,4, CD3,8, and T-Ly, with large amounts of macrophages.

Humoral Rejection

Humoral rejection, on the other hand, is the allograft destruction that results from specifically directed antibodies. This form of rejection occurs in two ways. If the recipient has preformed antibodies arising from previous blood transfusions or pregnancy, these antibodies may cross-react with alloantibodies on the endothelium of the new organ. This antigen–antibody combination, in turn, activates the complement system and attracts highly destructive neutrophils to the area. Hyperacute rejection ensues, and the organ is lost.

The second and more common form of antibody-mediated rejection occurs when allograft-specific antibodies arise after transplantation. These antibodies mediate graft destruction by infiltrating the organ, activating complement, and attracting tissue-destroying neutrophils to the site. Allospecific antibodies also coat allograft cells and make them attractive targets for killer macrophages and lymphocytes.

In reality, both cellular and humoral mechanisms operate in concert during graft rejection. The contribution of T and B cell systems varies with the transplanted organ and the recipient's genetic constitution.

Classifications of Rejection

Rejection is the body's normal protective response to a perceived threat. The body's usual response to a foreign substance (antigen) is to attack and destroy that antigen. Thus, when the immune system recognizes the transplanted organ as foreign, it seeks to destroy it. The body's ability to distinguish self from non-self is the basis for the rejection process (Fuller, 1985).

Rejection reactions have been classified as hyperacute, acute, and chronic. These rejections differ in their time of occurrence as well as their distinct pathology.

Hyperacute Rejection

Hyperacute rejection occurs from minutes to hours after the transplanted organ has been placed. The graft may fail immediately or may function well for a time. Before long, a massive immune response takes place, and perfusion of the organ dramatically decreases. The graft becomes ischemic and nonfunctional. This lack of perfusion is called white graft rejection.

Hyperacute rejection episodes occur because the recipient had preformed cytotoxic antibodies capable of reacting against antigens in the transplanted organ. These antibodies activate the complement system, attract phagocytes, and stimulate platelet agglutination. Phagocytes and platelets enhance blood coagulation. Immunoglobulin G (IgG) and sometimes immunoglobulin M (IgM) antibodies bind to the capillary walls and activate complement factors that, in turn, recruit various inflammatory cells such as neutrophils and platelets to the graft (Fuller, 1985).

The pathophysiology of hyperacute rejection can be visualized as a blood transfusion reaction. The transfused cells are eliminated when cytotoxic antibodies against A or B erythrocyte antigens bind to their surface and mediate their demise.

Potential transplant recipients may have antibodies against a transplanted organ due to previous exposure to a similar ABO- or HLA-type antigen. This presensitization can be caused by previous blood transfusions, multiple pregnancies (antibodies formed against paternal antigens), or previous transplants.

Fortunately, hyperacute rejection is now very rare. It is prevented by screening the potential recipient's blood groups and HLA antigens prior to transplant. A preformed reactive antibody (PRA) test is required particularly in renal transplant candidates. The recipient's serum is mixed with a random panel of leukocytes from multiple sources that contain all known Class I and Class II antigens. If the recipient's serum does not react (absence of antibodies) with the cells (antigens), transplantation can proceed without hyperacute rejection. If the recipient is reactive with more than one of the cells in the panel of leukocytes from random donors, a direct cross-matching of a potential recipient's serum with cells from the specific donor must be done. If that cross-match is negative (no antibodies present), transplantation can proceed; if positive (antibodies present), the risk of hyperacute rejection with this donor is high.

Acute Rejection

Acute rejection most frequently occurs weeks to months after transplantation and becomes progressively less common over time. Acute rejection remains a common cause of death or organ loss within the first year after transplantation.

Acute rejection begins when Class I and II HLA antigens in the transplanted organ are recognized as foreign and the recipient activates a cellular immune response. An interaction between macrophages (phagocytic cells) and helper T lymphocytes occurs, and IL-1 is released. The cell interaction causes the helper T lymphocytes to proliferate. These mature helper T cells release IL-2, which then causes proliferation of donor-specific cytotoxic T lymphocytes. Under the influence of IL-2, more IL-2 receptors are displayed and produced. An exponential increase in the allograft-specific cytotoxic T cells occurs, which destroys the target organ by attacking their surface membranes (Murdock et al., 1987). The accumulation of graft-specific cytotoxic T lymphocytes is the major basis of acute rejection. Cytotoxic T cells also cause the release of gamma interferon, which further activates macrophages, increases the display of Class II determinants in the donor graft, and accelerates rejection. In addition, helper T cells cause B cell differentiation, which produces graft-specific antibodies (see Figure 2.1.) and amplifies other cytotoxic mechanisms.

Chronic Rejection

Chronic rejection begins at a variable time after the transplant occurs and may progress inexorably for years. The function of the transplanted organ gradually deteriorates over time.

Chronic rejection results from humoral immune responses against the transplanted tissue. Sensitized B cells produce antibodies that activate complement and cause platelet aggregates at the site of the reaction. This leads to accumulation of fibrin on the endothelium and ultimately to stenosis and eventual occlusion of the organ vessels. Lack of blood supply to the organ leads to ischemia and eventual necrosis.

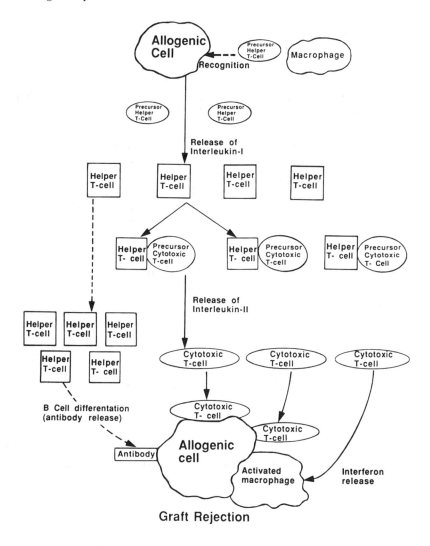

FIGURE 2.1 The acute allograft rejection process is demonstrated.

Rejection of Specific Organs

Heart

Hyperacute rejection of the transplanted heart is due to the presence of preformed cytotoxic antibodies generally directed against Class I antigens. Vessels that perfuse the heart are rich in Class I antigens. Coronary arteries are, therefore, early targets of this form of rejection. Thrombosis and ischemic heart failure are the ultimate results of hyperacute rejection.

Acute rejection of the heart occurs as early as 1 week after transplantation, when antigens on the surface cells of the transplanted heart are recognized as foreign. Initially, endothelium and dendritic cells that have been transferred into the recipient on the donor graft recruit recipient macrophages to attack it. Shortly thereafter, as Class I donor antigens are encountered, cytotoxic T cells also begin to attack it. Mononuclear cells in the myocardium are histologic evidence of acute rejection. The severity of rejection ranges from mild to severe; the presence of mononuclear infiltration without damage to the heart constitutes mild rejection. Myocyte necrosis as well as mononuclear infiltration is characteristic of moderate rejection. Severe rejection is characterized by varying degrees of intramyocardial edema, hemorrhage, or both , as well as macrophages, neutrophils, and eosinophils in the graft. (See Figure 2.2.)

Clinical manifestations vary. Some patients may be completely as-ymptomatic; other patients may show signs of congestive heart failure. Common symptoms include jugular venous distension, liver enlargement, presence of a third heart sound, decrease in blood pressure, and elevated hemodynamic pressures such as right atrial pressure, pulmonary artery pressures, and pulmonary capillary wedge pressure. Abnormalities in the electrocardiogram are decreases in voltage and poor R-wave progression. Echocardiograms may reveal poor wall motion and pericardial effusions. Chest x-ray may reveal cardiomegaly. (See Table 2.2.)

Chronic rejection is described as diffuse coronary artery disease resulting in ischemic organ damage. Since the donor heart is denervated, the patient does not experience angina; thus, this finding is usually documented during annual coronary angiography. Cross-sections of coronary arteries reveal internal hyperplasia with or without lipid deposition. Because of the diffuse nature of coronary artery disease, angioplasty or coronary artery bypass surgery is rarely effective. Retransplantation is the only therapeutic alternative.

Heart–Lung

Until recently, the surveillance protocol for heart–lung rejection was almost identical to that for patients who had undergone heart transplantation. Immunologists incorrectly predicted that pulmonary graft rejection and myocardial rejection occurred simultaneously. As experience has accumulated, however, this has proved not to be the case. Rejection in the heart is very rare in the heart–lung recipient; thus, heart rejection cannot predict pulmonary rejection. As a result, many large transplant centers have stopped doing endomyocardial biopsies for the detection of heart–lung transplantation rejection. The transplantation team detects rejection through clinical observation, monitoring of chest x-rays and pulmonary function, and identifying bronchial alveolar cell populations obtained by lavage and endobronchial biopsy. A unique problem in lung transplantation is the development of an early but reversible defect in pulmonary function characterized by

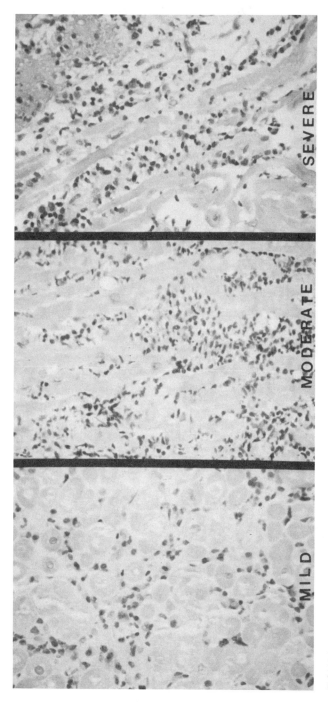

FIGURE 2.2 Rejection of heart allograft: Acute, *mild*, *moderate*, and *severe* heart transplant rejection. Note the progression from lymphocytic infiltration (mild), to myocyte necrosis (moderate), to edema and hemorrhage. (This figure is provided by Dr. Gayle Winters, Department of Pathology, Loyola University of Chicago.)

TABLE 2.2 Diagnostic Tests and Common Signs and Symptoms of Acute Rejection

	Heart	Heart–Lung	Liver	Kidney	Bone marrow (GVHD)
Diagnostic Tests	Endomyocardial biopsy	Endobronchial biopsy	Liver biopsy	Renal biopsy	Skin biopsy
	Measurement of hemodynamic pressures	Pulmonary function test	Elevated liver function tests (bilirubin, SGOT, SGPT)	Elevated BUN and creatinine	Liver function tests
	Electrocardiogram	Arterial blood gases			Immunologic blood testing
	Echocardiogram	Complete blood count			
	Chest x-ray	Chest x-ray			
Signs/symptoms	Fatigue	Dyspnea	Malaise	Oliguria	Maculopapular skin rash
	Decreased blood pressure	Sputum changes	Fever	Hypertension	Dry eyes and mouth
	Jugular venous distension	Fever	Abdominal discomfort	Graft tenderness	Diarrhea
	Presence of S3	Tachycardia		Fever	Jaundice
	Fluid retention				
	Cardiogenic shock				Joint pain

changes in gas exchange, vascular resistance, and airway compliance. The "shock-like-lung" syndrome, formerly known as "reimplantation response" usually occurs within 3 to 6 postoperative days but has been encountered up to 3 weeks after transplantation. This pulmonary interstitial response is apparently a mechanical one and is not based on specific immunologic rejection. True rejection responses in heart–lung transplantation are characterized by mixed cellular infiltrates with varying populations of CD3,4 and CD3,8 phenotypes and monocytes. They are initially encountered in the peribronchial submucosal areas with extension into the interstitium during severe reactions. Clinically, as in heart transplantation, the patient may be either asymptomatic or critically ill with severe loss of pulmonary function during the rejection process. The frequency and intensity of rejection episodes vary markedly from patient to patient. A general clinical impression is that rejection may be less frequent in pulmonary transplantation than in other organ transplantations.

An interesting phenomenon, bronchiolitis obliterans, can occur following heart–lung transplantation. Bronchiolitis obliterans is characterized by rhinitis, postnasal drainage, and cough production of mucopurulent sputum at the time of airway obstruction. Physical examination demonstrates bibasilar crackles in the lung fields (Burke et al., 1985). Transbronchial biopsy shows evidence of bronchiolitis. Bronchiolitis obliterans, evidenced by declining pulmonary function, is thought to be a manifestation of rejection. Early aggressive immunosuppressive therapy is indicated because this condition often progesses rapidly. Despite all efforts, it may be irreversible and fatal.

Liver

A fascinating aspect of the transplanted liver is its relative resistance to hyperacute rejection. Liver transplantation has been done successfully despite positive cross-matches between donor and recipient lymphocytes and also across ABO incompatibilities. A specific mechanism for this is as yet unknown (Duquesnay, Saidman, Markus, Demetris, & Zeevi, 1988).

Clinically, acute liver transplant rejection may be marked by malaise, fever, abdominal discomfort, and worsening liver function tests such as elevated bilirubin, serum glutamic oxaloacetic transaminase (SGOT), and serum glutamic pyruvic transaminase (SGPT). The graft may also become swollen and inflamed. Histologically, mononuclear cells migrate to the portal tract, and blood flow is disrupted. Necrosis of hepatocytes then ensues. Cholestasis becomes evident, and necrosis of small hepatic arteries occurs. Eventually, larger interlobular bile ducts may be damaged by progressive cellular infiltration and may subsequently disappear (Cuthbert, 1986).

Chronic rejection of the liver is characterized by a progressive thickening of the intima of the hepatic arteries and diminution of the bile ducts (so-called vanishing bile duct syndrome) seen on liver biopsy. Immunoglobins and complement are found in the vessel walls, suggesting a humoral response (Cuthbert, 1986).

Kidney

Hyperacute renal transplant rejection results in diffuse intrarenal thrombosis and permanent loss of graft function. Hyperacute rejection is diagnosed by the presence of anuria and the absence of renal flow. Histologically, there is evidence of renal infarction. Hyperacute rejection of the kidney occurs a few minutes to a few hours after implantation. The treatment is graft nephrectomy (Venkateswara Rao, 1984).

Clinical characteristics of acute cellular rejection include oliguria, hypertension, graft tenderness, and fever. Renal dysfunction may occasionally require temporary dialysis. Histologically, there are perivascular mononuclear cell infiltration, interstitial edema, and atrophy of tubular epithelium. The infiltrating cells are usually lymphocytes, but plasma cells, eosinophils, and polymorphonuclear cells may also be seen in the interstitium of the rejecting kidney.

Chronic renal rejection occurs months to years after transplantation. Generally, a slow decline in renal function is noted. Predominant clinical manifestations of chronic rejection are hypertension, proteinuria, and nephrotic syndrome. Renal biopsy reveals endothelial proliferation and obstruction of small arteries and arterioles. Medical management during chronic rejection is similar to managing patients in chronic renal failure. The chronically rejected kidney may or may not be removed, and the patient may be considered for retransplantation (Richard, 1984).

Bone Marrow

Graft rejection in bone marrow transplant recipients is characterized by the disappearance of an early grafting blood picture and recurrence of an aplastic state that follows immunosuppressive therapy.

Graft-versus-host disease (GVHD) is an immunologic reaction that occurs in bone marrow transplant recipients. The unique reaction is essentially the reverse of typical rejection in that the graft cells (stem cells that are the precursors of the key elements of the immune system) attack the host cells instead of the host attacking the graft. In most instances, the immune effector responses of the host have been ablated by chemotherapy prior to the transplant, and thus donor T lymphocytes are relatively unopposed as they react against antigens on the host. Recipient organs most frequently affected are the skin, liver, and gastrointestinal tract (Kamani & August, 1984). Efforts to ameliorate this formidable obstacle include meticulous cross-matching of donors and recipients. More recently, new techniques for purging aplastic cells from a patient's own collected marrow create a possibility for autologous bone marrow transplantation.

Acute GVHD usually develops within the first 100 days posttransplant. It generally presents as a maculopapular skin rash, diarrhea, and hepatic dysfunction. Skin biopsies usually show evidence of perivascular mononuclear cell infiltration in the dermis and degeneration of basal epidermal cells at the dermal-epidermal junction (Kamani & August, 1984). The severity of acute GVHD is determined by the degree of involvement of individual organ systems, ranging from mild to severe. Treatment of GVHD is similar to the treatment of other rejection processes.

Chronic GVHD begins 6 to 18 months after transplantation. Clinical manifestations are skin changes, dry eyes and mouth, jaundice, joint contractures, and weight loss. Specific immunologic abnormalities include hypergammaglobulinemia, eosinophilia, circulating antibodies, and immune complexes. Hypersplenism may occur, making patients more susceptible to infection.

IMMUNOSUPPRESSIVE THERAPIES

Immunosuppressive medications are used for long-term and short-term prevention and treatment of transplant rejection. Immunosuppressive protocols differ for each institution and with each specific organ. Immunosuppression begins prior to surgery and continues for the organ's life. An overview of five most common immunosuppressive medications follows.

Cyclosporine A

Cyclosporine A (Cy A) is a metabolite of two strains of *Fungi Imperfecti, Tolyplocladium inflatum gams* and *Cylindrocarpon lucidum*. It was discovered by Swiss scientist J. F. Borel in 1972 (Ota, 1983) while sampling soil in Southern Norway. Organ graft survival has improved dramatically since the introduction of Cy A in transplantation. Cy A suppresses the cell-mediated immune response. It prevents the proliferation of precursor T cells after alloantigen stimulation. This is accomplished primarily by inhibiting the release of IL-2 and perhaps also IL-1. It also affects the production of gamma interferon, causing the effector lymphocytes to recognize that the alloantigen(s) is foreign, but is unable to react to it. Cy A has little effect on phagocytosis and virtually no bone marrow suppression capability. Therefore, neutrophils are in good supply and effective, making the threat of infection much less. Cy A minimally affects humoral-mediated immunity.

Cy A helps prevent rejection but does not treat rejection once it has begun. Dosage is adjusted according to renal function. Many adverse side effects are related to Cy A use. More common effects include nephrotoxicity, hepatotoxicity, hypertension, tremors, burning of the hands and feet, hirsutism, gum hyperplasia, and an increased risk for infection and malignancy.

Corticosteroids

Corticosteroids (prednisone, methylprednisolone sodium, or Solu-Medrol®) were among the first antiinflammatory agents to be used as immunosuppressants in the prevention and treatment of allograft rejection. Steroids affect both the humoral- and cell-mediated immune response.

Corticosteroids hinder rejection by preventing macrophages from releasing IL-1 (Snyder & Unanve, 1982). They thereby block IL-1–dependent release of IL-2 from activated T cells (Busuttil, Goldstein, Danovitch, Ament, & Memsic, 1986). This blockage reduces the ability to produce cytotoxic T cells. In addition, by interfering with intracellular antigen processing and phagocytosis of macrophages, corticosteroids impair the lymphocyte's ability to recognize antigens (Snyder & Unanve).

At high doses, corticosteroids interfere with the function of the lymphocytic cell membrane. This effect stops the cytotoxic T lymphocyte from recognizing its target antigen. Thus, lymphocytes are no longer attracted to the graft, and those lymphocytes that have already accumulated are rendered ineffective (Murdock et al., 1987). All of the above effects make corticosteroids valuable in preventing and treating established rejection.

Corticosteroids have multiple side effects relating to other mechanisms of action. Effects include cushingoid appearance, glucose intolerance, sodium and water retention, increased appetite, osteoporosis, muscle wasting, gastric ulcers, exacerbation of infection, cataracts, and steroid psychosis. Many of the side effects of corticosteroids can be averted by using the lowest possible effective antirejection dose.

Azathioprine

Azathioprine (Aza) is an antimetabolite drug that theoretically prevents the rapid cell division necessitated by an immune response, thus blocking the ability to develop cytotoxic T cells. It also inhibits natural killer cell functions. The use of Aza for preventing rejection declined with the discovery of Cy A. Recently, Aza regained widespread use in organ transplantation after it was shown that combining Aza with Cy A and prednisone (known as triple therapy) further increased graft survival and patient survival rates. Dosage of Aza is adjusted according to the white blood cell count. Side effects of Aza are associated with suppression of other rapidly dividing cells. Bone marrow suppression, causing neutropenia, can make the transplant recipient more prone to infection. Aza can also cause gastrointestinal upset, hepatotoxicity, and tumors.

Antithymocyte Globulin

Antithymocyte globulin (ATG) is produced by immunizing either horses or rabbits with human thymocytes. It is therefore involved in the cell-mediated immune response. After injection, ATG binds to T-cell surfaces, changing their receptors and markers and neutralizing the ability of an antigen receptor to combine effectively with its antigen. It also makes lymphocytes more susceptible to phagocytosis. In the early transplant period, ATG can be used prophylactically to prevent rejection and later to treat established rejection. One drawback is that ATG contains more than anti-T-cell specificities. Antibodies present in ATG preparations can react with platelets, causing clinically significant thrombocytopenia. ATG also has the potential to cause a severe anaphylactic reaction. In addition, ATG potency may vary from lot to lot, and there is a clinical suspicion that lymphoproliferative diseases are more likely to occur when this agent is used repeatedly.

Orthoclone T-3 (OKT3)

OKT3 is the newest of the immunosuppressive medications used to prevent and treat transplant rejection. OKT3 is a murine (mouse-derived) monoclonal antibody produced through the application of genetic engineering to immunology. This monoclonal antibody reacts only with a specific receptor that is bound tightly to a T-cell-specific antigen receptor. After binding to the former, it blocks the generation and function of allospecific cytotoxic T cells by masking their antigen- specific receptors. Side effects associated with the drug include hypersensitivity; severe flulike symptoms, such as nausea and vomiting; bronchospasm; aseptic meningitis; lymphoma; and the development of antibodies against the medication. Approximately one third of patients receiving OKT3 will develop antibodies against the drug. These antibodies can cause rapid elimination and removal of OKT3 from blood after an intravenous infusion. This blunts the effectiveness of subsequent treatments of rejection episodes with OKT3.

NURSING CARE OF THE PATIENT IN REJECTION

Nursing care of the patient in rejection is complex and challenging. It requires expert knowledge of normal graft function and frequent and accurate assessments and intervention. Many times, astute observations of subtle changes by the nurse preserve graft function and may save the patient's life.

The overall nursing goal in caring for the patient in rejection is to preserve the graft with minimal compromise to the patient. Interventions include monitoring the patient for signs and symptoms of ensuing or worsening graft failure and prompt notification of the physician so that immediate treatment can begin. Treatment usually includes the adminstration of large doses of immunosuppressive medication. Patients may need to be artificially supported while the graft is undergoing treatment for rejection. For example, the heart transplant patient may need inotropes or, as a last resort, intraaortic balloon pump support. A heart–lung patient may need ventilatory support. The kidney transplant patient may require temporary dialysis.

The treatment of rejection can have adverse effects on other body functions. Because rejection treatment severely compromises the immune system, many posttransplant infections quickly follow. Monitoring a patient's vital signs, especially temperature, becomes extremely important. Alterations in any vital signs need to be promptly reported. Laboratory values such as white blood cell counts need to be astutely monitored. A sudden decrease in the white blood cell count can indicate a viral infection. An increase in bands and a decrease in segmented neutrophils can also indicate infection. Medications given for rejection also affect renal and hepatic functions. The transplantation team monitors kidney and liver function and adjusts medications appropriately.

Nurses can assist patients and families in dealing with the "realities" of transplantation. Because patients experiencing rejection can be extremely anxious, they need to vent their fears and frustrations. Many patients have false expectations following transplantation despite the most realistic and straightforward preoperative teaching. They hope to be the one patient transplanted who does not experience rejection. The recipient who is in rejection needs to be reminded that rejection does not necessarily mean death; it usually denotes that the immunosuppressant therapies need adjusting. Most rejection episodes are treated successfully with minimal damage to the graft, but when rejection episodes are severe, graft function may be compromised. For some patients, this may mean living with symptoms of congestive heart failure again; to others, it may mean returning to dialysis. In some cases, retransplantation must be considered. A small minority may face impending death.

Caring for patients in rejection requires compassion. It can be a long and tedious but rewarding task. Nurse managers need to realize the assignment's complexity. Many units that frequently care for posttransplant patients have "care for the caregiver" sessions with psychologists, psychiatrists, or psychiatric clinical nurse specialists providing assistance.

CONCLUSION

The human immune system is a complex network of organs, cells, and signaling systems. It does an amazing job of protecting the body against foreign invaders. Modifying such an intricate system to allow for allograft acceptance while maintaining protection from pathogens requires diligent patient monitoring. The discovery of Cy A and the advances in monoclonal antibody technology have provided some tools for selectively blinding the immune system and suppressing the immune response. A delicate balance must be struck. Inadequate immunosuppression can result in rejection; too much may cause infections and compromise other organ systems.

Nurses have the monumental task of monitoring and reporting responses to the above manipulations. The physical responses are many and complex. Nurses must remember the emotional needs of the patient and family who are faced with rejection and/or the myriad other potential side effects of immunosuppression.

The multiplicity of components and activities within the immune system seems staggering at first glance—even impossible, considering the enormous number of questions that are still unanswered. It is this complexity, however, that makes the future bright for increasingly successful organ transplantation. With new information about normal immune function comes a new opportunity for modifying the system. Advances, not only in drug therapy but in efficient cross-matching, donor selection, organ preservation, infection management and prevention, and many other areas, should make organ transplantation even more practicable over the next several years.

ACKNOWLEDGEMENT

Both authors wish to acknowledge the enormous assistance of John A. Robinson, M.D., Associate Dean for Research at Loyola University Medical Center, Chicago. He is the past Medical Director of Cardiac Transplant and continues as consultant for immunomodulation and infection problems in cardiac transplant patients. His willingness to share his wisdom, experience, expertise, and time has been essential to the completion of this chapter. We extend to him our deepest gratitude.

REFERENCES

Burke, C. M., Morris, A. J. R., Dawkins, K. D., McGregor, C. G. A., Yousem, S. A., Allen, M., Theodore, J., Harvey, J., Billingmam, M. E., Oyer, P. E., Stinson, E. B., Baldwin, J. C., Shumway, N. E., & Jamieson, S. E. (1985). Late airflow obstruction in heart-lung transplantation recipients. *The Journal of Heart Transplantation, 4*(4), 437–440.

Busuttil, R. W., Goldstein, L. I., Danovitch, G. M., Ament, M. E., & Memsic, L. D. F. (1986). Liver transplantation today. *Annals of Internal Medicine, 104*, 377–389.

Cuthbert, J. A. (1986). Southwestern internal medicine conference: Hepatic transplantation. *American Journal of Medical Sciences, 291*(4), 292.

Dinarello, C. A., & Mier, J. W. (1987). Current concepts: Lymphokines. *New England Journal of Medicine, 317*, 940–945

Duquesnay, R. J., Saidman, S., Markus, B. H., Demetris, A. J., & Zeevi, A. (1988). Role of HLA in intragraft cellular immunity in human liver transplantation. *Transplantation Proceedings, 20*(1), 724.

Fuller, B. F. (1985). Organ graft rejection: the The biological process. *Association of Operating Room Nurses Journal, 14*(4), 738–745.

Johnston, R. B. (1988). Current concepts: Immunology. Monocytes and macrophages. *New England Journal of Medicine, 318*, 747–752

Kamani, N., & August, C. S. (1984). Bone marrow transplantation: Problems and prospects. *Medical Clinics of North America, 68*(3), 662.

Kottra-Buck, C. (1986). Renal transplantation. In C.J. Richard (Ed.), *Comprehensive nephrology nursing* (pp. 408–423). Boston: Little, Brown.

Lafferty, K. J. (1988). The immunologic network. *Transplant Proceedings, 20*, 13–269 (suppl 2).

Murdock, D. K., Collins, E.G., Lawless, C.E., Molnar, Z., Scanlon, P.J., & Pifarre, R. (1987). Rejection of the transplanted heart. *Heart and Lung, 16*(3), 237–245.

Ota, B. (1983). Administration of cyclosporine. *Transplantation Proceedings, 15*(4), 3111–3123.

Richard, C. J. (1984). Renal transplantation. In *Comprehensive nephrology nursing* (pp. 408–423). Boston: Little, Brown.

Snyder, D. A., & Unanve, E. R. (1982). Corticosteroids inhibit murine macrophage Ia expression and interleukin 1 production. *Journal of Immunology, 129*, 1803.

Stobo, J. D. (1987). *Lymphocytes in basic and clinical immunology* (6th ed., pp. 65–81). Los Altos, CA: Lange Medical Books.

Venkateswara Rao, K. (1984). Status of renal transplantation: A clinical perspective. *Medical Clinics of North America, 68*(2), 427–453.

CHAPTER **3**

INFECTION IN IMMUNOSUPPRESSED PATIENTS

Elizabeth A. Collins
Bonnie B. Grusk
Eileen G. Collins

Organ transplant recipients are at high risk for infectious complications. Although recent evidence demonstrates that the number of infections has decreased since transplantation became a therapeutic modality in the early 1950s, infections continue to be the most significant cause of morbidity and mortality in organ transplant recipients (Garibaldi, 1983). Factors that have contributed to a decreased rate of infection are recognition of infection as a significant post transplant complication, aggressive identification and treatment of infection, titration of immunosuppressive therapy, and the use of cyclosporine A (Cy A) (Hofflin et al., 1987).

The potential for acquiring an infection is high in this population, and nurses must focus on critical time periods before, during, and after transplantation. Their interventions should be aimed at preventive measures by recognizing those situations and practices which contribute to the pool of potential risks. When possible, risks must be reduced or eliminated.

Throughout the transplant period, a major nursing focus is on patient assessment for infection and education of recipients and their families. Education includes recognition of situations and practices that have high potential for contributing to infection and the identification of measures to avoid or reduce the risks.

THE CHRONICALLY ILL PATIENT

Compromised Hosts

Transplant recipients are compromised hosts even before immunosuppressive therapy and the surgical transplantation procedures are used. In many cases, patients have had a chronic, debilitating disease. These patients are grouped into two categories: primary- and secondary- disease impairment.

Primary-Disease Impairment

The primary disease impairment directly alters the function of bone marrow, heart, liver, kidney, and/or lung function. Each of these organ systems contributes to host immune-defense mechanisms. Bone marrow produces both red and white blood cells, including neutrophils, which function as an integral part of the inflammatory response. The cardiovascular system, via the blood, transports nutrients, oxygen, and metabolic by-products to various parts of the body. Both specific and non-specific internal defense mechanisms are also transported to areas of infection via the cardiovascular system. Nonspecific defense mechanisms include macrophages, neutrophils, serum proteins, and complement. Antibodies and antitoxins are examples of specific internal defense mechanisms that are disseminated throughout the body. The liver also contributes to the immune system through phagocytosis by Kupffer cells and through detoxification of bacterial endotoxins. Urinary tract infections are prevented in the genitourinary system through micturition, which purges the bladder of invading organisms (DeGroot-Kosolcharoen, 1984). Multiple natural defense mechanisms in both the upper and lower respiratory tracts protect the lungs from infection. In the upper tract, dust particles and bacteria adhere to mucous membranes and may be expelled by sneezing; in the lower respiratory tract, organisms may be expelled via the cough reflex and upward movement of particles by the cilia.

Secondary-Disease Impairment

Secondary impairment of vital organ function may also be present. Each system and organ depends upon the proper functioning of all other systems. If one body system is affected by a disease process, a domino effect may functionally hamper or impair other systems. For example, if patients become anemic due to bone marrow depression from their primary disease, the cardiovascular system may be affected because the ability to transport red cells, and hence oxygenation is impaired. If the patient suffers from heart failure, perfusion to the kidneys may be reduced, predisposing the kidneys and bladder to infection through inadequate urinary flow. Decreased perfusion to the liver may also interfere with phagocytosis, severe reduction of toxin removal, and protein formation.

Nutrition in Prevention of Secondary-Disease Impairment

Adequate nutrition is also essential for preventing secondary impairment of organ function and infection. Malnourishment has a direct effect on morbidity and mortality after transplantation (DiCecco et al., 1989). Nutritional stores may be depleted in patients because of their primary disease, which can lead to a nitrogen imbalance and suppression of the antibody response (Axnick, 1984). If this is the case, the patient may need a special diet or nutritional supplementation prior to the transplant procedure to promote wound healing and general well-being after transplantation.

HOSPITALIZATION AS A RISK FACTOR

Hospitalization prior to transplantation is an extrinsic risk factor for the development of infections (Burke & Hildick-Smith, 1978). Colonization with nosocomial organisms rapidly occurs following hospital admission. Craven & Regan (1989) determined that nosocomial infection is a major complication of hospitalization, particularly in intensive care units. This group of patients, which may include organ transplant candidates and recipients, not only have a serious underlying disease, but may require treatments or devices while in the hospital that often alter their natural host-defense mechanisms. Clinical risk factors which contribute to colonization include: increasing severity of illness, duration of hospitalization, previous or concurrent antibiotic administration, intubation, alteration in gastric acidity, and major surgery (Craven & Reagan, 1989).

In addition to colonization of patients, pathogens may also colonize the hands of hospital staff and areas in the hospital environment. Inadequate hand-washing routines are associated with high rates of hand colonization, which then becomes a transferring vehicle for various organisms. Proper hand washing can reduce this process (Craven & Regan, 1989).

The duration of hospital stay prior to surgery has been associated with higher rates of wound infection (Axnick, 1984). Surgical wound infections directly influence not only patient morbidity and mortality, but the cost of hospitalization (due to the increased length of stay and necessity of further treatment). Numerous investigators (Cruse & Foord, 1980; Haley et al., 1981) have demonstrated that the risk of surgical wound infection rises for patients hospitalized preoperatively for 10 or more days. The lowest rates occur in patients undergoing surgery after only 1 day in the hospital. Therefore, because of the increased risk of infection, the patient awaiting transplantation should be hospitalized for as few days as feasible.

POSTTRANSPLANT PHASES OF INFECTIONS

Garibaldi (1983) has proposed three phases that occur in posttransplantation infections. The phases he described can be useful in predicting infectious complications in the transplant population, although each recipient must be individually evaluated. He categorized these phases according to time (1 month, 2–6 months, and more than 6 months) after transplantation, pathogenic organisms commonly seen in each phase, and risk factors developing in each phase.

Bacterial infections may occur at any time but are most common during the first month after transplantation. However, Rao and Anderson (1988) have noted bacterial infections as the most common infection experienced by renal transplant recipients as long as two decades after transplantation. Soon after transplantation, bacteria cause urinary tract infections, wound infections, and pneumonias (Counts, 1988; Ramsey et al., 1980). It is also common to see polymicrobial infections. Viral, fungal, and nocardial infections arise about 1 to 3 months after transplantation (Rifking, Marchioro, Schneck, & Hill, 1967). Cytomegalovirus (CMV) is the most common viral agent during this phase (Schumann, 1987).

Fungal and nocardial infections typically occur in the respiratory tract. The risk for developing fungal and nocardial infections extends throughout the posttransplantation period. Protozoal infections appear late in the first 6 months posttransplantation and are usually respiratory diseases such as *Pneumocystis carinii* pneumonia.

As in kidney transplant recipients, bacterial infections in the heart transplant recipient occur perioperatively and may involve the respiratory tract, blood stream, and surgical wound (Hofflin et al., 1987). Gentry and Zeluff (1986) noted that wound infections in cardiac transplant patients are relatively uncommon. Protozoal, viral, and fungal infections commonly emerge at 2 to 4 weeks after surgery (Luft, Naut, Arauso, Stinson, & Remington, 1983). CMV and *Aspergillus* organisms are major causes of morbidity and mortality in this patient population (O'Toole, Gary, Maher, & Wreghitt, 1986; Gurwith, Stinson, & Remington, 1971). Nocardial infections of the respiratory and integumentary systems are almost unique to the heart transplant recipient.

Heart–lung transplant infections are etiologically similar to those found in heart transplant recipients. However, pneumonia and other respiratory infections are most common in the heart–lung transplant recipient.

In the liver transplant recipient, the most common and severe infections are bacterial and are associated with intraabdominal abscesses, pneumonias, soft tissue infections, and cholangitis. Viral infections in liver transplant recipients, as with other solid-organ transplant recipients, emerge at 2 to 4 weeks after transplantation. The most common viral agent in this population is CMV. Kusne et al. (1988) described an 18% fungal infection rate in their series of liver transplants between 1984 and 1985. Wajszczuk et al. (1985) had previously described a 42% incidence of fungal infections in adult liver transplant patients in an era of intense immunosuppression in the early 1980s. Infections from such Protozoa as *P. carinii* and *Toxoplasma gondii* also occur about 8 weeks after transplantation.

In bone marrow transplantation recipients, the patients are at very high risk early after transplant because of a complete lack of white blood cells until marrow engraftment takes place. Bacterial infections are an important consideration in the early period after transplantation. Bacteremia is the most significant infection. Pirsch and Maki (1986) recently demonstrated an increased susceptibility to fungal infections in adults with bone marrow transplantation. Fungal and viral pathogens are most significant at about 1 month after transplantation (Peterson et al., 1983). *Aspergillus fumigatus, Candida albicans,* herpes simplex virus (HSV), and CMV are the most common examples of these pathogens (Thompson & Thomas, 1986). *P. Carinii* pneumonia is an uncommon infection but may emerge during a later stage, 6 months or more after transplantation.

The Centers for Disease Control (CDC) recently published an updated system for assessing nosocomial infections (Garner, Jarvis, Emori, Horan, & Hughes, 1988). This system uses a criterion-based, decision-tree method to define infections. Signs and symptoms normally associated with infections must be modified when assessing the immunodeficient host. These modifications may include a lower threshold for defining a febrile state or considering hypotension as a potential sign of sepsis. Subtle findings of disorientation and hypoxemia may also be important findings. It is best to establish criteria for defining infectious complications in the transplant recipient early in the program. This requires understanding and concurrence of the transplant team. These criterion-based definitions then become the basis for establishing diagnoses and for developing statistical analyses of infectious complications in the program.

One Month Posttransplantation

Infections in transplant recipients during this phase are not unlike those observed in other postoperative patients. Similar epidemiologic patterns emerge in terms of site of infection and causative agent. Bacterial infections are usually associated with hospital therapeutics, interventions, and monitoring procedures. Surgical wound infections may also be a problem during this early phase. Patient susceptibility, wound condition at the time of operative closure, and the magnitude of wound contamination at the time of operative closure are three factors cited by Simmons (1982) as influencing surgical wound infection rates. Invasive monitoring devices, ventilation equipment, intravascular-access catheters, and urologic instrumentation contribute to the incidence of pneumonias, bacteremias, and urinary tract infections seen in all hospitalized patients, but more important, they may contribute significantly to those seen in the transplant population. Infections occurring during this time period are typically attributable to nosocomial bacterial pathogens such as *Staphylococcus aureus*, *Pseudomonas* species, *Serratia marcescens*, *Enterobacteriaceae*, and *Legionella pneumophilia*. Legionnaire's disease has been reported as epidemic on some transplant units. Patients usually present with rapidly changing nodular or lobular consolidations on chest x-ray. Diagnosis of this disease process is made by culture or by demonstration of a rise in serum antibody titres.

Two to Six Months Posttransplantation

During the second to sixth month after transplantation, the transplant recipient is most vulnerable to infection. Opportunistic pathogens account for a large percentage of the infections encountered at this time. Viral, fungal, protozoal, and nocardial infections emerge. The pathogens commonly include *Pneumocystis carinii*, *Toxoplasma gondii*, *Aspergillus fumigatus* and other species, *Candida albicans*, *Torulopsis glabrata*, HSV, herpes zoster virus (HZV), and CMV.

Infections during this phase may be primary or reactivated. Primary infections are those infections without another underlying clinically evident site of infection. They may also be ones that patients have never experienced. Etiologic agents for primary infections may be traced to the organ donor, transfused blood products, environmental sources, or other exogenous sources. Primary infections tend to have a more virulent course than reactivated infections, although the latter also contributes to morbidity and mortality in transplant recipients.

Previously latent endogenous flora cause reactivation infections. Latent flora imply that at some time in the past the patient was infected with an organism which has then become part of the patient's endogenous flora. *P. carinii* is such an organism. The patient may also have experienced an asymptomatic primary infection in the past; the agent then persists in a dormant state in the body until immunosuppressive therapy stresses the host defenses. Viral organisms that commonly reside in a dormant stage after primary infection include Ebstein-Barr virus, HSV, HZV, and CMV. In addition, complications may develop. Neutropenia, for example, may reduce the immune response to infection. Requirements for intensified immunosuppression during rejection would predispose the patient to life threatening superinfections with other microbial agents. CMV is a particularly offending etiologic agent of this nature (O'Toole et al., 1986; Ramsey et al., 1980).

CMV is a very common posttransplant viral infection, especially if donors have been previously infected with CMV and recipients have not. CMV-positive donors are avoided whenever possible in heart, lung, and kidney transplantation. Infection with CMV can occur after transplanting an organ from a CMV-positive donor or using CMV-positive blood products. Diagnosis of CMV is made by isolating the virus, detecting its genetic characteristics in culture, by observing a fourfold or more rise in antibody titre between the previous and acute sera, or by localizing it in biopsy specimens. Patient presentation may be subclinical or so severe that the infection rapidly becomes fatal. Patients most often present with fever, leukopenia, and interstitial pneumonia. Diarrhea, ulceration, bleeding, and perforation may be observed if CMV invades the gastrointestinal tract. Retinitis, encephalitis, or various arthralgias may also be seen. The disease generally takes 3 to 6 weeks to run its course, and patients may or may not have to be hospitalized. A new antiviral medication, gancyclovir, can be effective in certain CMV infections.

HSV infection is often due to the reactivation of a latent virus. Infections usually begin as benign cold sores and may progress to a fatal illness. Common ulcerative sites are the lips, chest, back, and genitals. Lesions generally remain for 2 to 5 weeks. Treatment includes antiviral medications and pain control. It is important that nurses instruct the patient not to touch lesions since this can be a common mode of infectious spread to other parts of the body.

HZV infection presents as a painful skin rash distributed along the spinal nerve roots or the trigeminal nerve across the face. The rash usually subsides within 1 to 2 weeks. This is usually a reactivation of the varicella virus the patient was infected with as a child. Treatment includes the antiviral medication acyclovir, pain control, and possibly nerve blocks for analgesia. Again, nurses instruct patients not to touch the lesions. It is important to note that only those personnel, patients, or visitors who have had chicken pox can be in contact with the infected patient.

Candidiasis in the form of a white plaquelike thrush in the oropharynx is frequently seen in patients posttransplantation. Nystatin oral suspension swish-and-swallow may be given for 3 months after transplant to prevent and treat this complication. Occasionally, *C. albicans* may infect the gastrointestinal tract, skin folds, genitourinary tract, and the central nervous system. In these cases, more intense antibiotic treatment with amphotericin B or miconazole is necessary. Fungemias, which may develop after high doses of antibiotics for other infections, are extremely serious and can be fatal.

A. fumigatus is a very serious, and potentially fatal infection. Environmental perturbations, especially construction, may be the source of the organism. It usually presents as a localized lesion, an invasive pulmonary infection, or a disseminated disease. Diagnosis is difficult and may require transtracheal or transthoracic aspiration. Treatment of choice is amphotericin B. Favorable results from treatment are seen in those patients in whom the infection is confined to the lung and diagnosis is made early in a clinical situation when decreases in the intensity of the immunosuppressive therapy can be effective.

Clinically significant *P. carinii* and *T. gondii* infections occur almost exclusively in the immunocompromised host. Pneumocystis is generally limited to the lungs. Clinical manifestations include fever, nonproductive cough, dyspnea, cyanosis, and hypoxia. Physical findings are usually present on chest x-rays. Diagnosis is made by a transthoracic needle aspiration or surgical biopsy through bronchoscopy or open lung procedure. The treatment of choice, at present, is trimethoprim and sulfamethoxazole plus oxygen support. Sometimes infected patients will require intubation and ventilatory assistance.

Patients with toxoplasma pneumonia present very similarly to patients with pneumocystis pneumonia. The infection usually occurs after transplantation of a *Toxoplasma*-infected organ, especially the heart, into a *Toxoplasma*-naive recipient. Reactivated *Toxoplasma* organisms in a donor heart can be severe and unfortunately may mimic the histology of rejection on endomyocardial samples. Thus comparisons of pre and postoperative *Toxoplasma* antibody titres may be helpful. Treatment of choice at this time is sulfadiazine and pyriamethamine.

Hooten et al. (1981) describe the association of risk factors with the occurrence of nosocomial infections. They cite previous infection, active rejection, and administration of steroids or other immunosuppressive therapy as those risks that place patients in the highest intrinsic risk category for nosocomial infection. It is not uncommon for patients to be at high levels of immunosuppression in this time period. Immunosuppressive therapy depresses both humoral and cellular immunity. Therefore, the body's ability to mount an inflammatory response is impaired. Neutropenia may be at its nadir, and the mononuclear cell system is inhibited. Manifestations of these alterations include depressed phagocytosis, leukocyte dysfunction, and in extreme instances decreased immunoglobulin production. Advances in pharmacotherapeutics and frequent assessment of rejection status facilitate titration of immunosuppressive therapy to lowest possible levels. This allows a careful balance to be maintained between prevention of organ rejection and an adequate immune response to invading pathogens.

More Than Six Months Posttransplantation

During this phase, opportunistic organisms are commonly encountered and, in addition to those previously cited, may include *Nocardia* and *Mycobacteria* species. Infections are often related to the frequency and degree of organ rejection and the subsequent level of immunosuppressive therapy required to treat that rejection. The more often a patient experiences rejection the greater the use of immunosuppression and the more likely he is to develop infectious complications.

Patients are also at high risk for developing infections that are pandemic or epidemic in the community. Influenza, during its seasonal presentation, is one example of this exogenous risk factor. Due to a patient's immunocompromised state, this virus may cause a disseminated infection or severely impair the function of a transplanted lung that is undergoing rejection or proliferate unchecked in the normal lungs of other organ recipients.

Nocardial infections may be encountered at this time. These infections are primarily located in the lung, although disseminated nocardiosis involving skin, muscle, lymph nodes, and liver has been reported. Patients usually present with a dry cough or fever and a solid or cavitating lung nodule on chest x-ray. Definitive diagnosis is made by transtracheal or transthoracic aspiration or biopsy of new skin or subcutaneous nodules.

Table 3.1 lists the most common opportunistic pathogens encountered by organ transplant recipients after transplantation. Bacterial organisms have not been included in this table, although they may be considered opportunists. The route of infection or the cause of disseminated disease is cited, and the usual method of treatment is identified. Nurses observe for the side effects of drugs and other potential problems, including alteration of host metabolism or pharmacologic interactions with other medications. It is important to particularly note the potentially graft threatening interactions that occur with immunosuppressive medications.

TABLE 3.1 Common Non-bacterial Pathogens In Immunosuppressed Hosts

Organism	Source	Treatment
Aspergillus species	Inhalation of spores	Amphotericin B
Herpes simplex Type 1 & 2	Direct transfer / Reactivation of latent virus	Acyclovir
Varicella Zoster	Reactivation of latent virus	
Cytomegalovirus	Blood and body fluids / Transplanted organs / Reactivation of latent virus	
Pneumocystis carinii	Activation of endogenous flora	Trimethoprim Sulfamethoxazole Pentamidine
Nocardia species	Inhalation	Sulfadiazine
Candida species	Activation of endogenous flora	Amphotericin B
Hepatitis A	Fecal-oral contamination	—
Hepatitis B	Blood and body fluids	—
Hepatitis C	Blood and body fluids	—

PRETRANSPLANT NURSING EVALUATION FOR INFECTION

When patients are evaluated by the transplant team as candidates, assessment of the potential for infection begins. A thorough history of previous infectious diseases is elicited and documented. This history becomes the basis for future evaluation of primary versus reactivated infections and for assessing the patient's susceptibility to pathogens. The history includes an assessment of "childhood" diseases such as measles, mumps, rubella, and chickenpox. The patient should be queried about whether the disease was actually present or whether a vaccine was administered to establish resistance.

Vaccination History

The patient's vaccination history is important. The history includes the age at which the initial vaccination and subsequent boosters were given for diptheria, pertussis, tetanus (DPT); measles, mumps, and rubella (MMR); polio, hemophilus influenza; and hepatitis B. If the patient was born in a foreign country, bacille Calmette–Guérin vaccine (BCG) for tuberculosis immunization may have been given. This immunization can cause a positive tuberculin test. Serologic testing may be warranted to establish the presence or absence of adequate antibodies.

Previous History of Infection

The presence or absence of Hepatitis B antigen or antibody, *Toxoplasma* organisms, and human immunodeficiency virus (HIV) antibody are part of the evaluation. Traditionally, active systemic viral disease has precluded transplantation. Presence or absence of serologic markers for diseases endemic to the geographic area or institution may be valuable to establish prior to transplantation. These serologic markers may include *Histoplasma*, *Coccidiomycosis*, and *Legionella*.

Cytomegalovirus (CMV) status is well recognized as important in matching donors and recipients. Matching a CMV-negative donor with a CMV-negative recipient decreases but does not eliminate the probability of a significant CMV infection in the posttransplant period. Primary CMV infections are more virulent than recurrent or latent infections. CMV infections usually occur 1 to 3 months after the transplant procedure.

Family History of Infection

Evaluation of the candidates' family may be important at this time. The communicable-disease history elicited from the patient should also be obtained from household members. Many organ recipients are in their childbearing years; thus, the vaccine status of children is important. Household members, especially children, may represent sources for infection after transplantation. Household members may acquire endemic or epidemic diseases, such as influenza, and transmit them to the transplant recipients. Therefore, this is an ideal time to assess sanitation habits and to initiate comprehensive educational intervention.

INFECTION CONTROL DURING THE PREOPERATIVE PERIOD

The goal of preoperative patient preparation focuses on limiting microbial contamination, thereby reducing the risk for developing a subsequent wound infection. Nursing interventions include preoperative bathing of the patient with an antiseptic solution (Cruse & Foord, 1980). The antiseptic inhibits or kills the growth of cutaneous microorganisms for a specified time. Because the integrity of the skin as a barrier to microbial invasion is also important, abrasive scrubbing should be avoided. If the patient is ambulatory and stable, a shower with the antiseptic solution may be taken.

Assessment of the infection potential in recipients and donors must be considered. Principles to minimize infection and infectious risks apply to both donors and recipients. Strict attention is given by nurses to preventing nosocomial infections. Invasive hemodynamic monitoring, therapeutic and diagnostic interventions, and respiratory support place both the recipient and the donor at high risk for microbial invasion by overcoming natural mechanical barriers. They also provide access for direct inoculation of pathogens through improper and careless techniques. Hospital infection-control policies provide standard principles for preventing nosocomial infections, through equipment sterilization and disinfection standards, and techniques for the insertion and care of urinary tract catheters, intravenous catheters, and intraarterial lines. *One of the most vital and effective preventive measures is frequent, thorough handwashing by all health care givers.*

Donors are at additional risk for pathogenic invasion if neurologic function is absent. Brain death precludes normal defense mechanisms such as the gag and cough reflex and enhances the development of pneumonia, urinary tract infection, and mucositis. Extended hospitalization of donors contributes to colonization with nosocomial organisms and may lead to occult infections. These organisms may have developed high-level resistance to traditional antibiotic therapy. The goal of nursing interventions is to maintain life-support measures while controlling infectious risks.

Evaluating the organ donor's infectious status is necessary. Organ donation centers have established a standard battery of tests to be performed on the organ donor prior to transplantation. This battery includes hepatitis and HIV serology. Timing of serologic testing may be problematic, as the donated organ may be available prior to obtaining results.

INFECTION CONTROL DURING THE OPERATIVE PERIOD

Sterile technique is observed in the removal and transplantation of organs. If the organ is recovered at a distant site, it is transported quickly and in a sterile fashion.

During the transplant procedure, post-operative hospital accommodations are arranged. Institutional policies regarding the use and extent of post-operative protective isolation vary. If protective isolation is used, the room is prepared during the transplant procedure. This preparation entails thorough cleaning of the entire room with special attention to sources of dust and spores, such as ventilation systems and little-used horizontal surfaces that attract and retain lint and dust.

Special Considerations

On site construction, air ventilation systems, and water systems may present special problems for immunosuppressed patients. If there is construction in the hospital or problems arise with the air ventilation or water systems, special evaluation measures and barriers may need to be implemented to control environmental pathogens.

Aspergillus species are ubiquitous organisms and are noted by Herman (1980) to be one of the four most common fungi in the environment. The spores of *A. fumigatus* are 2.0 to 3.0 µm in size and are readily found in lint and dust, carpeting, soil, and compost. Aisner, Schimpff, Bennett, Young, and Weirnik (1976) also noted a significant correlation between *Aspergillus* species infections and fireproofing materials. Air currents easily disturb these spores, resulting in airborne contamination. Arnow, Anderson, Mainous, and Smith (1978) cited a dose–response relationship between the number of *Aspergillus* colonies recovered by environmental settle plates and the endemic rate of nosocomial aspergillosis.

Special measures have been recommended to reduce the incidence of aspergillosis in hospitals (Rhame, Streifel, Kersey, & McGlave, 1984; Rotstein et al., 1985). As mortality due to invasive aspergillosis is significant in the transplant recipient population, environmental surveillance (by air sampling) and decontamination should be routinely done in any hospital area housing these patients (Lentino et al., 1982). Hospital construction contributes to contamination with *Aspergillus* species spores. Control measures to minimize associated morbidity and mortality from this type of infection include airtight barriers between construction and patient care areas and negative-pressure ventilation in the construction zone. Fungicidal treatment with copper-8-quinolinolate as a decontamination agent is recommended for fireproofing and air ventilation systems (Opal et al., 1986).

Increased frequency in environmental housekeeping is also a consideration. Horizontal surfaces should be damp-dusted frequently, the scheduled time of dusting corresponding to peak periods of construction and air turbulence. The goal of this activity is to minimize the potential for infection by controlling recognized risk factors.

Cooling water systems, such as air conditioning units, and water sources, such as tap water, showers, and hot water storage tanks, have been identified as sources of *Legionella* organisms (Myerowitz, 1983). The immunocompromised patient is at high risk for acquiring legionellosis; therefore, exposure of transplant recipients to tap water and tap water aerosolization should be minimized. Using sterile water to fill and clean all respiratory therapy equipment is advised, and bathing may be preferable to showering to minimize aerosolization.

Environmental surveillance for *Legionella* organisms may be warranted if a clinical problem exists. Hospital staff may conduct periodic culturing and water treatment. Water treatments include periodic superheating of the hot water system and hyperchlorination.

INFECTION CONTROL DURING THE ACUTE POSTOPERATIVE PERIOD

Nurses play an important role in preventing infection during the first month after transplantation, while the patient is hospitalized. Nurses encourage early discontinuation of invasive devices such as ventilators, endotracheal tubes, Foley catheters, and multiple, deep, intravenous access catheters. Patients are instructed and expected to participate in measures to prevent the development of atelectasis and stasis complications and to resume eating and taking medications by mouth as soon as possible. Simple interventions such as early and frequent ambulation, turning, coughing, deep breathing, and/or incentive spirometry prevent infectious complications. During this period, meticulous handwashing is essential because of frequent patient contact and invasive procedures. Prior to skin puncture, nurses must give careful attention to cleansing the skin with an iodophor preparation.

The nursing staff also monitors health care workers and visitors for communicable diseases. This is accomplished through visual observation of personnel entering the patient's room and by formal and informal education of hospital staff and visitors. This educational opportunity initiates or reinforces hygiene principles that the recipients and their families need to learn before leaving the hospital. No one with an active infection should come in contact with transplant recipients at this time.

Protective Isolation

Protective isolation affords a significant but incomplete reduction in the incidence of serious infections. If protective isolation is observed, it is instituted during the immediate postoperative period. Various regimens have been suggested, but the most complete measure is reverse, or complete protective isolation. This regimen entails a single room for the patient and requiring all persons who enter the room to wear gown, gloves, mask, booties, and cap. Air filtration systems may be added to complete protective isolation precautions. High-efficiency particulate air (HEPA) filters and laminar air flow rooms reduce deposits of organisms when environmental air culturing is performed. HEPA filters are 99.7% efficient in filtering particles greater than 0.3 µm. They effectively decrease turbulence and reduce the risk for airborne infections, such as aspergillosis.

Additionally, oral absorbable and nonabsorbable antibiotic regimens have been used to reduce or eliminate endogenous gastrointestinal flora, particularly in bone marrow transplant recipients. The ultimate protective isolation regimen consists of all of the above practices in addition to disinfection or sterilization of everything which is brought into the room, sterile water, and semisterile food. Pizzo (1981) calls this a total protected environment. Bone marrow transplant recipients who have experienced extended, severe granulocytopenia benefit from a totally protected environment. Skinhoj et al. (1987) reported that the use of a protected environment in allogeneic bone marrow transplantation ensures a low frequency of early infectious complications but that this type of environment does not prevent posttransplant fever or graft-versus-host disease (GVHD).

The use of protective isolation in other transplant populations is controversial (Nauseef & Maki, 1981). Reports about protective isolation precautions for kidney and liver transplant recipients are limited. In the heart transplant population, complete protective isolation appears to have no impact on incidence, morbidity, or mortality resulting from infection in the early postoperative period (Gamberg, Miller, & Lough, 1987). A simplified procedure of combining private room, strict handwashing, and masks (modified protective isolation) may be more beneficial in this patient group because it not only appears to be as effective as complete isolation but is easier to enforce and less traumatic to patients and their families (Hess, Brooks-Brunn, Clark, & Joy, 1985).

The burdens associated with a totally protected environment must be assessed and weighed against the benefits of real or potential infection reduction. The most obvious benefit would be a decreased risk of infection. The potential burdens include psychosocial isolation of the recipient and his family, high cost, and the need for specially trained personnel in nursing, dietary and housekeeping staffs, maintenance and operations, and laboratories.

INFECTION CONTROL DURING RECOVERY

Three to Six Weeks

While patients usually require less intensive medical and nursing intervention during this period, they are receiving high doses of immunosuppressants and therefore are at great risk for developing infectious complications. The nurse's primary role is to assess the patient for early signs of infection. This prompts aggressive diagnostic procedures and early appropriate therapy.

Infection

Infection signs and symptoms may mimic the symptoms of an acute rejection process; this makes the diagnosis of infection even more difficult. Therefore, evaluation for infection and rejection are often performed at the same time. The symptoms may be subtle and include fever, fatigue, anorexia, malaise, and weakness. Bacterial and viral cultures are obtained when symptoms develop. Appropriate biopsies or laboratory studies are also performed as indicated. The immune response is iatrogenically suppressed; therefore, patients may be unable to respond to microbial invasion with an elevated temperature or elevated white blood count. Conversely, an elevated white blood cell count may be artifactitious and attributable to steroid therapy. Laboratory results need to be followed carefully, and any alteration or abnormality in laboratory findings warrants a thorough investigation.

Initiation of empiric antimicrobial therapy is often indicated and may be continued until a more definitive diagnosis is made. The selection of antibiotics is often based upon nosocomial organisms unique to or frequently encountered in the hospital, or upon organisms previously colonizing the recipient that were documented during the pretransplant workup. Aggressive diagnostic measures will be performed if the episode's etiology is elusive because specific clinical findings may be very subtle or even not apparent. Unfortunately, many of the infections encountered during this phase are diagnosed postmortem.

Education

Many patients and families do not understand the basics of infection prevention. Therefore, nurses must educate them about preventing and detecting infectious complications. Immunocompromised patients need to be taught the signs and symptoms of infection, such as fever, chills, red and inflamed wounds, cough, and burning on urination. They should be instructed that ignoring a potential infection causes serious complications and that they must report signs of a potential infection immediately to their physicians.

Oral Hygiene

Good oral hygiene is essential because normal flora in the mouth are altered by immunosuppressive therapy, thus predisposing patients to infection. Some oral hygiene protocols use a Betadine® mouthwash, while others use an antibiotic mouthwash. In general, patients should brush and floss after each meal and visually inspect their mouths for sores daily (Crow, 1983). If their mouths injure easily, a soft sponge or other soft material could be used instead of a brush.

Skin Care

Skin care helps prevent infection. Routine general hygiene is usually sufficient. Dry skin should be avoided. Skin sores or lesions on the skin should be reported. If the patients experience skin lacerations, they should cleanse them thoroughly and watch for any signs of infection such as redness, tenderness, or discharge from the affected area. If any of these occur, he should inform his transplant physician immediately.

Hand Washing

Patients should be encouraged to use good handwashing practices, including the following:

  Washing hands before eating.
  Washing hands after using the bathroom.
  Washing hands when they are visibly soiled.
  Washing hands if they feel they have been in contact with a contaminated environment such as wiping up a spill from the floor.

Nutrition

Adequate nutrition is essential for preventing infection. Many patients are nutritionally depleted prior to transplantation and may need special diets to promote tissue healing after the transplant surgery. Encouraging nutritious food as well as having the family bring food in from home may increase the patients' appetites. Occasionally, smaller feedings instead of three large meals may also be helpful. Some programs encourage patients to eliminate fresh fruits and vegetables to avoid gram-negative colonization. Others, however, suggest to patients that washing the fruits and vegetables is sufficient.

Six Weeks and Later

Once recipients are stable and no longer require inpatient hospital services, they are followed as outpatients at varying intervals. The intervals will depend upon their course of rejection, infection, and overall health status. Interventions to control infectious complications during this phase include continued patient education, reinforcement of information provided while the patient was in the hospital, and recognition of unusual or occult infections. The patient is encouraged to resume normal, daily activities. Everyday situations such as housecleaning, home repairs, construction, or gardening may present potential risks because of spores released from the environment. Without the intensive support provided in the hospital environment, the recipient may forget much of what he has learned. Thus, reinforcement of previously learned principles is essential.

TEAM APPROACH TO INFECTION CONTROL

A multidisciplinary team is responsible for infection control in organ transplantation. Infection control extends from pretransplant evaluations through the rest of the patients' lives. Nurses must know what to anticipate, including what aspects of infection control should have been addressed and resolved and by whom, and where responsibilities lie in infection control problem identification and resolution.

The following outlines some key members of the multidisciplinary infection control team and suggests responsibilities for each.

Attending Physician. Physicians and their teams are responsible for directing patient care, including decisions about implementing diagnostic procedures and instituting antimicrobial treatment. They establish policy about the extent of protective isolation measures and, based on hospital experience, order prophylactic antiinfectives. They also monitor hospital-generated reports for potential risk factors to their patient population.

Primary and Associate Nurse. Nurses provide direct patient care using aseptic technique when necessary, teach patients to recognize and avoid potential risks, teach patients signs and symptoms of infection, provide family education, and when to call the physician after discharge, and monitor infection control activities in the patients' rooms.

Transplant Coordinator. Coordinators act as case managers for the transplant program, coordinate the multidisciplinary team, assure that the educational content is appropriate, and reinforce education to the patient and the family (Grady, 1985).

Infection-control Nurse. Infection-control nurses act as consultants in establishing policies and procedures for organ transplantation programs, monitor infectious events, and assure compliance with infection-control policies in all hospital departments.

Housekeeping. The housekeeping staff provides thorough, extensive room cleaning in preparation for organ transplant recipients, and provides daily thorough cleaning activities using disinfectant agents.

Infectious Disease and/or Microbiology, Virology, Pathology Laboratories. The laboratories act as consultants for infectious disease events. They facilitate diagnosis and treatment by identifying complex pathogens.

Operations and Maintenance. Operations and maintenance personnel monitor environmental sources of potential pathogens (ventilation and water systems) and assist in recognizing potential environmental risks to immunosuppressed patients.

Personnel Health. The personnel health staff establishes and implements personnel policies consistent with infection-control standards.

The multidisciplinary team may also include any individual or department with an interest in controlling infections in this special patient population. Each member makes valuable contributions to the transplant program's success.

CONCLUSION

Because of an immunocompromised state, transplant recipients are especially vulnerable to infectious complications. This chapter provided information about the unique infectious threats occuring in the phases after transplant. It also presented an overview of the organisms to which transplant patients are susceptible. Although progress in diagnosis and treatment of infection has improved over the years, infectious complications remain a significant cause of morbidity and mortality in the immunosuppressed host (Garibaldi, 1983). Nurses are in a key position to help improve patient survival after transplantation through (a) ongoing assessment of donors and recipients for infectious signs and symptoms, (b) providing education to recipients and their families about infection prevention and surveillance, (c) maintaining the team approach of infection control, and (d) conducting nursing research in infection control.

Conducting nursing research in infection and the immunocompromised host is extremely important. Potential areas for future research include evaluation of isolation practices and educational techniques nurses use in caring for these patients. Through continued observation and monitoring of infectious complications in transplant recipients, additional insights will be gained. New methods of infection control and risk reduction will be developed. Searching for and developing new practices is a collaborative effort in which nurses play an important role.

ACKNOWLEDGEMENT

We wish to extend our gratitude to John A. Robinson, MD, for his assistance in completing this chapter. Dr. Robinson is the Associate Dean for Research and past Medical Director of the Cardiac Transplant Program at Loyola University Medical Center. His willingness to share his experience and expertise in the area of infection and the immunocompromised patient is greatly appreciated.

REFERENCES

Aisner, J., Schimpff, S., Bennett, J., Young, V., & Weirnik, P. (1976). *Aspergillus* infections in cancer patients, associated with fireproofing materials in a new hospital. *Journal of the American Medical Association, 235,* 411–412.

Arnow, P., Anderson, R. Mainous, P.D., & Smith, E. (1978). Pulmonary aspergillosis during hospital renovation. *American Review of Respiratory Diseases, 118,* 49–53.

Axnick, K.J. (1984). Knowledge base: Integumentary system. In K.J. Axnick & M. Yarborough (Eds.), *Infection control: An integrated approach* pp. 456–463(1). St. Louis: C.V. Mosby.

Burke, J., & Hildick-Smith, G. (1978). *The infection-prone hospital patient.* Boston: Little Brown.

Counts, G. (1988). Infection risk in organ and bone marrow transplant units. *APIC Curriculum for Infection Control Practice, 3,* 1246–1258.

Craven, D.E., & Regan, A.M. (1989). Nosocomial pneumonia in the ICU patient. *Critical Care Nursing Quarterly, 11*(4), 28–44.

Crow, S. (1983). Nursing care of the immunosuppressed patient. *Infection Control, 4*(6), 465–467.

Cruse, P.J.E., & Foord, R. (1980). The epidemiology of wound infection: A ten year prospective study of 62, 939 wounds. *Surgical Clinics of North America, 60* 27–40.

DeGroot–Kosolcharoen, J. (1984). Knowledge base: Genitourinary system. In K.J. Axnick & M. Yarborough (Eds.), *Infection control: An integrated approach* (pp. 334–363). St. Louis: C.V. Mosby.

DiCecco, S.R., Wirners, E.J., Weisner, R.H., Southorn, P.A., Plevak, D.J., & Krom, R.A.F. (1989). Assessment of nutritional status of patients with end stage liver disease undergoing liver transplantation. *Mayo Clinic Proceedings, 64,* 95–102.

Gamberg, P., Miller, J.L., & Lough, M.E. (1987). Impact of protective isolation on the incidence of infection after heart transplant. *The Journal of Heart Transplantation, 6,* 147–149.

Garibaldi, R. (1983). Infections in organ transplant recipients. *Infection Control, 4,* 460–464.

Garner, J.S., Jarvis, W.R., Emori, T.G., Horan, T.C., & Hughes, J.M. (1988). CDC definitions for nosocomial infections. *American Journal of Infection Control, 16*(3), 128–140.

Gentry, L., & Zeluff, B. (1986). Diagnosis and treatment of infection in cardiac transplant patients. *Surgical Clinics of North America, 66,* 459–465.

Grady, K. (1985). Development of a cardiac transplantation program: Role of the clinical nurse specialist. *Heart and Lung, 14,* 490–494.

Gurwith, M., Stinson, E., & Remington, J. (1971). *Aspergillus* infection complicating cardiac transplantation, report of five cases. *Archives of Internal Medicine, 128* 541–545.

Haley, R.W., Hooton, T.M., Culver, D.H., Stanley, R.C., Emori, T.G., Hardison, C.D., Quade, D., Schachtman, R.H., Schaberg, D.R., Shah, B.V., & Schatz, G.D. (1981). Nosocomial infections in U.S. hospitals, 1975–1976: Estimated frequency by selected characteristics of patients. *American Journal of Medicine, 70* 947–959.

Herman, L. (1980). *Aspergillus* in patient care areas. *Annals of New York Academy of Science, 353,* 140–146.

Hess, N.J., Brooks-Brunn, J.A., Clark, D., & Joy, K. (1985). Complete isolation: Is it necessary? *The Journal of Heart Transplantation, 4*(4), 458–459.

Hofflin, J., Postasman, I., Baldwin, J., Oyer, P., Stinson, E., & Remington, J. (1987). Infectious complications in heart transplant recipients receiving cyclosporine and corticosteroids. *Annals of Internal Medicine, 106,* 20–216.

Hooton, T., Haley, R., Culver, D., White, J., Morgan, W.M., & Carroll, R. (1981). The joint association of multiple risk factors with the occurrence of nosocomial infection. *American Journal of Medicine, 70,* 960–970.

Kusne, S., Dummer, J.S., Singh, N., Iwatsuki, S., Makowka, L., Esquivel, C. Starzl, T., & Ho, M. (1988). Infections after liver transplantation: An analysis of 101 consecutive cases. *Medicine, 67,* 132–143.

Lentino, J., Rosenkranz, M.A., Michaels, J., Kurup, V., Rose, H., & Rytel, M. (1982). Aspergillosis: A retrospective review of airborne disease secondary to road construction and contaminated air conditioners. *American Journal of Epidemiology, 116,* 430–437.

Luft, B., Naut, Y., Arauso, F., Stinson, E., & Remington, J. (1983). Primary and reactivated toxoplasma infection in patients with cardiac transplants. *Annals of Internal Medicine, 99,* 27–31.

Myerowitz, R. (1983). Nosocomial Legionnaires disease and other nosocomial *Legionella* pneumonias. *Infection Control, 4,* 107–110.

Nauseef, W., & Maki, D. (1981). A study of the value of simple protective isolation in patients with granulocytopenia. *New England Journal of Medicine, 304,* 448–453.

Opal, S., Asp, A., Connady, P., Morse, P., Burton, L., & Hammer, P. (1986). Efficacy of infection control measures during a nosocomial outbreak of disseminated aspergillosis associated with hospital construction. *Journal of Infectious Diseases, 153,* 634–670.

O'Toole, C., Gary, J., Maher, P., & Wreghitt, T.G. (1986). Persistent excretion of cytomegalovirus in heart transplant patients correlates with inversion of the ratio of T helper/T suppressor cytotoxic cells. *Journal of Infectious Diseases, 153,* 1160–1162.

Peterson, P., McGlave, P., Ramsay, N., Rhame, F., Cohen, E., Perry, G., Goldman, A., & Kersey, J. (1983). A prospective study of infectious diseases following bone marrow transplantation: Emergence of *Aspergillus* and cytomegalovirus as the major causes of mortality. *Infection Control, 4,* 81–89.

Pirsch, J., & Maki, D. (986). Infectious complications in adults with bone marrow transplantation and T-cell depletion of donor marrow, increased susceptibility to fungal infections. *Annals of Internal Medicine, 104,* 619–631.

Pizzo, P. (1981). The value of protective isolation in preventing nosocomial infections in high risk patients. *American Journal of Medicine, 70,* 631–670.

Ramsey, P., Rubin, R., Tolkoff-Rubin, N., Cosimi, A.B., Russell, P., & Greene, R. (1980). The renal transplant patient with fever and pulmonary infiltrates: Etiology, clinical manifestations, and management. *Medicine, 59,* 206–222.

Rao, K.V., & Anderson, R. (1988). Long-term results and complications in renal transplant recipients. *Transplantation, 45,* 45–52.

Rhame, F., Striefel, A., Kersey, J., & McGlave, P. (1984). Extrinsic risk factors for pneumonia in the patient at high risk of infection. *American Journal of Medicine, 43,* 28–38.

Rifking, D., Marchioro, T., Schneck, S., & Hill, R. (1967). Systemic fungal infections complicating renal transplantation and immunosuppressive therapy. *American Journal of Medicine, 43,* 28–38.

Rotstein, C., Cummings, K.M., Tidings, J., Killion, K., Powell, E., Gustafson, T., & Higby, D. (1985). An outbreak of invasive aspergillosis among allogeneic bone marrow transplants: A case control study. *Infection Control, 6,* 347–355.

Schumann, D. (1987). Cytomegalic virus infection in renal allograft recipients: Indicators for intervention in the SICU. *Focus on Critical Care, 14*(3), 41–47.

Simmons, B.P. (1982). CDC guidelines for prevention of surgical wound infection. *Infection Control, 3*(Suppl), 187–196.

Skinhoj, P., Jacobsen, N., Hoiby, N., Faber, V., & Copenhagen Bone Marrow Transplant Group. (1987). Strict protective isolation in allogeneic bone marrow transplantation: Effect on infectious complications, fever and graft versus host disease. *Scandinavian Journal of Infectious Disease, 19,* 91–96.

Thompson, C.B., & Thomas, E.D (1986). Bone marrow transplantation. *Surgical Clinics of North America, 66*(3), 589–601.

Wajszczuk, C.P., Dummer, J.C., Ho, M., Van Thiel, D.H., Starzl, T.E., Iwatsuki, S., & Shaw, B., Jr. (1985). Fungal infections in liver transplant recipients. *Transplantation, 40,* 347–353.

PART II

Nursing Care of Specific Transplant Recipients

CHAPTER **4**

KIDNEY TRANSPLANTATION

Pamela K. Jacobsson
Janet L. Cohan

Kidney transplantation evolved through the work of researchers who were determined to alter the course and outcome of end-stage renal disease (ESRD). In 1936 a Russian surgeon performed the first kidney transplant by placing a kidney in a young woman's thigh. From 1936 to 1954 improvements in surgical techniques, appropriate placement of the graft, and a beginning understanding of the immune process occurred. In 1954 the prototype operation for human kidney transplant was performed in Boston, Massachusetts. Since then, advances have been made in organ preservation techniques, dialytic approaches, immunosuppression, and governmental financial support.

Nursing care of the kidney transplant patient can be exciting and challenging. It is a dynamic field in that new knowledge with respect to immunology, nephrology, and pharmacology is continually being acquired. This chapter will discuss the preoperative, postoperative, and outpatient nursing care of the kidney transplant patient.

SELECTION CRITERIA

Both kidney transplantation and hemodialysis are recognized as acceptable modes of therapy. Both therapies also pose risks. The focus of transplantation must be more than giving an individual additional time to live. Annas (1985) supports the concept that the initial screening process should be based exclusively on medical criteria that measure the probability of a successful transplant.

Indications for Kidney Transplantation

The indication for kidney transplantation will ultimately be determined by the particular disease process. Refer to Table 4.1 for a list of etiologic pathologies leading to ESRD.

TABLE 4.1   Etiologic Pathologies Leading to ESRD

Diabetic nephropathy
Glomerular disease
   Membranous nephropathy
   Membranoproliferative glomerulonephritis: Type I and Type II (dense deposit disease)
   IgA nephropathy (Berger's disease)
   Focal segmental glomerulosclerosis
   Rapidly progressive crescentic glomerulonephritis
   Antiglomerular basement membrane disease
Interstitial disease (primary, secondary, idiopathic)
   Acute renal failure
   Analgesic nephropathy
   Chronic pyelonephritis
   Oxalosis hyperoxaluria
Nephrosclerosis
   Idiopathic or essential hypertension
   Malignant hypertension
Urologic diseases
   Chronic infection with nephrolithiasis
   Idiopathic stone disease
   Ileal conduit
   Staghorn calculi
   Cystinuria
   Chronic obstruction
   Urethral valves
   Ureteropelvic junction obstruction
   Neurogenic bladder
   Retroperitoneal fibrosis
Systemic disease
   Systemic lupus erythematosus
   Amyloidosis
   Fabry's disease
   Cystinosis
   Henoch-Schönlein purpura
   Polyarteritis nodosa
   Scleroderma

(continued)

TABLE 4.1. Etiologic Pathologies Leading to ESRD (continued)

Hereditary disease
  Polycystic kidney disease
  Alport's syndrome   Congenital
Nephronophthisis (medullary cystic disease)
  Aplastic kidneys

From "Evaluation and Selection of Candidates for Renal Transplantation" by D. Steinmuller, 1983. *The Urologic Clinics of North America, 10*(2) p. 219. Copyright 1983 by W.B. Saunders Co. Reprinted by permission.

Potential Contraindications

Potential contraindications may include age, substance abuse, end-organ damage, HIV-positive status, and functional retardation and psychosis. The following pages amplify each of these potential contraindications.

Age

The number of individuals over age 65 entering the ESRD program is increasing each year. The age of 65 as an arbitrary number was established, based on the retirement age years ago, but retirement age and physiological age are not synonymous.

Substance Abuse

Kidney transplantation for an individual who admits to or who tests positive for substance abuse (i.e., alcohol, cocaine, heroin, crack, codeine, marijuana, etc.) generally is inappropriate. A return to addictive behavior posttransplant with a high incidence of graft loss, is common, especially if environmental and lifestyle habits do not change. Successful completion of a drug rehabilitation program and randomly drawn toxicology-negative serums for a specified time would indicate continuation of the workup.

End Organ Damage

Overall end organ damage is seen in poorly controlled and malignant hypertension, advanced age, diabetes mellitus, and other chronic and acute diseases. Transplantation of patients with underlying diseases requires careful scrutiny, and the risk/benefit ratio of transplantation must be closely weighed. Kidney transplantation can reverse certain sequelae of uremic-induced organ pathologies but not organ damage secondary to other chronic pathologies.

The following questions must be addressed:

1. Can the potential candidate safely undergo anesthesia and the surgical procedure?

2. Will the candidate be able to tolerate aggressive immunosuppressant therapy if rejection should occur?
3. How well is the candidate going to tolerate long-term immunosuppression?
4. What are the projected long-term outcomes of the underlying disease?
5. Will transplantation provide a reasonable level of functioning for a number of years, or will the already failing systems further degenerate posttransplant with concomitant morbidity and/or mortality?

HIV Positive Status

HIV-positive candidates have undergone kidney transplantion in the past. A recent study of 26 such individuals revealed a 50% survival rate of 3.84 years (Tzakis, Cooper, & Starzl, 1989). Seven of the 13 survivors have either AIDS-related complex (ARC), lymphocytic interstitial pneumonia, or recurrent cytomegalovirus (CMV) and invasive candidiasis. Of the 13 patients who succumbed, 7 of the deaths were directly attributed to the complications of being HIV-positive. With these statistics in mind, each transplant team needs to develop protocols to determine if individuals should be HIV-tested as part of the pretransplant workup and, if positive, whether or not to transplant.

Functional Retardation and Psychosis

Neither mental retardation nor psychosis is an absolute contraindication to transplantation. Physical parameters and the availability of support systems must be evaluated. Transplantation can free family members from the rigid schedules that maintenance dialysis requires; however, a strong support system is still a prerequisite to transplantation for individuals who are unable to function independently. Thorough psychological evaluation is necessary to ascertain the appropriateness of transplantation for a psychotic patient. Availability of psychiatric backup posttransplant is another important consideration. The concomitant administration of antipsychotic medication with immunosuppressants is not contraindicated.

PRETRANSPLANT WORKUP

Thorough assessment of potential transplant candidates is a time-consuming process requiring data from a variety of sources. Recording and maintaining information in a central location facilitates data retrieval for prospective and retrospective research studies. Some centers maintain data in computer banks.

Because every candidate being considered for kidney transplantation needs to have a workup file, forms such as the following could be developed:

1. Medical history and interventions.
2. Consultations and procedures.

3. Hemodynamic assessments and laboratory tests.
4. Kidney donor matching and screening.

Form 1: Medical History and Interventions

The clinical nurse specialist or pretransplant coordinator guides the workup. Test results that deviate from acceptable parameters for a uremic individual must be reviewed with the medical staff for further guidance and workup direction. Potential recipients set the pace of the workup, and their physical and emotional tolerance determine the number of procedures and the time frame for performing them.

Data Collection

Nurses gather relevant historical data from the nephrologist and from the dialysis and professional staff and use the patient's chart as the first screening step. (See Table 4.2a.) If the transplant team discovers contraindications, the workup does not proceed. For example, a 43-year-old patient with severe chronic obstructive pulmonary disease, coronary artery disease, and a previous stroke is not an appropriate candidate. Proceeding with a workup gives individuals false hope and makes individuals endure unnecessary testing.

Candidate Interview

If the initial screening process is favorable, the nurse interviews the transplant candidate. A face-to-face meeting is ideal, and when family members are present, the nurse evaluates family dynamics.

Special interview problems arise with uremic patients on dialysis. They are in a "captive" position and cannot easily terminate the interview. They may not be feeling well, not tolerating the dialytic procedure well, or may not be able to concentrate and retain data. Therefore, the interviewer must keep the initial interview simple, explain the pretransplantation process and the individual's goals and expectations in the workup phase; answer questions, and give explanatory literature along with a professional business card.

Form 2: Consultations and Procedures

The following section discusses the necessary testing procedures for a kidney transplant workup using a systems approach. (See Table 4.2b.)

Cardiopulmonary System

Chest x-ray. Posterior-anterior (PA) and lateral (LAT) views are taken. Left ventricular hypertrophy (LVH) is a common finding in individuals with ESRD secondary to anemia and/or fluid overload.

TABLE 4.2a Pretransplant Recipient Workup
(an Example)

Form 1: Medical History and Interventions

NAME_____SEX_____RACE_____BIRTHDATE_____
ADDRESS_____PHONE[a]_____
SS#_____UIH#_____PHONE_____
OCCUPATION_____EDUCATION_____PHONE_____
DIALYSIS UNIT_____REFERRING M.D._DAYS DIALYZED_____
PRIMARY DIAGNOSIS_____SECONDARY DIAGNOSIS_____
DATE OF 1ST DIALYSIS_____LOCATION OF 1ST DIALYSIS[b]_____
PRESENTATION DATE[c]_____DATE SEEN[d]_____
TISSUE TYPE: DATE_____ABO_____HLA_____
                                                                       DR_____

ACTIVE PROBLEM LIST   INACTIVE PROBLEM LIST

_____   _____
_____   _____
_____   _____
_____   _____
_____   _____

MEDICATIONS   Smoking History_____
_____   Drinking History_____
_____   Drug Abuse History_____
_____
_____   Pregnancies: G_____
_____   P_____
_____
_____   ALLERGIES
_____
_____   _____
_____   _____

[a]Three phone numbers are requested to facilitate locating an individual once a cadaver kidney becomes available.
[b]Specific location, i.e., name of hospital or dialysis center.
[c]Date case presentation made to transplant team or transplant surgeon.
[d]Date of information-sharing session between potential candidate and transplant surgeon.

Electrocardiogram (ECG). An ST-T wave abnormality secondary to uremic electrolyte imbalance and LVH are common results and are within "normal" parameters for uremic individuals. Any serious cardiopulmonary problems warrant clearance from a cardiologist before proceeding with the workup.

Purified Protein Derivative (PPD). A 12-fold increase in the incidence in tuberculosis (TB) occurs in the uremic population (Andrew, 1980) immediately prior to and during the first 6 months of dialysis. This is thought to be a consequence of azotemia-induced depressed cell-mediated immunity. To determine the presence of TB, it is necessary to place a PPD concomitantly with an anergy battery. An anergy battery consists of subdermal injections of

TABLE 4.2b Pretransplant Recipient Workup
(an Example)

Form 2: Consultations and Procedures

	DATE	RESULTS
A. CARDIOPULMONARY		
Chest x-ray	_____	_____
ECG	_____	_____
Echocardiogram	_____	_____
PFTs	_____	_____
PPD with anergy battery	_____	_____
Pneumovaccine	_____	_____
B. GASTROINTESTINAL		
Stool guaiac x 3	_____	1.__ 2.__ 3.__
Upper GI	_____	_____
Endoscopy	_____	_____
Lower GI	_____	_____
Flexible sigmoidoscopy (over age 45)	_____	_____
Barium enema	_____	_____
GI motility studies	_____	_____
Gallbladder studies	_____	_____
C. UROLOGIC		
VCUG	_____	_____
Ultrasound	_____	_____
Biopsy	_____	_____
Renins	_____	_____
Nephrectomy	_____	_____
D. OTHER		
Dental	_____	_____
Gyn (Pap smear)	_____	_____
Ophthalmology (diabetics)	_____	_____
Psychological	_____	_____
Interview	_____	_____
E. ADDITIONAL PROCEDURES		
_____	_____	_____
_____	_____	_____
_____	_____	_____

mumps skin-test antigen, purified extract of *Candida albicans*, and *Trichophyton inguinale.* If the PPD is positive, sputum should be cultured for *Mycobacterium tuberculosis* and checked for acid-fast bacilli (AFB). Urine, if available, may be tested simultaneously. Testing three times on the early morning sputums and urine is most appropriate. A diagnosis of TB necessitates stopping the workup process until at least a full-year course of anti-TB drug therapy is completed.

Pulmonary Function Tests (PFTs). PFTs are performed on individuals with positive histories of asthma, smoking, or COPD. Performing a PFT on an asthmatic patient pre- and posttreatment with a bronchodilator can ascertain the degree of asthma control and reversibility. For individuals with COPD and/or smoking history, PFTs can estimate the degree of pulmonary dysfunction. Baseline information determines candidacy appropriateness and risk factors for the operative and postoperative period.

Pneumovaccine. Injecting Pneumovax® prevents pneumococcal pneumonia posttransplant. Revaccination should be done every 5 years.

Gastrointestinal System

Stool for Guaiac. Giving the individual three guaiac cards to test for occult blood in the stool is safe, noninvasive, and effective. Nurses instruct patients on appropriate collection. Once completed, the cards are mailed to the professional in charge of the workup.

Upper Gastrointestinal Series (UGI) and Gallbladder (GB) Ultrasound. These two tests are standard screening procedures in many centers, and if cholelithiasis is identified, a cholecystectomy prior to transplantation should be performed. A UGI with small-bowel follow-through may reveal strictures, tumors, hiatal hernia, diverticula, varices, and ulcers. This is valuable information for the pre- and posttransplant period.

Lower Gastrointestinal Series (LGI). LGI is done to rule out polyps, diverticula, and structural changes in the large intestine. This may be warranted in the elderly and in those with positive guaiac cards, or a history of diverticulitis. Diverticulitis posttransplant is frequently accompanied by perforation and a high mortality rate. Therefore, its presence is an indication for elective partial colectomy pretransplant.

Endoscopy. Individuals with uremic gastritis and/or peptic ulcer disease need to undergo endoscopy. If an ulcer is present, appropriate medical drug management with re-endoscoping to ascertain resolution is necessary. Failure of the ulcer to heal, however, justifies operative intervention (truncal vagotomy and pyloroplasty or antrectomy) because posttransplant recurrence is frequent and carries a high risk of mortality.

Proctoscopy. This definitive procedure aids in diagnosing inflammatory, infectious, or ulcerative diseases and can aid in diagnosing malignant and benign neoplasms, hemorrhoids, hypertrophic anal papillae, polyps, fissures, fistulas, and abscesses. Any candidate over 45 years of age or presenting symptoms should be scheduled for this procedure.

Renal/Urologic System

Kidney Biopsy (performed by abdominal laparoscopy). When a diagnosis of ESRD is made, a biopsy is frequently performed to determine the cause of failure. However, biopsy is often of little help when the disease is detected at a late stage. The kidney may be too scarred and atrophied to afford much information. Nevertheless, if a biopsy yields a diagnosis, this information must be used as part of the pretransplant evaluation. Because many of the glomerular diseases have a high rate of recurrence the choice for using a living related donor must be carefully considered. If a living donor is considered in the scenario of possible recurring disease, the donor must be made aware of the statistical likelihood for recurrence.

Voiding Cystourethrogram (VCUG). All potential candidates need to have a VCUG done to rule out any obstructive, infective, malignant, or dysfunctional parameters. Any evidence of reflux must be corrected prior to transplantation. If transurethral bladder catheterizing is part of the VCUG procedure, antibiotic coverage with 1 tablet of trimethoprim/sulfamethoxazole 1 hour prior to the VCUG is appropriate.

Ultrasound. Patients with polycystic kidney disease (PKD) may need to have an ultrasound done to ascertain the size of the kidneys.

Nephrectomy. Several situations warrant nephrectomy prior to transplantation. These include:

- Polycystic kidneys with significant infection and/or significant hemorrhage.
- Renal tumors.
- Renin-dependent hypertension that cannot be controlled medically.
- Chronic pyelonephritis with or without severe reflux.
- Kidneys diverted into conduits.
- Heavy proteinuria refractory to attempts with chemical nephrectomy.

Other Testing

Dental. Every transplant candidate needs dental clearance prior to the operative procedure; the mouth can be a source of severe infection problems.

Gynecological. All female candidates need a thorough pelvic examination and Pap test. Obviously, any pathologies need to be corrected prior to transplantation.

Psychological Interview. Obtaining a consult for evaluation and documentation of an individual's psychological profile is important. If the psychological evaluation indicates a need to reconsider candidate appropriateness, a team meeting should be held to discuss the case and its attendant concerns.

Special Evaluation for Diabetic Recipients

Approximately 25% of the ESRD population are diabetics. Diabetes mellitus damages the entire body vasculature and therefore requires additional studies.

Ophthalmologic studies are conducted on all potential recipients with diabetes to assess degree of retinopathy. A gastric emptying study can provide useful information in evaluating somatic complaints in the pretransplant period. The nephrologist routinely orders an evaluation of a diabetic recipient's peripheral neuropathy and circulation. This pretransplant evaluation can decrease the incidence of limb loss. Because of the high incidence of coronary artery disease (CAD), ventricular dysfunction, and subsequent high mortality rates, some transplant centers are now requiring cardiac catheterization, when indicated, as a requirement for transplantation in the diabetic population. Finally ascertaining functional bladder capacity by cystometrogram determines severe bladder pathologies that may precipitate urinary retention and sepsis after transplant surgery.

Form 3: Hemodynamic Assessments and Laboratory Tests

The third section of the workup (Table 4.2c) involves obtaining information about vital signs, urine testing and blood work.

Hemodynamic Assessments

Obtaining data regarding dry weight, interdialytic weight gains, and pre- and postdialysis blood pressures can indicate overall fluid restriction compliance. Malignant hypertension warrants renin determinations. High renins and malignant hypertension may necessitate nephrectomy prior to transplantation.

Laboratory Tests

Urine Testing. Gross proteinuria (several grams) in a 24-hour specimen needs consistent and periodic evaluation. Before transplantation, determination for surgical or chemical nephrectomy must be made. However, after transplantation the shunting of blood to the new organ sometimes causes a cessation in the proteinuria that would obviate the need for nephrectomy. The surgeon decides about the necessity for and timing of a nephrectomy. Positive urine cultures (or positive bladder washings) need fastidious intervention and follow-up cultures. Repeated UTIs need further workup as to etiology. Referral to a urologist is appropriate.

Coagulation. Uremic patients experience bleeding tendencies even though they may have normal coagulation studies. Platelets may aggregate abnormally.

Virology Titers. Baseline data on the sero status of the herpes family of viruses such as herpes simplex virus (HSV), Varicella zoster (VZ), CMV, and Epstein-Barr virus (EBV) are important. Almost every individual who is CMV-

TABLE 4.2c Pretransplant Recipient Workup (an Example)

Form 3: Hemodynamic Assessments and Laboratory Tests

A. VITAL SIGNS	DATE	DATE	DATE
Height			
Dry Weight			
Predialysis wt.			
Postdialysis wt.			
B/P predialysis			
B/P postdialysis			

B. URINALYSIS			
24-hr urine output			
24-hr urine protn			
Urine bladder C&S			

C. HEMATOLOGY			
WBC			
Hematocrit			
Platelet			
Sickle cell prep[a]			
Hgb elec.[a]			

D. COAGULATION			
Bleeding time[a]			
PT/control[a]			
PTT/control[a]			

E. HEPATITIS			
HBsAg[a]			
HBsAb[a]			
Other[a]			

F. VIROLOGY			
CMV titer[a]			
HSV titer[a]			
HZV titer[a]			
EBV titer[a]			
HIV titer[a]			

G. IMMUNOLOGY	DATE	DATE	DATE
C3[a]			
C4[a]			
IgA[a]			
IgG			
IgM[a]			
LE prep/ANA[a]			
Anti-DNA[a]			

H. CHEMISTRY			
BUN			
Creatinine			
SGOT			
SGPT			
Bilirubin			
Alk phos			
LDH			
Total protein			
Albumin			
Glucose			
Uric acid			
Calcium			
Phosphorus			
Cholesterol			
Triglycerides			
Amylase			

I. OTHER			
PTH[a]			
VDRL			

[a]These laboratory tests need to be done only once and repeated only as abnormal values indicate.

seropositive pretransplantation reactivates the virus posttransplantation; 20% become clinically ill (Cerilli, 1988). Theoretically, kidneys from CMV seropositive donors should not be transplanted in seronegative recipients. However, recent studies show that the use of high-dose acyclovir for 90 days posttransplant provides adequate prophylaxis against severe CMV infection in seronegative recipients (Balfour, Chace, Stapleton, Simmons, & Fryd, 1989).

Hepatitis

Hepatitis B is usually acquired secondary to frequent blood transfusions. Considerable debate exists about whether to perform transplantation on individuals before they seroconvert because once transplantation has taken place these patients remain antigen-positive. Statistics have shown that, 1 to 2 years posttransplant, these individuals begin to present with signs and symptoms of far-advanced cirrhosis and/or hepatocellular carcinoma (Cerilli, 1988). Non-A, non-B hepatitis, also acquired primarily from blood transfusions, is associated with a high posttransplant morbidity and mortality. Chronic hepatitis in these individuals eventually leads to cirrhosis and, ultimately, death.

Immunologic Tests

C_3 and C_4 are two of 11 serum proteins that constitute complement and play a key role in antibody-mediated immune reactions. The complement system enables the body to destroy cells that it recognizes as alien. Antibodies IgA, IgG, and IgM are also part of the humorally mediated immune system and can mediate complement fixation. The immunodeficiency observed in chronic kidney failure is predominantly cell-mediated rather than humoral, so normal values would be expected unless another condition existed. These parameters are useful in evaluating some of the immunologically based nephropathies.

Systemic lupus erythematosus (SLE) prep to diagnose or monitor SLE is less sensitive and reliable than the antinuclear antibody (ANA) test. SLE is not known to recur in the transplanted kidney, but transplanting when the disease is quiescent or "burned out" is more advisable.

Chemistries

In ESRD the creatinine and blood urea nitrogen (BUN) obviously are going to be elevated, even with dialytic intervention. Severely elevated BUNs can indicate high intake of protein and therefore noncompliance with the dietary regimen or severe muscle wasting.

Calcium, phosphorus, alkaline phosphatase, and parathyroid hormone (PTH) levels are monitored in ESRD secondary to the kidneys' inability to excrete phosphorus and a decreased intestinal absorption of calcium (resulting from decreased conversion of vitamin D to the physiologically inactive form). These imbalances set off a negative feedback loop with the parathyroid gland, which, in turn, secretes PTH. Elevated PTH levels ultimately result in demineralization of the bones. If individuals are noncompliant in taking phosphate binders and are not restricting dietary phosphorus, this situation is further aggravated. Hand and clavicle films assess the presence of kidney osteodystrophy. Parathyroidectomy with autoimplants may ultimately be necessary. This procedure permits ready diagnosis of recurrent secondary hyperparathyroidism by measuring PTH concentration in blood obtained from a vein in the forearm, where the parathyroid gland is implanted.

Serum uric acid levels are characteristically elevated in predialyzed ESRD secondary to impaired kidney excretion. Adequate dialysis clears this substance from the blood with a return to normal levels. Elevated uric acid levels, despite regular dialysis, require further evaluation for the possibility of gout.

Cholesterol levels are usually normal in uremic patients whereas triglyceride levels are often elevated due to high levels of very low density lipoproteins (VLDLs), which are triglyceride rich. The mechanism of this abnormality is unclear, but it may be a combination of increased production by the liver, decreased lipoprotein lipase, and hyperinsulinism (Knochel & Seldin, 1981). This elevated triglyceride level accelerates atherosclerotic disease, especially with concomitant hypertension.

Amylase, an enzyme synthesized in the pancreas and salivary glands, is elevated in cases of pancreatic disease. Slight elevations in uremia are not abnormal, but considerable elevations warrant a physician's evaluation.

The Venereal Disease Research Laboratory (VDRL) test screens for primary and secondary syphilis. A reactive VDRL occurs in 50% of individuals with primary syphilis and in all individuals with secondary syphilis. Biologic false-positive tests occur in individuals with SLE; therefore, a rapid plasma reagin (RPR) should be performed. Biologic false-positives can also occur in hepatitis and rheumatoid arthritis.

Monitoring serum glutamic-oxaloacetic transaminase (SGOT), serum glutamic-pyruvic transaminase (SGPT), and lactic dehydrogenase (LDH) is important, especially in the presence of serum positive for hepatitis B or suspected non-A, non-B hepatitis. Prolonged elevated enzymes with fractionation of LDH, indicating liver pathology as the source, may necessitate liver biopsy prior to transplantation to determine etiologic pathology and probable prognosis.

The uremic patient's serum total protein and serum albumin, which composes 50% of all serum proteins, is almost universally depressed secondary to poor nutrition and disordered protein metabolism or nephrotic syndrome. Markedly depressed levels of serum albumin combined with high fluid intake results in the edema seen in ESRD. If albumin levels are very low at the time of the transplant surgery, albumin may be infused to facilitate interstitial fluid mobilization to the vascular compartment, resulting in improved renal perfusion. Adequate levels of serum proteins bind and detoxify drugs; facilitate wound healing; synthesize antibodies, enzymes, and hormones; and act as blood buffers in maintaining acid–base balance. Therefore, the low-protein diet must be of high biologic value.

Form 4: Kidney Donor Matching and Screening

The fourth and final section of the recipient pretransplant workup involves recording the names of potential living donors (obtained in the initial interview) and the general family disease history (See Table 4.2d). Reviewing the family history gives valuable information that guides part of the recipient's workup. For example, a strong family history of diabetes not currently present in potential recipients may indicate a chance for steroid-induced diabetes mellitus in the posttransplant period. A strong family history of hypertension may exclude family members younger than 25 years from donating organs.

If living donors are used, the donor names, dates of tissue typing, and mixed lymphocyte culture and monocyte cross-matching results are recorded.

TABLE 4.2d Pretransplant Recipient Workup (an Example)

Form 4: Kidney Donor Matching and Screening

FAMILY HISTORY AND
   POTENTIAL DONORS: DONOR:_____
_____   TISSUE TYPE: DATE:_____ABO_____
_____   HLA_____
_____   DR_____
_____   MATCH_____

	MLC	*DATE*	*RESULT*
	#1	_____	_____
	#2	_____	_____

_____   MONOCYTE CROSSMATCH
_____   DATE_____RESULT_____
DONOR-SPECIFIC TRANSFUSIONS: #1 Date_____#2 Date_____#3 Date____
                            WBC_____WBC_____WBC_____
                            Imuran_____Imuran_____Imuran____
BLOOD TRANSFUSION RECORD: TOTAL # OF UNITS_____

Date	*Type*	*#Units*	*Location Given*
_____	_____	_____	_____
_____	_____	_____	_____
_____	_____	_____	_____
_____	_____	_____	_____
_____	_____	_____	_____

Work completed by:_____
Workup approved by:_____M.D.
Date:_____
Date placed on ready list and UNOS registry:_____

Monocyte cross-matching is done in many transplant centers on all living related (but not living nonrelated) donor–recipient pairs. In many centers positive monocyte cross-match necessitates canceling donation by those individuals and locating other living donors or choosing the cadaver donor option.

Recording of blood transfusions as to type, number of units, and the institution where transfused is important. Comparing the number of transfusions and percentage of reactive antibody (PRA) can indicate whether individuals are high or low responders, which ultimately gives parameters for waiting time on the cadaver list. Individuals who have received 40 units of packed red blood cells and have a low PRA will not be as difficult to match as individuals who are highly sensitized. Space is also provided for recording dates of donor-specific blood transfusions (DSBT) and mixed lymphocyte culture results.

CARE OF CANDIDATES AWAITING TRANSPLANT

Once the pretransplant evaluation process is completed, the candidates' files are reviewed with the transplant surgeons. If all test results are acceptable, approval is given for individuals' names to be placed on the transplant center "ready" list and on the UNOS computer registry. Because several months can pass before suitable donors are found, the pretransplant nursing coordinator updates the workup form with laboratory values, listing any hospitalizations, infections, or blood transfusions. Temporary removal from the ready list may be necessary until a candidate's physical condition permits relisting.

Every month the dialysis unit nurses draw serum samples from recipients and send them to the appropriate tissue-typing laboratories. The PRA is measured in the serum; then a small aliquot of this serum is placed in a tissue-typing tray to be thawed and used for cross-matching with potential donors. The longer potential recipients remain on a waiting list, the more serum samples will be tested with potential donors. It is imperative that monthly samples be sent in a timely fashion, with notification of any blood transfusions within that month.

Notification of Candidate

The actual procedure for notifying recipients of available cadaver kidneys varies. Discussion with nephrologists about physical clearance for hospital admission, date of last dialysis, and date of last blood transfusion are important variables. If individuals had blood transfusions after the last submitted serum sample, cross-matches must be performed on current serum. The presence of active infections is an immediate disqualifier. Ascertaining when individuals were last dialyzed determines the need for preoperative dialysis. Getting clearance from nephrologists for admittance before contacting the recipients is not always possible. In such situations, recipients are called into the transplant unit and evaluated at that time.

Also varied are recipients' responses to the news that kidneys are available. The responses range from joyous and elated acceptance to fearful refusal. A person who knows the recipient should make the phone call. In situations in which callers are unknown, a professional approach is necessary. When recipients agree to come to the hospital, the following questions are asked:

1. How are you feeling now?
2. Have you had any fevers or infections recently?
3. When was your last dialysis treatment?
4. When was the last time you ingested food or fluid? (Then they are told not to drink or eat anything from that moment on.)
5. How long will it take you to get to the hospital?

All of the above information is noted, and the surgeons and transplant units are notified.

LIVING RELATED DONORS

For some, the decision to donate a kidney to a family member is easy. These individuals have close emotional ties with the family member in need. For others, the decision to donate is more difficult. These individuals are often subject to family pressure that results in feelings of guilt if they do not offer to donate during the interview process. Getting to know donors and their families affords clinicians insight into their motives and fears regarding donation.

A classic behavior pattern is that the potential donor's spouse vigorously protests the donation. Often the spouse expresses feelings that potential donors are unable to express. Individuals with ambivalent feelings predonation are at high risk for negative feelings postdonation, especially if the graft fails. If poor self-esteem or poor self-image motivates donation, these feelings will not be corrected postdonation.

Selection Criteria

The following are indications for living donor transplant:

- Ages 18 to 55.
- Matched tissue typing.
- Absence of hypertension, diabetes, thromboembolic disease, heart disease, renal disease, severe obesity, positive HIV antibody, positive HB Ag, or a psychiatric disorder.

Living Donor Workup and Tissue Typing

The living donor workup process includes:

- Tissue typing.
- Noninvasive studies.
- Invasive studies.
- Donor-specific blood transfusions (DSBTs).
- Preoperative teaching.

Each step of the process continues unless contraindicated by the preceding steps.

Tissue Typing

Potential donors who intend to donate will first be tissue-typed. One-year graft survival, using prednisone and azathioprine (Aza), is 90% to 95% when the donor is HLA-identical, 70% to 80% when haploidentical, and 60% to 70% when totally mismatched (Morris, 1988). DSBTs and cyclosporine A (Cy A) have dramatically improved the success rates of both haploidentical and totally mismatched living donor grafts to the 90% to 95% rates seen with HLA-identical donors (Sollinger, Burlingham, Spaeks, Glass, & Belzer, 1984).

Noninvasive Studies

A nursing clinician qualified in physical assessment can adequately complete the donor workup, a history and physical, laboratory tests, and ECG. If any parameter on this initial visit is abnormal, a review of findings with the transplant surgeon is necessary. The following situations require further special testing before advancing to the more invasive phase of the workup:

1. Glucose tolerance testing (GTT) for a potential donor from a family with juvenile-onset diabetes mellitus (JODM) or a strong family history of diabetes.
2. DNA analysis for presymptomatic testing of a potential donor from a polycystic kidney family. (Blood samples from at least two family members are necessary for confirmation of diagnosis.)
3. Pulmonary function tests on all asthmatics and/or smokers.
4. Stress thallium tests for males over 45 years and females over 50 years if evaluation of cardiopulmonary status indicates.
5. Beta human chorionic gonadotropin (BHCG) testing for all females of child-bearing age.
6. Proctoscopies for anyone 45 years or older.
7. Pap smears for all women.
8. Dental clearances.
9. Psychological evaluation.

Invasive Studies

The donor workup progresses to more invasive parameters when all of the foregoing noninvasive parameters are acceptable. An intravenous pyelogram (IVP) and chest x-ray are scheduled on an outpatient basis to determine the presence of two kidneys, a normally functioning urological system, and a normal chest roentgenogram.

Referral to specialists for review and clearance of abnormal findings is appropriate. Precautions for a thorough and safe preoperative evaluation is mandatory to prevent possible adverse sequelae postoperatively.

Donor-Specific Blood Transfusions

If all of the workup parameters are within normal limits, DSBTs are scheduled. HLA-identical donor–recipient parents do not require DSBTs. Menstruating women who are to be living donors need to take ferrous sulfate supplements during the workup process and up to the time of surgery.

DSBTs are time-consuming and require strict adherence to the infusion and cross-match schedule. Records are kept of when the transfusions are given, what type of blood tubes are drawn, and from whom they are drawn. One unit of blood from donors will be withdrawn and one third of the packed red blood cells (PRBCs) will be transfused into recipients on three separate occasions at 2-week intervals.

The volume of packed cells necessary to evoke sensitization or graft enhancement in an adult ranges from 50 to 100 cc. Therefore, donors may need to donate a 240-cc to 480-cc unit of whole blood, which will be separated into three equal aliquots for infusion. If, after the DSBTs, the cross-matches are positive, the transplant is canceled and another donor source is sought.

Beginning 1 to 2 days before potential recipients receive the initial DSBT, Aza is begun. The dose is titrated to the recipient's white blood cells (WBCs). If the WBC count declines below $5,000/\mu l$ despite decreasing the Aza dose, discontinuing the drug is appropriate to prevent possible infectious complications.

Cross-matches are performed 2 weeks after each transfusion. Antibodies to the cells that are reactive at 37°C are most likely to be harmful, while those directed to B-cells, especially those reactive at 4°C, are innocuous (Opelz, Graver, Mickey, & Terasaki, 1981). If the T-cell or warm B-cell cross-matches become positive, no further DSBTs are done; the transplant is canceled, and another donor source is sought. If none of the three cross-matches is positive, the transplant is scheduled for 4 weeks after the last DSBT, with the final cross-match scheduled for 5 to 7 days prior to the scheduled day of surgery. No blood transfusions are to occur during this time.

One to 2 weeks prior to the operation date, an autologous unit of blood is obtained from the donor. Use of an autologous unit can prevent contraction of HIV, hepatitis, or a transfusion reaction. If surgery is canceled for longer than 30 days, the blood bank should be notified to freeze the autologous unit. If the surgery is canceled for longer than 6 months, the blood bank may be notified to release the unit for general use.

Preoperative Teaching

Patient education is an ongoing component of living donor workups. The transplant nurse must realize that assessment of information is as important as the content discussed. Repeating information in different formats is appropriate because anxiety blocks information retention.

As the workup phases become more invasive, the preparatory teaching needs to become more thorough because most living donors have never been hospitalized. A tour of the hospital unit and introduction to nursing personnel help prepare them for the admission. Including key family members in the preoperative tour and teaching helps alleviate anxiety.

Teaching Checklist for Donor Preoperative teaching for the living related donor is conducted by the staff nurse the day prior to surgery. The following is a sample checklist of the topics discussed:

Respiratory:	Rationale, importance
	Incentive spirometer
	Cough, turn, deep breath
	No smoking
	Abdominal splinting
	Out-of-bed technique
	Ambulation
Gastrointestinal:	Rationale, importance
	Tap water enemas
	NPO after midnight
	Clear liquids advanced as tolerated once passing flatus and bowel sounds present
Genitourinary:	Foley catheter location, rationale
	Length of placement
Integumentary:	Incision location and size
	May shower once sutures removed
	Intravenous lines
Senses:	Pain
	Frequency and type of analgesia
Medications:	Antibiotics
	Laxatives

LIVING-DONOR NEPHRECTOMY

On the morning of surgery, the donor and recipient are placed in adjoining operating rooms. Communication between the two teams allows the least amount of warm ischemia time between the donor's nephrectomy and the recipient's anastomosing.

After endotracheal intubation and Foley catheter placement, the donor is positioned on the opposite side to the kidney that is to be removed. Then the table is flexed to extend the presenting flank. An NPO status since midnight necessitates infusing a fluid bolus. Usually, 500 cc is infused over a few minutes; then a liberal drip rate continues to assure good hydration and renal perfusion. The infusion of an autologous unit of blood is performed if warranted during the procedure.

Operative Techniques

Two surgical approaches for the donor's nephrectomy are possible. The most common one is the retroperitoneal, or flank, approach; the other is the anterior transperitoneal approach. (Morris, 1988; Toledo-Pereyra, 1988). The incisions are made from the tip of the 11th or 12th rib to the lateral border of the rectus sheath. The incision is deepened through all layers, but the peritoneum is not entered. Removal of the distal portion of the 12th or 11th rib facilitates dissection and removal of the kidney. Gerota's fascia is incised, and the kidney is bluntly dissected free. Care is taken not to enter the peritoneal and pleural cavities. The surgeon next dissects the renal vessels and ureter. No dissection is done in the renal hilus to protect the blood supply to the renal pelvis and ureter. Once urinary output is assured from the cut ureter, the renal vessels are clamped and ligated. The removed kidney is perfused with chilled, heparinized electrolyte solution. The wound is closed without drains. Then the donor is taken to the recovery room, where a chest x-ray excludes the possibility of a pneumothorax.

Postoperative Care of Living Donor Nephrectomy

Nurses manage donors postoperatively in the same manner as any other individual who has undergone a nephrectomy. Potential complications after living-donor nephrectomy are enumerated in Table 4.3. Donor deaths occurred approximately 20 times in the worldwide experience estimated at 40,000 (Starzl, 1987). Pulmonary embolus was the primary cause of those deaths.

Within days of the nephrectomy, the glomerular filtration rate of the remaining kidney increases so that 1 week after nephrectomy the creatinine clearance is about 70% of the prenephrectomy value. Renal

TABLE 4.3 Complications of Living Donor Nephrectomy

Procedure and complications	Incidence (1000 cases) (%)
Aortogram	
Prolonged discomfort	0.5
Femoral thrombosis or aneurysm	0.4
Nephrectomy wound	
Prolonged discomfort	3.2
Infection	2.1
Hernia	2.0
Hematoma	0.5
Pulmonary	
Atelectasis	13.5
Pneumothorax or pneumomediastinum	9.1
Pneumoitis or pleural effusion	4.3
Urinary tract	
Infection	8.6
Retention	1.6
ATN	0.9
Late proteinuria	3.0
Other	
Prolonged ileus	2.6
Thrombophlebitis with or without pulmonary embolus	1.9
Peripheral nerve palsy	1.1
Hepatic dysfunction (late)	0.9
Hypertension (late)	15.0[a]

[a]Similar to general population (Levey et al., 1986)
From *Organ Transplantation and Replacement* (chapter 5), by J.G. Cerilli (Ed.), 1988, Philadelphia: J.B. Lippincott. Copyright 1988. Reprinted by permission.

functional reserve has been demonstrated to be good many years after nephrectomy in kidney donors following a high-protein meal and during pregnancy. This renal reserve is only slightly reduced, however, compared to individuals with two kidneys (Weiland et al., 1984). Levy, Hou, and Bush (1986) and Spital (1988) indicate the following long-term effects on donors:

1. Urinary excretion of protein increases slightly (50–100 mg/day).
2. Blood pressure may be slightly higher than before nephrectomy in a small percentage of cases (by approximately 5 mmHg). This incidence of hypertension is similar to that seen in the general population.

3. Creatinine clearance postdonation stabilizes at approximately 80% of the prenephrectomy level.
4. Donors from a wide variety of occupations agreed almost universally that their organ donation did not affect their earning capacity and ability to carry out their occupational responsibilities.

Donors are discharged approximately 4 to 6 days postoperation. A return clinic appointment is scheduled for 1 to 2 weeks postoperation to evaluate wound integrity, remove staples (if not done before discharge), and assess overall physical status. Succeeding donor checkups are done at 6 weeks, 6 months, and 12 months postoperation. Checkups generally include complete physical examinations and appropriate laboratory studies.

Prior to discharge from the hospital, donors are advised to force fluids, restrict major physical exertion such as lifting or housework, and to call immediately if they develop a fever. Generally, donors may resume sexual activity as tolerated at 3 weeks, drive a car at 3 weeks, and return to work at 6 weeks (provided it is not heavy physical labor, which requires a longer period of healing).

NURSING CARE OF RECIPIENTS

The arrival of potential kidney transplant recipients in the transplant unit precipitates a flurry of activity. Protocols and standing orders streamline the preoperative period and help assure a systematic and thorough approach to assessment and preparation. The transplant nurse is instrumental in the coordination of this preoperative sequence of events.

Laboratory studies and a cross-match (if required) are the first tasks to be accomplished. Chemistry results determine the need for preoperative hemodialysis, and the cross-match results determine whether or not the transplant will take place. A urine culture is sent off, and a peritoneal fluid culture if the patient is on chronic ambulatory peritoreal dialysis (CAPD). In addition, a baseline chest x-ray and ECG are done. The resident on call obtains the surgical consent.

The nurse then conducts a patient history and physical assessment. A preoperative weight and assessment of vascular access are of particular importance. Tap water enemas are given until clear, and the patient is instructed to take a Phisohex shower. Immunosuppression is administered orally before surgery or intravenously during surgery as ordered.

Due to the time constraint, the transplant nurse provides preoperative teaching throughout the admission process. The following is a sample checklist of the topics discussed:

Preoperative Teaching Checklist for Recipients

Respiratory:
  Rationale, importance
  Incentive spirometer
  Cough, turn, deep breath
  No smoking
  Abdominal splinting
  Out of bed technique
  Ambulation
Gastrointestinal:
  Rationale, importance
  Tap water enemas
  NPO after midnight
  Clear liquids advanced as tolerated
    once passing flatus and bowel sounds present
  Possible sodium, potassium, and
    fluid restrictions
Genitourinary:
  Foley catheter location, rationale
  Length of placement
  Hematuria
  Irrigation technique
  Bladder spasms
  Catheter care
  Frequency of voiding after removal
    of catheter
Integumentary:
  Incision location and size
  Intravenous lines
  Shower once sutures removed
  Position on back or operative side
Senses:
  Pain
  Frequency and type of analgesia
Medications:
  Immunosuppressants
  Antibiotics
  Antacids
  Antihypertensives
Postoperative Complications:
  Acute tubular necrosis
  Rejection
  Dialysis
  Infection

Intraoperative Phase

Preparation of Recipients

Recipients are taken to the operating room and placed in a supine position. A peripheral IV is started, and anesthesia is induced. Most commonly, general anesthesia is used, but under certain circumstances spinal anesthesia may be preferred, using an epidural or a combination of epidural and light general anesthesia.

Upon induction of anesthesia, individuals are prepped and draped. A large-gauge Foley catheter is gently inserted into the bladder. The bladder is then irrigated with an antibiotic solution to reduce wound contamination at the time of ureteral implantation (Cerilli, 1988).

Preparation of Donated Kidneys

The donated kidney is closely examined, and any dissection of perinephric fat or vascular reconstruction is completed. Prior to its implantation, the kidney is maintained at a temperature of 5° to 7°C.

Surgical Placement and Anastomosis

The transplanted kidney is placed in either the right or left iliac fossa. Regardless of side, either the right or left kidney can be used. In primary transplants, placement of the left kidney in the right iliac fossa is preferred. This allows for ease in visualizing the renal pelvis and ureter of the transplanted kidney if repeat surgical procedures are required. Also, the sigmoid colon lies close to the transplanted kidney, and the iliac vein runs deeper on the left. The kidney is placed extraperitoneally; therefore, individuals maintained with chronic peritoneal dialysis may continue using peritoneal dialysis if delayed renal function occurs. However, most surgeons prefer to remove the peritoneal catheter because of the risk of infection with subsequent immunosuppression posttransplant.

The most commonly used incision line starts 3 to 4 cm above the iliac crest, extends down to the inguinal ligament, and ends near the midline just above the pubis (Cerilli, 1988). The result is a curvilinear incision extending approximately 20 cm. The skin, subcutaneous, and musculofascial layers are incised. The peritoneum is reflected medially and retracted, allowing for a pocket to accommodate the kidney in the iliac fossa. Tissues and lymphatics overlying the iliac vessels are ligated to lessen lymph leakage. In males, the spermatic cord is dissected from the surrounding structures and carefully retracted, allowing the ureter to pass below when implantation into the bladder occurs (Calne, 1985).

Identification and dissection of the vessels is done meticulously, keeping involvement of perivascular structures to a minimum. Two techniques are commonly used for vascularization of the transplant graft. The choice of vessels is determined by the recipient's anatomy, the degree of atherosclerotic disease present in the required vessels, and the anatomy of the donor organ. Most commonly, an end-to-side vascular anastomosis of the donor's renal artery and the recipient's external iliac artery is performed. (See Figure 4.1.) The end-to-end vascular anastomosis involves suturing of the donor renal artery to the end of the recipient's internal iliac artery. The venous anastomosis is performed by attaching the end of the donor renal vein to the side of the external iliac vein. (See Figure 4.2.)

When the vascular anastomoses are completed and the vessels unclamped, attention is directed to the kidney. In an uncomplicated transplant, the kidney quickly "pinks up" and urine begins to flow through the still unattached ureter. Aggressive fluid management in combination with diuretics is imperative at this point in the procedure. Mannitol and/or furosemide may be administered to promote diuresis.

Ureteral Implantation

Attention is now turned to anastomosis of the ureter into the bladder. The most common method for attachment is the tunnel technique.

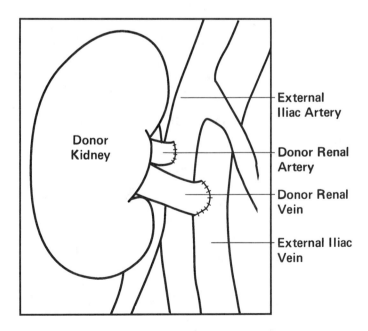

FIGURE 4.1 Illustration of end-to-side vascular anastomoses of donor renal artery to recipient's external iliac artery and donor renal vein to external iliac vein.

The Tunnel Technique Because the ureter is delicate, great care must be taken to avoid any trauma to it caused by excessive handling. Adequate circulation also must be provided and preserved to the transplanted ureter. In the native kidneys, multiple sources provide the blood supply. In the transplanted kidney, the primary blood supply is via the renal vessels. Therefore, at the time of the harvest, tissue surrounding the renal vessels medial to the lower pole and proximal to the ureter is also reserved in order to preserve small periuretic branches that aid in feeding the ureter (Toledo-Pereyra, 1988). Circulation to the ureter is restored at the time that the renal artery anastomosis is performed. Careful inspection of the ureter for areas of poor blood supply is completed before the ureter is attached to the bladder. The bladder is entered through an incision in the dome slightly lateral to the midline. Working from both inside and outside the bladder, a submucosal tunnel is created, with eventual placement of the new transplanted ureteral orifice just lateral and superior to the organ. The end of the ureter is then spatulated and secured to the bladder with absorbable sutures. This method

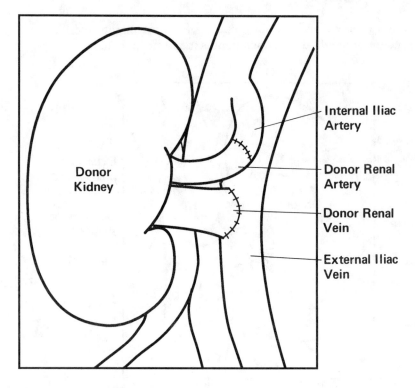

FIGURE 4.2 Illustration of end-to-end vascular anastomosis of donor renal artery to recipient's internal iliac artery and end-to-side anastomosis of donor renal vein to external iliac vein.

of anastomosis has the important advantage of being antireflux. That is, as the bladder contracts upon emptying, the ureter is compressed by the bladder wall, preventing reflux of urine into the kidney.

The kidney's position in the iliac fossa is then examined. Care is taken to assure that no kinking or tension of the ureter or vessels occurs. Any areas of bleeding are ligated. The wound is liberally irrigated with an antibiotic solution, and then the wound is closed. A few centers advocate using drains to prevent perinephric fluid collections. These are usually placed in the upper aspect of the incision and are removed in the early posttransplant period. Anesthesia is then reversed, and the recipient is taken from the operating room.

Intraoperative Recipient Management

Alteration of Fluid Balance

Vigorous intraoperative hydration maintains perfusion and function in the transplanted kidney. Maintenance of adequate circulating volume and blood pressure also aids in preserving the recipient's hemodialysis access. Fistula thrombosis secondary to hypotension is a common transplant complication. This complication distresses recipients and creates a major logistical problem for the transplant team if the kidney fails to function, necessitating hemodialysis. The most commonly used IV solutions are 5% dextrose with 45% normal saline and lactated Ringer's. Intravenous fluids are infused at a rate sufficient to maintain central venous pressure (CVP) readings just above normal range.

Diuretics, in combination with aggressive fluid replacement, are always administered to assure perfusion and filtration in the transplanted kidney. Mannitol and furosemide are the diuretics of choice.

Postoperative Nursing Care of Recipients

The postoperative care of kidney transplant recipients presents many nursing challenges. Managing instability of hemodynamics, diabetes mellitus, and fluid and electrolytes are just a few examples. The following discussion describes these postoperative problems in greater detail. A sample nursing care plan is included at the end of this chapter.

Creatinine

The serum creatinine is the primary marker of renal transplant function. In living related transplants, the serum creatinine normalizes around Day 3. In cadaver donations, the course is more variable. If acute tubular necrosis (ATN) is not a major factor, normalization occurs between the 10th and 15th posttransplant day. Several factors may cause a transient rise in serum creatinine; these include Cy A toxicity, dehydration, and laboratory error or variation. These possible causes must be ruled out to identify changes that indicate rejection. A rapidly rising hematocrit in combination with decreased body weight, elevated BUN, and urine output that exceeds intake indicates dehydration. Cy A toxicity may be suspected as the cause of dysfunction if blood concentration of Cy A is high or if there are other indications of nephrotoxicity such as hyperkalemia or acidosis.

Electrolytes

Renal failure is a disease of imbalances. Hyperkalemia, hypokalemia, hyperphosphatemia, acidosis, anemia, and fluid overload are all major sequelae inherent in the disease process. In instances of nonfunction, all of these imbalances continue or may be exacerbated. Aggressive fluid replacement places recipients at high risk for overload. Blood transfusions, the trauma of surgery, and the nephrotoxic effects of Cy A may aggravate hyperkalemia. Kayexalate® enema, dextrose 50% and insulin, or hemodialysis can correct these imbalances until renal function resumes.

When immediate kidney function returns, recipients are prone to imbalances. Hypokalemia secondary to aggressive diuresis or diuretics is common; dehydration may also occur. Cy A's effects on renal tubules are associated with hypomagnesemia, hypophosphatemia, acidosis, hyperkalemia, and sodium retention. Supplementation with oral magnesium, phosphorus and correction of acidosis with bicarbonate may be warranted. Hyperkalemia is controlled with low-potassium diet and, if necessary, Kayexalate®, a potassium-exchanging resin. Reduction in Cy A dose can often improve these sequelae.

Hematology

Complete reversal of anemia is not observed until approximately 6 weeks of normal renal functioning has been achieved. Changes in hematocrit are usually not marked in the immediate posttransplant period. Significant rises indicate dehydration. Conversely, significant falls may indicate fluid overload or bleeding.

Aza, antilymphocyte globulin, (ALG), and OKT3 also significantly influence circulating leukocytes. All three are associated with leukopenia, and they may cause thrombocytopenia. Significant leukopenia or thrombocytopenia may necessitate lowering the dose or discontinuing these drugs.

Hypertension

Instability in blood pressure is common during the operative period. In general, the initial effects of anesthesia and vigorous fluid removal prior to surgery cause blood pressure to fall. However, by the end of surgery, most recipients have elevated blood pressure (Toledo-Pereyra, 1988). Therefore, antihypertensive medications should be continued prior to and after surgery. This is especially important in individuals taking clonidine and beta blockers, as withdrawal of these drugs may precipitate a rebound-worsened hypertension.

Diabetes Mellitus

Diabetic patients undergoing surgery are at risk for developing hypo- and hyperglycemia. Therefore, it is difficult to predict insulin requirements intraoperatively. In general, regular insulin is withheld preoperatively, and long-acting insulin dosage is reduced. The administration of prednisone will also affect serum glucose levels in some diabetic patients. Nurses are particularly attentive to the potential instability of these patients. Frequent serum and capillary glucose monitoring is conducted, along with routine assessment for signs and symptoms of hypo- and hyperglycemia. Some diabetic recipients may require continuous insulin drips for adequate glucose control.

Infection

Infectious complications are a major cause of morbidity and mortality in the transplant population. The highest incidence occurs during periods of aggressive immunosuppression in the early posttransplant period or as a result of immunosuppression given to treat rejection. In the immediate posttransplant period, urinary tract infections (UTIs) wound infections, and sepsis related to IV lines are the most commonly observed causes of bacterial infection (Flye, 1989).

Early removal of IV lines and Foley catheter helps reduce the incidence of infection from these sources. In many cases, though, it is necessary to maintain IV access and Foley catheters. While these remain in place, meticulous care using aseptic technique is prescribed. Foley catheter care with warm soap and water is indicated twice a day. IV site dressing changes are done every 48 hours; IV tubing changes, every 72 hours. Careful nursing assessments of IV insertion sites and character of urine for signs and symptoms of infection are essential.

UTIs continue to arise with great frequency in renal transplant recipients. Up to 42% of recipients develop UTIs within the first year posttransplant (Flye, 1989), and many will be asymptomatic. Frequent monitoring of urine cultures is indicated with aggressive treatment of infections as they arise. Once-a-day administration of a prophylactic antibiotic reduces the incidence of urinary tract infections.

Aggressive immunosuppression is also associated with a high incidence of viral infections. These include CMV, EBV, HSV, and VZ. Other viruses that may occur include adenovirus and influenza (Flye, 1989).

HSV most often occurs within the first 1 to 2 months posttransplant. The prophylactic administration of low-dose acyclovir significantly reduces its recurrence in recipients who have a positive HSV titre prior to transplantation (Seale et al., 1985). Acyclovir is usually prescribed for the first month posttransplant. A half dose is prescribed if the serum creatinine is greater than 3.0 mg/dl. Routine nursing assessment of the patient's oral cavity for herpes lesions is common.

CMV is another viral pathogen affecting renal transplant recipients. CMV infections most often occur between the first and fifth months posttransplant, with varying degrees of severity. The infection may represent a recurrence of latent CMV in recipients with prior exposure to the virus, or it may be a primary infection. The source of a primary infection is usually the donor organ, and primary infections tend to be severe. The signs of infection include fatigue, headache, arthralgias, fever, and leukopenia. CMV may cause pneumonia, gastrointestinal bleeding, hepatitis, or retinitis and may increase superimposed bacterial or fungal infections. In some studies, CMV has also been associated with graft rejection, although graft rejection can be secondary to obligatory reduction or discontinuation of immunosuppression during significant infections (Flye, 1989). The prophylactic use of CMV-immune globulin reduces the incidence of significant CMV infection in recipients who are at high risk for primary infection (Snydman et al., 1988).

The clinical effectiveness of high-dose administration of acyclovir in prophylaxis against CMV is also under investigation. Acyclovir has been tested in bone marrow transplant recipients and has not been found to be effective against reactivation of CMV, but it does delay its manifestation (Migliori & Simmons, 1988). High-dose oral administration of acyclovir is being evaluated as prophylaxis against primary CMV in renal transplant recipients.

Fungal infections are also observed in transplant recipients. Colonization of the oropharynx and gastrointestinal tract with *Candida* organisms may be avoided by using antifungal agents such as nystatin or Mycelex®.

Immunosuppression

Immunosuppressant therapies vary from center to center. The choice of agent depends on a variety of factors, including donor source, tissue match, the presence of a high level of preformed antibiotics, suspected ATN posttransplant, and high-risk status. Individuals may be considered high risk for medical or immunological reasons. An example of immunologically high risk is rejection of a previous transplant.

Methylprednisolone is always administered intravenously when the transplant procedure is initiated.

Cyclosporine A (Cy A) is routinely used with cadaver and mismatched living related transplants. IV Cy A is associated with significant nephrotoxicity; consequently, many centers have switched to oral administration.

The ultimate goal of immunosuppressive protocols is to maximize protection against rejection while minimizing side effects. Cy A, a mainstay of most immunosuppressive protocols, is unpredictably absorbed and metabolized. Blood levels must be maintained within a closely monitored therapeutic range to assure adequate immunosuppression but avoid the multiple sequelae associated with this drug. Two methods for monitoring Cy A are high-performance liquid chromatography (HPLC) or radioimmunoassay (RIA). HPLC measures only parent Cy A, whereas RIA detects both Cy A parent compound and its numerous metabolites. Within the first 2 months posttransplant, the therapeutic range of trough levels using HPLC is 100 to 150 ng/ml or, when using RIA, 300 to 800 ng/ml (blood) or 100 to 250 ng/ml in serum (Maddeux, 1989).

Azathioprine (Aza): Because successful outcomes are so high using a combination of Aza and prednisone, very few centers use Cy A with HLA-identical sibling grafts. Some centers also advocate using Aza when postoperative ATN is deemed likely. This is done because the nephrotoxic effects of Cy A prolong ATN. When normal renal function is achieved, Cy A is added.

Many centers advocate using a combination of Aza, prednisone, and Cy A, commonly called triple therapy, in the initial period and as maintenance immunosuppression.

DIAGNOSTIC STUDIES

In addition to physical findings and laboratory results, diagnostic studies are an integral component in evaluating renal function and, when indicated, in determining appropriate intervention.

Because nurses prepare kidney transplant patients for the following diagnostic studies, they must know how the studies are conducted, whether the studies are invasive or noninvasive, how results affect patients' well-being, and how to plan postprocedural nursing care.

Ultrasonography is a noninvasive technique for evaluating the transplanted kidney and the surrounding spaces. Ultrasonography is most commonly employed to assess for obstruction, hydronephrosis, and fluid collections. The ultrasound is done by removing the abdominal dressing, placing a transmission gel on the skin, and moving a smooth instrument across the area of the kidney transplant until an image is located on the viewing screen.

Renal scan has long been an important tool in assessing immediate and long-term renal function, providing information regarding both renal blood flow and tubular function and bladder emptying. This test, conducted in the department of nuclear medicine, takes approximately 30 minutes. Radioactive isotopes are injected intravenously, and every 5 minutes the scanner takes an image for a total of six images. Prior to the last image, the patient is asked to void so that bladder emptying can be evaluated. Because patients excrete the radioactive isotopes in their urine following a urine scan, it is imperative that nurses wear gloves when handling patients' urine.

Percutaneous needle biopsy is the definitive test for evaluating kidney function. However, risks include damage to the renal vessels, fistula formation, infarction, or hemorrhage that could result in losing the transplant kidney. To reduce these risks, biopsies are performed using ultrasonography. Local anesthesia is injected, and a small nick is made in the skin where the needle is to be inserted. The specimen is obtained, the needle withdrawn, and direct pressure is applied over the puncture site for 10 to 15 minutes. A 5-lb sandbag is then placed over the biopsy site for 2 to 4 hours. Urine output is closely monitored for hematuria, the biopsy site is observed for signs of bleeding, and pedal pulses are palpated for disturbances in circulation. The patient remains on strict bedrest for 4 to 6 hours, and analgesia may be required.

Both the prospect of a renal transplant biopsy and the potential results of that biopsy often frighten recipients. Therefore, it is important that nurses not only explain the procedure and the degree of discomfort that can be expected but provide emotional support as well.

Diagnosis and Treatment of Rejection

The rejection process results from the reaction of the recipient's immune system to the antigens present in the donor kidney. The rejection response can be humoral, cellular, or mixed. Despite a greater understanding of immunology, refinement in tissue typing and cross-matching techniques, and improvements in immunosuppressants, rejection continues to be the major limiting factor to successful transplantation. Although 1-year graft survival for cadaver renal transplants is reported to be as high as 90% in some centers, 5-year graft survival continues to hover around 50% to 60%, with rejection causing the major number of failures.

Additionally, survival has become more difficult in the Cy A era. Scans are now of less value in detecting rejection. Cy A nephrotoxicity can mimic rejection, and the classic symptoms of rejection (i.e., fever, pain, weight gain, decreased urine output, and elevated creatinine) are often less dramatic. Therefore, despite the inherent risks, biopsies are often necessary to yield a diagnosis in a clinically clouded picture.

The following is an overview of the four types of rejection patterns and their histological appearance as found upon kidney biopsy. Additional information on this subject is addressed in Chapter 2 "Immunological Aspects of Organ Transplantation."

Hyperacute Rejection

Hyperacute rejection is a violent humoral response that occurs when recipients have been presensitized to antigens present on the donor kidney. Presensitization can result from previous transplantation, pregnancy, or prior blood transfusion. The recipient's antibodies react to antigens on the endothelial cells of the donor organ capillaries. Complement is activated, leukocytes attach at the site, and the endothelial cells are destroyed. Platelets then attach to the capillaries, forming a clot and obstructing the vessel (Toledo-Pereyra, 1988).

Within minutes of revascularization of the kidney, the formerly pink, firm kidney is flaccid and cyanotic. Damage is irreversible, and the kidney must be removed. Upon biopsy, the peritubular capillaries are clumped with red cells, and frank thrombosis of the small vessels is observed. Fortunately, this type of rejection can be avoided by cross-matching prior to the transplant.

Accelerated Rejection

Accelerated rejection normally occurs between the second and fifth days posttransplant. It is both a cellular and a humoral response. The abrupt decline in urine output associated with accelerated rejection may be confused with ATN. Therefore, a biopsy may be necessary to make a diagnosis. This type of rejection is difficult to reverse and often resists treatment with high-dose steroids. ALG or OKT3 are therefore often prescribed. Even with aggressive immunosuppression, accelerated rejection is associated with significant graft loss.

Acute Rejection

Acute rejection occurs most commonly within the first 2 weeks after transplant but can occur many years later. The clinical signs associated with acute rejection include oliguria, rising creatinine, worsening hypertension, weight gain, fever, and pain over the kidney. Unfortunately, in many instances, the clinical picture may be as benign as a slowly climbing creatinine that initially appears to improve with reduction in Cy A dosage but then begins rising again. In order to rule out Cy A nephrotoxicity and confirm acute rejection, a biopsy is warranted.

Acute rejection may damage any structure within the kidney. The biopsy findings in acute rejection vary according to its severity, the length of time since the transplant, and the nature of the immune response. In general, when glomerular or arterial changes predominate, the rejection is humoral or antibody mediated. When interstitial changes are prominent, the rejection is cellular. In many cases, the picture is mixed, especially when the biopsy is performed several months posttransplant and chronic rejection is superimposed.

In mild or early rejection, interstitial swelling and edema of the peritubular capillaries are present. The tubular endothelium is normal, and the small arteries and arterioles are unchanged. There is cortical infiltration with lymphocytes. As rejection progresses, interstitial hemorrhages may be seen. Fibrin clots are formed that block the peritubular capillaries, which may result in vessel wall rupture. The tubules become dilated, and focal areas of necrosis may develop. Infiltration with mononuclear cells is often prominent. Small arteries and arterioles become swollen secondary to lymphocyte invasion. These changes are usually reversible. However, if necrosis develops in the small vessels, rejection cannot be reversed (Morris, 1988).

Chronic Rejection

Chronic rejection may occur within weeks to years posttransplant. Although the exact cause is still not clearly understood, it appears to be primarily a humoral response. In general, the clinical signs of chronic rejection mimic those of ESRD. Proteinuria may be the first indication. Rising serum creatinine, decreased creatinine clearance, worsening hypertension, and fluid weight gain from sodium retention may be present. As renal function continues to deteriorate, anemia, acidosis, and hyperphosphatemia are observed.

Biopsy findings indicative of chronic rejection include interstitial fibrosis, glomerular lesions, tubular atrophy, basement membrane thickening, and destruction of the peritubular capillaries. These changes are irreversible. Renal function can remain quite stable, although at a lower level, for many years despite findings of chronic rejection on renal biopsy. However, when chronic changes are significant, a rapid decline in renal function may ensue. In these instances, plans for retransplantation or dialytic intervention should be addressed.

Kidney Transplant Dysfunction versus Rejection

Biopsy of a transplanted kidney is used for differential diagnosis of rejection from ATN, nephrotoxicity, and recurrent disease.

Acute Tubular Necrosis

ATN is the major cause of early nonfunction in cadaver kidney transplants. Between 35% and 45% of cadaver transplant recipients experience some degree of delayed function; whereas delayed function is rarely observed in living donation recipients (Morris, 1988). Cy A appears to increase the incidence and duration of ATN. Other factors associated with the increased likelihood of ATN include donor factors such as pulmonary and cardiac arrest, multiple fractures, multiple organ donation, prolonged preservation time, prolonged warm ischemia, and reperfusion injury.

Clinically, ATN is characterized by oliguria and a failure of patients' creatinine levels to decline. Usually a renal biopsy will not be performed until 2 weeks posttransplant if ATN has not resolved or if renal function declines after a transient improvement. Biopsy results vary according to the severity and duration of nonfunction. Tubular dilation with simplification of the tubular epithelial layer is seen, and interstitial and intratubular oxalate crystals are often present. In some instances, coagulation necrosis with sloughing into the tubular lumen occurs. If ATN is prolonged, significant interstitial edema and fibrosis and tubular atrophy may occur. Concomitant findings of lymphoid infiltrates and tubulitis may also be observed. These are suggestive of superimposed acute rejection (Cerilli, 1988).

ATN is associated with an increased incidence of graft loss, presumably secondary to rejection. The reason for this remains unclear. In addition to its association with increased graft failure, ATN results in increased hospital stays, prolonged need for maintenance dialysis, and dietary restrictions. ATN is a profoundly disappointing experience for many transplant recipients. In an effort to reduce the incidence and severity of ATN, great care is taken to minimize preservation and warm ischemia time as well as to avoid unnecessary handling and injury to the kidney. Some centers delay introduction of Cy A into the immunosuppressive regimen when ATN is considered likely, and most centers avoid the use of intravenous Cy A.

Nephrotoxicity

Nephrotoxicity secondary to Cy A remains a major complication in managing renal transplant recipients. An acute onset nephrotoxic response to Cy A may occur in the immediate postoperative period in association with ATN or the use of IV Cy A. A more insidious form of nephrotoxicity is observed in the majority of transplant recipients. In these cases, a rise in serum creatinine equal to or greater than 25% above baseline levels occurs. Additional indications of nephrotoxicity include hyperkalemia, hyperuricemia, hyperchloremic renal tubular acidosis, and hypertension (Kahan, 1986).

The usefulness of percutaneous biopsy in diagnosing Cy A nephrotoxicity in these instances remains controversial. Acute toxicity is not associated with biopsy changes, but is rather a diagnosis of elimination. If no other causes, such as acute rejection, are identified, Cy A is considered the likely cause of dysfunction. A reduction in the Cy A dose will result in a return to normal renal function.

A chronic form of nephrotoxicity is associated with histological findings. These changes are most prevalent with long-term use of high-dose Cy A. Findings for chronic nephrotoxicity are variable but may include diffuse interstitial fibrosis, toxic tubulopathy, peritubular capillary congestion, arteriolopathy, and tubular atrophy (Cockburn, Gotz, Gülich, & Krupp, 1988). The clinical picture of chronic toxicity is one of a chronically elevated creatinine. Maintaining Cy A levels within a tight therapeutic window with frequent monitoring of serum levels may help minimize these changes.

Recurrent Disease

In addition to ATN and Cy A toxicity, kidneys are also at risk of developing de novo disease or recurrence of the original disease process. Recurrent disease occurs in approximately 5% to 10% of transplant grafts and accounts for less than 2% of all failures (Matthew, 1988). Histological findings via percutaneous biopsy distinguish these disorders from other causes of dysfunction. Any glomerular disease can recur in the transplanted kidney (Cerilli, 1988). The incidence, extent, and rapidity of decline in transplant function varies according to the specific disease process. Therefore, it is important to ascertain the cause of renal failure before transplantation. Knowing the causes of kidney failure aids in determining the appropriateness of living donation and in assessing changes in function during the posttransplant period. The most commonly reported de novo disease is membranous glomerulonephritis (Flye, 1989), which is associated with significant proteinuria but does not usually lead to graft failure.

Various complications may arise that affect the renal vessels, ureter, or allograft itself. The sequelae of these events often require surgical intervention and may result in graft loss. Table 4.4 outlines the more common postoperative complications and treatments.

DISCHARGE PLANNING AND TEACHING

The average hospital stay following an uncomplicated renal transplant ranges from 7 to 10 days. Because the hospital stay is normally short, patient teaching begins as quickly as possible. Written materials aid in the learning process. An educational packet provides detailed information that recipients can use in the initial posttransplant period to supplement verbal instructions. The packet also serves as a reference when questions and problems arise after discharge. The text includes information about medications, including their purpose, side effects, and proper method of administration. An explanation of blood tests and their normal values is included. This information helps recipients understand the level of their renal function as well as the clinical significance when abnormal values arise. The common signs and symptoms of rejection are also described along with instructions for contacting the transplant team. A list of telephone numbers for the physician, clinical nurse specialist, social worker, psychologist, and other members of the transplant team is helpful. Guidelines regarding activity and dietary restrictions are included as well.

Recipients' participation in the teaching program is essential to a successful posttransplant course. During the hospital stay, the need for consistency and proper timing and administration of medications is stressed by the nursing staff. Self-administration of medications, under the supervision of a primary nurse, expedites pill recognition and ease in drawing up Cy A. A card that includes all medications, prescribed dosage, and time of administration may be given at the time of discharge to help recipients and practitioners keep track of frequently changing drug regimens in the early posttransplant period.

TABLE 4.4 Postoperative Complications of Kidney Transplantation

1. VASCULAR SYSTEM: A. RENAL ARTERY THROMBOSIS

Etiology	Almost always due to surgical/technical error such as anastomoses of thin-walled vessel to thick-walled vessel, anastomoses of multiple vessels with disparity in size or intimal damage during harvesting procedure
Onset	Immediately postoperative to 1–2 days postoperative
Frequency	Rare
Signs and symptoms	Intraoperatively, nonpinking of kidney; Postoperatively, sudden cessation of urine output
Diagnosis	Catheterizing the bladder—fluid challenge and diuretics; renal scan or arteriography
Treatment	Surgical reexploration with thrombectomy and anastomoses correction or nephrectomy; usually ischemia time to renal parenchyma too long before surgical reexploration

B. RENAL ARTERY STENOSIS[a]

Etiology	Anastomotic surgical technique: Suture line stenosis is probably due to reaction with suture materials; use of synthetic versus silk suture material has decreased the incidence; technical surgical errors such as kinking secondary to poor positioning of the kidney or poor intimal anastomosing can also cause stenosis Generalized renal artery vessel stenosis probably secondary to immunologically mediated mechanisms (frequently associated with rejection) Inherent atherosclerotic plaque formation—incidence may increase in frequency as more diabetics and elderly receive transplants
Onset	Variable—months to years posttransplant
Frequency	0.6 to 25% occurrence
Signs and symptoms	Denovo hypertension, severe hypertension refractory to drug therapy; denovo bruit or change in previously present bruit, diminished renal function (i.e., increasing creatinine and BUN with decreasing creatinine clearance and increasing renin levels)
Diagnosis	Intraarterial DSA, selective renin elevations, and angiography stenosis > 50% are considered hemodynamically significant
Treatment	Percutaneous transluminal angioplasty (PTA), surgical reentry through transplant incision and employing allograft vessel bypass or reanastomosing the vessels

(continued)

TABLE 4.4   (continued)

C. RENAL ARTERY RUPTURE/HEMORRHAGE[b]

Etiology	Bleeding from arterial anastomoses; perinephric abscesses, mycotic (infected) aneurysms from hematoma infections at the suture line; nonanastomotic bleeding from untied or torn hilar vessels
Onset	Intraoperatively or postoperatively
Frequency	Rare
Signs and symptoms	Drop in hematocrit, vascular collapse, intense graftsite pain, back pain radiating to flank or rectum; anuria, hematuria; rise in temperature, elevated white blood count.
Diagnosis	Accurate and frequent monitoring of vital signs, complete blood count, urine output postoperatively; appropriate culturing; arteriogram to diagnose anastomotic aneurysm; sonography to detect mycotic aneurysm
Treatment	Appropriate intraoperative hemostasis; prompt return to operating room for reexploration to correct bleeding; transfusing as appropriate; nephrectomy in cases of mycotic aneurysm.

D. RENAL VEIN THROMBOSIS

Etiology	Intimal injury during organ retrieval; vessel kinking; extension of thrombus from the iliac-venous system; pressure from lymphoma, uroma, or hematoma; severe rejection; Questionable role of Cy A
Onset	Days to years posttransplantation
Frequency	1 to 4% (rare)
Signs and symptoms	Oliguria, anuria, kidney function, graft swelling, proteinuria, hematuria, ipsilateral leg swelling
Diagnosis	Venography; anuria post–fluid bolus and diuretics
Treatment	Thrombectomy; nephrectomy

2. UROLOGIC SYSTEM: A. KIDNEY RUPTURE

Etiology	Kidney biopsy, ischemic damage at time of harvest or implantation, accelerated acute rejection
Onset	Within first 2 weeks after surgery
Frequency	Rare
Signs and symptoms	Pain, swelling over graft, oliguria, massive hematuria, vascular collapse
Diagnosis	Sonography and biopsy if time permits
Treatment	Early diagnosis and treatment of rejection episodes; surgical repair of rupture or nephrectomy.

B. URETERAL NECROSIS, STENOSIS, OBSTRUCTION

Etiology	Major cause of ureteral necrosis postoperatively is damage to artery supplying blood to the implanted ureter; ureteral stenosis can be secondary to surgical-technical error and obstructive secondary to blood clots or edema.

(continued)

TABLE 4.4 (continued)

Onset	Days for necrosis and resultant urine leak; days to months to years for stenosis
Frequency	2%
Signs and symptoms	*Necrosis:* Fever, allograft tenderness, fluid collection around graft, wound drainage, decreased urine output, edema of leg on side of transplant, decreased graft function
	Stenosis: Usually no overt symptoms but decreased renal function and hydronephrosis on ultrasound
Diagnosis	Sonography with aspiration of fluid, CT scan, renal scan, percutaneous antegrade pyelography
Treatment	Placement of percutaneous nephrostomy tube with surgical repair; percutaneous dilation or surgical intervention for stricture

C. BLADDER LEAKAGE

Etiology	Surgical technical error, inadequate bladder decompression postoperatively
Onset	Hours to days postoperatively
Signs and symptoms	Suprapubic pain or mass
Diagnosis	Ultrasonography, surgical exploration
Treatment	Surgical repair

3. WOUND INFECTION

Etiology	Microorganism contamination during surgery, poor intraoperative hemostasis combined with uremia, poor nutritional status and immunosuppressives; other variables such as age, diabetes and obesity increase the likelihood of occurrence
Frequency	1 to 10%
Onset	Within a few days postoperatively
Signs and symptoms	Wound drainage, poor closure, fluctuance around wound, fever, pain in incisional area
Diagnosis	Direct visualization of drainage, culturing, sonography with aspiration
Treatment	Evacuation of pus or hematoma; Drainage of lymphocele; packing of wound with wet-to-dry normal saline or quarter-strength Dakins solution when appropriate; antibiotics as indicated

4. PERIRENAL AREA FLUID COLLECTION

Etiology	Technical error during surgery; lymphatic vessels must be carefully ligated at the time of operation; otherwise lymphatic spillage will not be absorbed and will accumulate

(continued)

TABLE 4.4   (continued)

Onset	Days posttransplant
Frequency	2% to 18%
Signs and symptoms	Diminished renal function, edema of leg on side of transplant. Sensation of fullness in rea of fluid accumulation. Urinary frequency or constipation due to compression on bladder and rectosigmoid colon.
Diagnosis	Sonography
Treatment	Internal or external drainage

5. GASTROINTESTINAL SYSTEM
A. PANCREATITIS

Etiology	Post-CMV infection or other viral infection; questionable etiologic role of cyclosporine and prednisone.
Onset	Months to years posttransplant
Frequency	Rare
Signs and symptoms	Increased serum amylase, abdominal and back pain
Diagnosis	Ultrasonography and CT scans to detect commonly occurring sequelae of pancreatic pseudocysts and abscess. Serum monitoring of amylase levels.
Treatment	Adequate pain management; parenteral nutrition with vigorous fluid replacement, especially in the first 48 hrs; NG tube placement; reduction in steroid dosage; discontinuance of Aza and cyclosporine as warranted; necessity for nephrectomy is not uncommon.

B. DIVERTICULAR-COLONIC PERFORATION

Etiology	Renal failure with associated constipation paired with poor healing and poor tissue integrity. There may be a correlation with high doses of steroids. Preexisting diverticulitis, CMV infections
Onset	Any time posttransplantation
Frequency	Very rare, but mortality is high
Signs and symptoms	Constipation, pain, no bowel movements
Diagnosis	X-rays with water-soluable contrast media preceded by abdominal CT scan.
Treatment	Surgical correction with appropriate antibiotic coverage; reduction in immunosuppression

[a]The use of ace inhibitors with this condition is associated with graft failure secondary to diminished kidney perfusion.
[b]Potential cadaver donors who are septic must not be accepted as candidates as mycotic aneurysms are the likely sequelae. Posttransplant positive cultures from a cadaver donor necessitate immediate antibiotic prophylaxis for the recipient of such a kidney.
[c]Cecal rupture can occur posttransplant and secondary to the cecum's being cut or stapled during the operative procedure.
Source: Cerilli, 1988; Morris, 1988; Toledo-Pereyra, 1988.

Nurses further involve patients in their care by having them measure their own temperature and weight, measure and record their intake and output, and document their laboratory values on a daily basis.

At the time of discharge, recipients and/or their families must demonstrate correct administration of prescribed medications, recognize symptoms requiring intervention, and be aware of any restrictions in activity. A formal test, given verbally or in written form prior to discharge, measures recipients' knowledge of past transplant care.

Discharge Follow-up

Posttransplant follow-up care includes detection and treatment of rejection, evaluation and adjustment of immunosuppression, screening for and treatment of infection, and stabilization of hypertension, diabetes, and other medical problems. Another essential component of posttransplant care is evaluating recipients' understanding of and ability to adhere to prescribed treatment modalities. The clinic nurse allots time at each visit to review laboratory results, discuss medications, and address recipients' questions and concerns.

Most transplant programs have protocols outlining the frequency of clinic follow-up. Most centers monitor recipients on a twice-a-week schedule initially, when the majority of problems are likely to occur. The frequency of visits is then gradually reduced.

Teaching and Counseling

Recipients must realize that experiencing rejection is not synonymous with graft loss. Frequent clinic follow-up at a center with experience in managing transplant recipients favors early detection and treatment of rejection episodes. With overall first-year graft survival at 90%, recipients can be realistically assured that graft loss and an episode of rejection are not synonymous. The gray cloud of possible graft loss follows every recipient, whether 1 month or many years posttransplant. Sometimes this emotional burden becomes debilitating, and professional counseling is necessary. Posttransplant support groups may aid recipients in coping with this and other concerns.

There appears to be a correlation between HLA matching and recipient as well as graft survival, with the lowest mortality rates in HLA identical transplants and the highest in cadaver recipients. This effect seems to disappear after 10 years of successful renal function (Opelz, Mickey, & Terasaki, 1977). How well individual recipients fare is unpredictable. Underlying disease processes, such as diabetes, affect survival rates, as does compliance with medical management. Recipients can honestly be told that, although life expectancy is difficult to predict, many recipients are now more than 20 years beyond successful renal transplant and doing very well.

NURSING CARE PLAN FOR KIDNEY TRANSPLANT RECIPIENT

Nursing diagnoses	Nursing assessment	Nursing interventions
RESPIRATORY: Decreased lung expansion and airway clearance related to Anesthesia Fluid administration Decreased mobility Incisional pain	Diminished and/or adventitious lung sounds Increased respiratory rate Decreased respiratory depth Elevated temperature Inability of patient to expectorate secretions Large quantity of respiratory secretions Tenacious green or yellow sputum Subjective complaint of "pain," and/or "shortness of breath"	1. Measure respiratory rate and temperature every one hr for 24 hr, then every 2 hr for 48 hr, then every 4 hr. 2. Auscultate lung sounds every 4 hr and prn. 3. Elevate head of bed. 4. Turn every 2 hr for 24 hr, then out of bed to chair and ambulate tid. 5. Incentive spirometry every 1 hr. 6. Cough every 1 hr. 7. Assess and document character and amount of respiratory secretions. 8. Medicate with analgesia as ordered prn.

Nursing goal:
Patient will have improved lung expansion and airway clearance as measured by
    Clear lung sounds
    Normal temperature
    Normal respiratory rate and depth
    Clear respiratory secretions

                *   *   *   *

Nursing diagnoses	Nursing assessment	Nursing interventions
FLUID BALANCE: Fluid volume excess related to: Intraoperative fluid administration Rejection Acute tubular necrosis (ATN)	Edema Jugular venous distention (JVD) Elevated CVP Increased blood pressure Increased heart rate Increased respiratory rate Decreased urine output Adventitious lung sounds Pink, frothy sputum Subjective complaint of "fullness," "puffiness," and/or "shortness of breath"	1. Maintain strict intake and output. 2. Measure daily weight. 3. Measure blood pressure, heart rate, respiratory rate, and urine output every 1 hr for 24 hr, then every 2 hr for 48 hr, then every 4 hr. 4. Auscultate lung sounds every 4 hr and prn. 5. Measure CVP every 4 hr and prn. 6. Assess presence and degree of edema and jugular venous distension (JVD).

(continued)

NURSING CARE PLAN FOR KIDNEY TRANSPLANT RECIPIENT (continued)

Nursing diagnoses	Nursing assessment	Nursing interventions
		7. Administer and record response to diuretics if ordered by physician.
		8. Elevate head of bed.

Nursing goal:
Patient will return to normovolemic status as measured by
  Postoperative weight equivalent to preoperative weight
  Intake equivalent to output
  Normal heart rate, blood pressure, and respiratory rate
  Clear lung sounds
  Subjective indication of decreased fluid volume
  Absence of edema

*   *   *   *

PAIN:

Nursing diagnoses	Nursing assessment	Nursing interventions
Patient with complaint of pain related to:	Subjective complaint of "pain" over surgical incision site	1. Administer analgesia/antispasmodics as ordered by physician.
Surgical incision	Subjective complaint of "pain" around Foley catheter insertion site	2. Evaluate and document effectiveness of analgesia/antispasmodic.
Bladder spasms	Facial grimacing	3. Provide position of comfort.
	Guarding	4. Assist patient with abdominal splinting.

Nursing goal:
Patient will experience relief of pain as measured by subjective indication of pain
  relief.

*   *   *   *

ELIMINATION:

Nursing diagnoses	Nursing assessment	Nursing interventions
Decreased urinary elimination related to	Fluid intake greater than urinary output	Maintain patency of Foley catheter.
Obstruction of Foley catheter	Sudden cessation of urinary output	Measure and record urine output every 1 hr for 24 hr, then every 2 hr for 48 hr, then every 4 hr.
Ureteral obstruction	Hematuria	
Bladder leak	Palpable bladder distention, subjective complaint of "bladder fullness"	Irrigate Foley catheter to remove clots obstructing urinary flow prn.

(continued)

NURSING CARE PLAN FOR KIDNEY TRANSPLANT RECIPIENT (continued)

Nursing diagnoses	Nursing assessment	Nursing interventions

Nursing goal:
Patient will eliminate urine without difficulty as measured by
    Patent Foley catheter
    Clear urine (absence of clots)
    Absence of bladder distention

*   *   *   *

IMMUNOSUPPRESSION:

Nursing diagnoses	Nursing assessment	Nursing interventions

Infection related to:
   Immunosuppression
   Hospitalization
   Surgery
   ESRD
   IV lines
   Foley catheter
   Diabetes mellitus
	Redness, swelling, or
	   drainage from IV
	   insertion sites
	Cloudy or foul
	   smelling urine
	Elevated temperature
	Tenacious green
	   or yellow sputum
	   production
	Oral cavity with
	   thrush or lesions
	Redness, swelling, or
	   drainage from
	   surgical incision site
	Subjective complaint of
	   "pain" or "burning"
	   upon urination
		1. Measure temperature
		   every 1 hr for 24 hrs,
		   then every 2 hrs for 48 hrs,
		   then every 4 hrs.
		2. Assess and document
		   appearance of IV and
		   surgical incision sites.
		3. Assess and document char-
		   acter of urine and sputum.
		4. Foley catheter care
		   with warm soap and
		   water bid
		5. IV tubing change every
		   72 hrs
		6. Prepare all central line ports
		   with Betadine prior to
		   adding IV medication
		7. Cultures as indicated

Nursing goal:
Patient will remain free of infection as measured by
    Normal temperature
    Clear urine
    Clear respiratory secretions
    IV and surgical incisions remain dry and clear

*   *   *   *

EDUCATION:

Nursing diagnoses	Nursing assessment	Nursing interventions

Lack of knowledge
regarding kidney
transplant related to
   Immunosuppression
   Nutritional changes
   Activity limitations
	Age and educational
	   level
	Physical deficit,
	   i.e., paraplegia
	Sensory deficit,
	   i.e., blindness
		1. Instruct and involve patient in
		   daily weight, temperature,
		   and intake and output
		   measurements.
		2. Observe patient preparation
		   and administration of
		   medication.

(continued)

NURSING CARE PLAN FOR KIDNEY TRANSPLANT RECIPIENT (continued)

Nursing diagnoses	Nursing assessment	Nursing interventions
Signs and symptoms of rejection	Presence of support system Motivation toward learning and self-care Language barrier Cultural and religious background	3. Instruct patient on the signs and symptoms of rejection. 4. Instruct patient on the purpose and side effects of his/her medications. 5. Instruct patient on postrenal transplant nutrition, activity, infection, and sexuality. 6. Involve support persons in the teaching process. 7. Positively reinforce patient/ family learning efforts.

Nursing goal:
Patient and support system will demonstrate increased knowledge of kidney transplant as measured by
   Observation of self-care during hospitalization
   Patient's ability to state signs of rejection accurately

*   *   *   *

PSYCHOSOCIAL:

Anxiety related to:
  Rejection
  Hospitalization
  Financial concerns
  Family issues
  Life-style changes
	Subjective statement of "anxiety," "fear," "depression," "sadness"
	Tearful
	Withdrawn
	Decreased appetite
	Decreased involvement in learning activities
		1. Encourage verbalization of feelings.
		2. Provide emotional support.
		3. Obtain social service and/or chaplain referral.

Nursing goal:
Patient will experience decreased anxiety as measured by subjective indication of resolved anxiety.

Nursing Care Plan written by Kimberly Stephens, RN, MSN.

Given an uncomplicated posttransplant course, recipients are usually instructed that they may resume sexual relations at 3 weeks posttransplant. The degree and timing of return of normal sexual function is unpredictable. Therefore, practitioners must allow recipients an opportunity to voice concerns and problems. Referrals to specialists in urology, gynecology, obstetrics, or family planning should be obtained as problems arise.

Questions regarding life expectancy must also be addressed. Mortality rates following renal transplant have significantly improved over the last decade primarily because of reduction of aggressive use of steroids and more selective immunosuppression since earlier periods. The highest mortality rates occur within the first year posttransplant. Survival rates decline more slowly thereafter (Flye, 1989). The major causes of death are cardiovascular disease and sepsis.

ACKNOWLEDGEMENTS

Grateful acknowledgment to Patricia Barber, BSN, FNP, Clinical transplant coordinator at the University of Illinois Medical Center, for her contributions in editing, illustrating, and providing her significant expertise in completing this chapter.

Further appreciation for contributions by Kimberly Stephens, RN, MSN. Ms. Stephens has extensive experience in the area of kidney transplantation, as a staff nurse on the kidney transplant unit at the University of California, San Francisco, and as a kidney transplant clinical nurse specialist at Stanford University Medical Center.

Special thanks to Oscar Salvatierra, MD, Professor of Surgery and Urology, Chief of Transplant Service, University of California, San Francisco, for reviewing the surgical part of this chapter.

REFERENCES

Andrew, O. T. (1980). Tuberculosis in patients with end-stage renal disease. *American Journal of Medicine, 68*(1), 59–65.

Annas, G. (1985). The prostitute, the playboy, and the poet: Rationing schemes for organ transplantation *American Journal of Public Health, 75*(2), 187–189.

Balfour, H., Chace, B., Stapleton, J., Simmons, R., & Fryd, D. (1989). A randomized placebo-controlled trial of oral acyclovir for the prevention of CMV disease in recipients of renal allografts. *New England Journal of Medicine, 320*(21), 1381–1387.

Calne, R.Y. (1985). Organ transplantation: From laboratory to clinic. *British Medical Journal, 291 (6511)*, 1751-1754.

Cerilli, J. G. (Ed.). (1988). *Organ transplantation and replacement.* Philadelphia: J. B. Lippincott.

Cockburn, I., Gotz, E., Gülich, A., & Krupp, P. (1988). Nephrotoxicity pathogenic mechanisms: Hypertension and renovascular disease. *Transplant Proceedings, 20*(Suppl. 3), 519–529.

Flye, M. W. (Ed.). (1989). *Infectious complications in renal transplant patients.* Philadelphia: W. B. Saunders.

Kahan, B. D. (1986). Cyclosporine nephrotoxicity: Pathogenesis, prophylaxis, therapy and prognosis. *American Journal of Kidney Disease, 8*(5), 323–331.

Knochel, J. P., & Seldin, D. W. (1981). The pathophysiology of renal disease. In B.M. Brenner & F.L. Rector (Eds.), *The kidney* (2nd ed.). Philadelphia: W. B. Saunders.

Levy, A. S., Hou, S., & Bush, H. L. (1986). Kidney transplantation from unrelated living donors. *New England Journal of Medicine, 314,* 914–916.

Maddeux, M. S. (1989). The pharmacology and complications of immunosuppressive therapy. *Problems of General Surgery, 6*(2), 368–387.

Mathew, T. (1988). Recurrence of disease following renal transplantation. *American Journal of Kidney Disease, 12*(2), 85–96.

Migliori, R., & Simmons, R. L. (1988). Infection prophylaxis after organ transplantation. *Transplantation Proceedings, 20*(3), 395–399.

Morris, P. J. (Ed.). (1988). *Kidney transplantation principles and practice* (3rd ed.). Philadelphia: W. B. Saunders.

Opelz, G., Graver, B., Micker, M. R., & Terasaki, P. (1981). Lymphocytotoxic antibody responses to transfusions in potential kidney transplant recipients. *Transplantation, 32,* 177–183

Opelz, G., Mickey, M. R., & Terasaki, P. I. (1977). Calculations on long-term graft and patient survival in human kidney transplantation. *Transplantation Proceedings, 9*(1), 27–30.

Seale, L., Jones, C., Kathpalia, S., Jackson, G., Mozes, M., Maddeux, M., & Packham, P. (1985). Prevention of herpes virus infections in renal allograft recipients by low-dose oral acyclovir. *Journal of the American Medical Association, 254*(24), 3435–3438.

Snydman, D., Werner, B. G., Heinze-Lacey, B., Tilney, N. L., Berardi, V., Kirkman, R., Milford, E., Cho, S., Bush, H., Levey, R., Harmon, W., Logerfo, F., Idelson, B., Schröter, G., Levin, M., McIver, J., Leszczynski, J., & Grady, G. (1988). A further analysis of primary CMV disease prevention in renal transplant recipients with a CMV immune globulin: Interim comparison of a randomized and an open-label trial *Transplantation Proceedings, 20*(Suppl. 8), 24–30.

Sollinger, H. W., Burlingham, W. J., Spaeks, E. M., Glass, N. R., & Belzer, F. O. (1984). Donor specific transfusions in unrelated and related HLA-mismatched donor-recipient combinations. *Transplantation, 38*(6), 612–615.

Spital, A. (1988). Living kidney donation: When is it justified? *Nephrology Letter, 5*(1), 1–15.

Starzl, T. E. (1987). Living donors. *Transplantation Proceedings, 19*(1), 174–176.

Steinmuller, D.R. (1983). Evaluation and selection of candidates for renal transplantation. *The Urologic Clinics of North America, 10* (2), 217–229

Toledo-Pereyra, L. H. (1988). *Kidney transplantation.* Philadelphia: F. A. Davis.

Tzakis, A.G. Cooper, M.H. Dummer, J.S., Ragni, M., Ward, J.W., & Starz L.T.E. (1989, December) Transplantation in HIV+ patients. Paper presented at the annual meeting of the American Society of Tranplant Surgeons, Chicago.

Weiland, D., Sutherland, D. E. R., Chavers, B., Simmons, R. L., Ascher, N. L., & Najarian, J. S. (1984). Information on 628 living-related kidney donors at a single institution with long term followup in 472 cases. *Transplantation Proceedings, 16*(1), 5–7.

CHAPTER 5

HEART AND HEART-LUNG TRANSPLANTATION

Barbara A. Williams
Doris M. Sandiford-Guttenbeil

HISTORY OF HEART TRANSPLANTATION

The first human heart transplantation was performed in 1967 by Christiaan Barnard in Cape Town, South Africa (Shinn, 1980). This event encouraged medical teams at many medical centers worldwide to pursue heart transplantation. Poor survival statistics for the first year after transplantation (22%), in addition to the complexities of immunosuppression, contributed to a decline in performing this procedure (Funk, 1986; Shinn, 1985).

In January 1968, at Stanford University Medical Center (SUMC), Dr. Norman E. Shumway and his team accomplished the first adult heart transplant in the United States. SUMC was one of the few centers that continued with their program despite low survival numbers (Grady, 1985).

SURVIVAL STATISTICS

A report from the International Society for Heart Transplantation Registry indicates that since 1987 more than 12,631 heart transplants were performed worldwide. As of 1989, 1,673 of them were performed in 148 centers in the United States. The first-year survival is approximately 81%, and the 5-year survival for all recipients is approximately 72% (Kriett & Kaye, 1990). The United Network of Organ Sharing (UNOS) reveals that as of May 1990 there were 1,626 people waiting for heart transplants (American Council on Transplantation, 1990).

RECENT ADVANCES IN TRANSPLANTATION

Heart Transplantation

Recent advances in transplantation have occurred with the development of new therapies for improved allograft survival. The latest developments are in new immunosuppressive drugs, improved detection and monitoring of rejection, and changes in isolation techniques.

The introduction of a new immunosuppressant, cyclosporine A (Cy A), in 1980 has had major impact. This drug, which specifically suppresses T cells, was the key to spurring renewed global interest in performing heart transplantation. It became possible for transplantation to be performed on a wider range of patients, most notably in the pediatric and neonate population. One of the benefits of Cy A is the ability to prescribe lower doses of supplementary immunosuppression with corticosteroids. Successful treatment of rejection and infection have added to improved survival rates (Oyer et al., 1983). Overall, Cy A has contributed to increased survival, a reduced incidence of severe acute rejection, and decreased rates of infection. Another important benefit of Cy A is that it has decreased the hospital length of stay and overall cost.

Heart–Lung Transplantation

Prior to the introduction of Cy A, heart–lung transplantation in humans had been unsuccessful. In 1968, Cooley et al. performed the first heart–lung transplantation in a human (Lekander, 1988) followed by Lillehei in 1970 and Barnard in 1971 (Reitz, 1982). All recipients succumbed shortly after surgery due to respiratory insufficiency, pneumonia & bronchial disruption (Lekander, 1988).

After the introduction of Cy A a renewed interest in heart–lung transplantation occured. Heart-lung transplantation was successfully accomplished in a woman at SUMC in 1981. Since 1981, more than 785 heart–lung transplantations have been accomplished worldwide, with a 1-year survival of about 60% and a 2-year rate of about 52% (Kriett & Kaye, 1990). UNOS reported that a total of 70 heart–lung transplants were performed in 1989 in 79 centers in the United States, a 43% increase over the reported 43 in 1987 (American Council on Transplantation, 1989).

Pioneering efforts at SUMC under the direction of Dr. Norman E. Shumway in 1981 set the foundation for further exploration in the field of heart–lung transplantation. Successful primate survival, development of surgical techniques, administration of Cy A, and improvement in immunological monitoring have added to the success in this dynamic field (Reitz, Pennock, & Shumway, 1981).

Physicians have been able to decrease the dose of corticosteroids previously administered for primary immunosuppression. Therefore, healing proceeds normally at the bronchial anastomotic site, and there is reduced risk of graft infection (Covner & Shinn, 1983; Reitz, Stinson, Oyer, Jamieson, & Shumway, 1982).

Advances in Noninvasive Monitoring Tools for Rejection

Since the introduction of Cy A, other challenges have become the focus of heart and heart–lung transplantation. Further research is needed in detecting and monitoring cardiac and pulmonary allograft rejection. For example, right ventricular endomyocardial biopsy (EMB) is the standard, most reliable procedure for the diagnosis of acute cardiac rejection. Studies in the United States and abroad are being conducted to find reliable noninvasive monitoring tools to decrease the frequency of EMBs. Cytoimmunological monitoring (CIM) and echocardiograms are among the most promising noninvasive methods, in conjunction with EMB, to detect cardiac rejection (Dawkins et al., 1984; Hammer et al., 1984; Haverich et al., 1987).

Nurses have always participated in change based upon the development of new therapies. This chapter addresses how change influences nursing care. Additional discussion focuses on current nursing care from acceptance into the transplant program through discharge.

PREOPERATIVE NURSING ASSESSMENT AND CARE

Patients who meet the criteria for heart and heart–lung transplantation have end-stage disease and are unresponsive to further conventional medical or surgical treatments. Criteria for acceptance into the transplant program have changed over the years.

The current medical criteria for cardiac transplantation are as follows:

- End-stage cardiac disease, not correctable by medical or surgical therapy.
- New York Heart Association functional class III–IV.
- Good health except for end-stage cardiac disease.
- Emotional stability with a strong will to live.
- Willingness to comply with a complex medical regimen for the rest of his/her life.
- Age up to 60 years with occasional exceptions.

Contraindications to cardiac transplantation include:

- Severe pulmonary hypertension (greater than 6–8 Wood units).
- Irreversible hepatic or renal dysfunction.
- Active systemic infection.
- Unresolved pulmonary infarction.
- Severe peripheral or cerebrovascular disease.
- Diabetes mellitus requiring insulin (this is being evaluated at various medical centers).
- Active peptic ulcer disease.
- Obesity (this is evaluated on an individual basis).

- History of substance abuse or mental illness (this is evaluated on an individual basis).

The current medical criteria for heart–lung transplantation are:

- End-stage cardiopulmonary disease not correctable by medical or surgical therapy.
- Good health, except for end-stage cardiopulmonary disease.
- Age under 45 years (greater survival rate in younger candidates).
- Stable psychosocial status.

The contraindications to heart–lung transplantation are:

- Systemic disease, i.e., peripheral vascular disease, diabetes mellitus, autoimmune illness.
- Active systemic infection.
- Moderate to severe renal or hepatic dysfunction.
- Obesity (this is evaluated on an individual basis).
- History of substance abuse or mental illness (this is evaluated on an individual basis).

In addition patients must be ABO compatible with the donor heart and lung. If necessary, a direct cross-match of the recipients' serum with cells from the specific donor will be done.

Most candidates for heart transplantation have been diagnosed with dilated cardiomyopathy (DCM) or end-stage coronary artery disease (Jamieson et al., 1984). The cause of DCM is often unknown but alcohol abuse, a history of viral infection and pregnancy have been associated with it (Mersch, 1985).

Briefly, DCM is a primary heart muscle disease characterized by enlargement of the cardiac chambers with normal ventricular wall thickness and poor systolic function (O'Connell & Gunnar, 1982). Medical treatment is palliative and includes the use of a low-salt diet, inotropes, diuretics, preload and afterload reducing agents, and anticoagulants (O'Connell & Gunnar, 1982). The disease progresses from fatigue, weakness, and dyspnea to congestive heart failure; and the prognosis is poor (Mersch, 1985). Often, 50% of patients die within 2 years of diagnosis. Cardiac transplantation offers a therapeutic alternative for patients with DCM.

Most candidates with end-stage coronary artery disease have already undergone one or more revascularization operations. However, they too have very poor systolic function, in spite of previous surgery, because of the damage to the heart from one or more myocardial infarctions.

The heart–lung candidate's underlying disease usually is some form of pulmonary hypertension; for example primary or secondary pulmonary hypertension in conjunction with congenital heart defects such as Eisenmenger's syndrome. In addition, patients diagnosed with cystic fibrosis have recently undergone successful transplantation.

Evaluation of Candidates

Acceptance into a transplant program requires extensive and thorough testing with a multidisciplinary approach. The team members participating in candidate evaluation include a cardiologist, a transplant surgeon, transplant nurses, and social workers. The evaluation includes a complete medical, family, financial, and psychological history. The candidates also undergo thorough physical assessment/testing to determine if they meet the criteria for transplantation and to rule out potential contraindications to heart or heart–lung transplantation. During the preliminary evaluation, nurses begin teaching the candidate about the procedures. Nursing responsibilities include monitoring vital signs, assessing physical condition, and scheduling and compiling laboratory studies, electrocardiogram, chest x-ray, blood typing and cross-matching, tissue typing, determination of reactivity to antigens (HLA antibody screen), and cultures from blood, urine, and sputum. These important tests provide baseline data on potential transplant candidates.

After acceptance into the program, if the candidates do not live in the area, they must move to a location near the transplant center. They are given a radio pager so that they may be contacted when a donor becomes available. Transplantation candidates who are hemodynamically unstable requiring continuous monitoring and multiple therapies are taken care of in the intensive care unit (ICU). Nursing care centered around the critically ill and unstable potential recipient is specifically addressed in Chapter 11, on mechanical assist devices for the failing heart.

Preparations for Transplantation

When a candidate matches a donor, the immediate preoperative preparation begins. The surgical ICU is notified that a heart or heart–lung transplant is in progress. The transplant room is cleared of all supplies and cleaned with a bactericidal agent by the housekeeping staff. The room is restocked with sterile disposable supplies when possible. Nondisposable supplies are cleaned with a bactericidal agent or gas-autoclaved (Lough & Williams, 1985). A nurse is assigned to set up the isolation room and to provide immediate preoperative teaching, continuing the teaching process. The immediate preoperative teaching of the candidate and family focuses on the following:

- Tour of ICU (if time permits).
- Review of heart or heart–lung transplant surgery and postoperative care (including tubes that will be present immediately after surgery).
- Routine surgery preparations: consents, shave, scrub, preoperative medications.
- Review of protective isolation, infection, immunosuppression, and rejection
- First dose of immunosuppressants, (Lough & Williams, 1985).

SURGICAL PROCEDURE

The duration of surgery for heart or heart–lung transplantation is usually 4 to 6 hours. The most common intraoperative complication is hemorrhage. Heart and heart–lung candidates are more prone to coagulation deficiencies because of long-standing right heart failure and hepatic congestion. If recipients have had previous pericardiotomy, adhesions are frequently present and require careful dissection during surgery. The adhesions represent scarring and increase the risk of hemorrhage. Postpump syndrome after a long surgery can also potentiate postoperative coagulopathy.

Briefly, heart transplant surgery is performed via a median sternotomy incision. After induction of anesthesia, the recipient's body temperature is cooled to below 34°C and cardiopulmonary bypass (CPB) is begun. Hypothermia is necessary to reduce the body's metabolic needs during surgery. The recipient's heart is removed, leaving only the posterior walls of the atria and portions of the aorta and pulmonary artery in place. Prior to this, the donor heart has been prepared for suturing, beginning with the left atrium, right atrium, pulmonary artery, and finally the aorta. Protection of the donor sinoatrial (SA) node, located in the right atrium, is important to maintain normal pacemaking action.

In cardiopulmonary transplant surgery, the heart and lungs have been excised from the donor's chest cavity as a combined unit. The three major sites of anastomosis are the trachea just above the carina, the right atrium, and the aorta. The most important aspects of the recipient's operation are to remove the heart and lungs without injury to the phrenic, vagus, or recurrent laryngeal nerves. Figures 5.1 and 5.2 show the sites of anastomoses in heart and heart–lung transplantation.

At the end of surgery, the heart is defibrillated, the lungs are reinflated, and each is tested for optimum function. Two temporary atrial or ventricular pacing wires are placed in case of bradycardia. The recipient is slowly removed from CPB and given methylprednisolone 500 mg intravenously. Mediastinal chest tubes are inserted, and the chest is closed. During surgery, the heart has been traumatized by ischemia and hypothermia, which contribute to a decrease in cardiac output. In addition, the heart is *denervated* (without autonomic nervous system control). The nurse therefore administers inotropic drugs (dopamine and dobutamine) and vasodilators (sodium nitroprusside, trimethaphan, esmolol) as needed. Low-dose dopamine may also be started to maintain renal perfusion. Isoproterenol is often necessary for the first few postoperative days. It is regulated to maintain a heart rate between 100 and 120 beats per minute in the denervated heart to further enhance cardiac output. Sodium nitroprusside is prescribed to decrease systemic vascular resistance and facilitate rewarming. The ICU nurse is notified of the recipient's impending transfer from the operating room and the anesthesiologist informs the nurse of lines and continuous intravenous medications that the recipient requires.

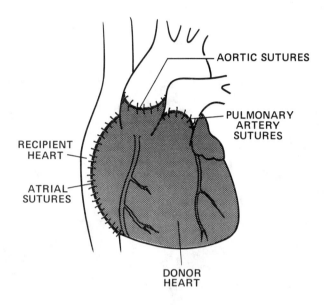

FIGURE 5.1 Cardiac transplantation suture lines: atrial, pulmonary artery, aortic anastomoses. Drawing by Bayard Colyear, medical illustrator.

Intravenous arterial lines and tubes required for heart and heart–lung transplantation are the same as for routine cardiac surgery.

They include the following:

- Endotracheal tube.
- Central venous pressure (CVP) line, left internal jugular vein site preferred and double- or triple lumen catheter suggested.
- Peripheral intravenous line (1 or 2).
- Arterial pressure line.
- Nasogastric tube.
- Chest tubes (2 or 4).
- Indwelling catheter (Foley).
- Atrial or ventricular pacing wires (2).

POSTOPERATIVE NURSING CARE

The immediate postoperative care of the heart and heart–lung transplant recipient is similar to care for other cardiosurgical patients (Sandiford, 1976). The nurse carefully assesses the patient and watches for signs of:

- Hemorrhage.
- Cardiac tamponade.
- Low cardiac output.

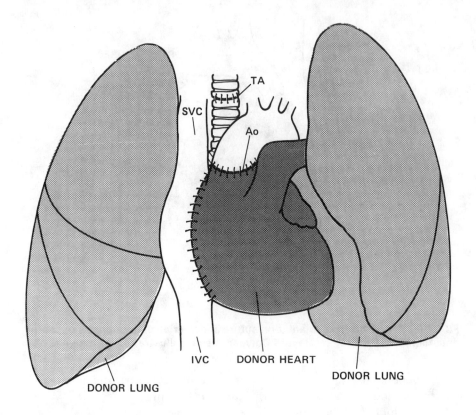

FIGURE 5.2 Cardiopulmonary transplantation suture lines: atrial, aortic, and tracheal anastomoses. TA=tracheal anastomosis; AO=aorta; SVC=superior vena cava; IVC=inferior vena cava. Drawing by Bayard Colyear, medical illustrator.

- Hypovolemia.
- Coagulopathy.
- Rewarming problems.
- Dysrhythmias.
- Renal dysfunction.
- Hypertension.
- Imbalance of fluid, electrolytes, and acid/base.
- Adverse neurological changes.

Immediate Postoperative Complications of Heart Transplantation

The following complications may occur more commonly after heart transplantation: hemorrhage, dysrrhythmias, renal dysfunction, hypertension.

Hemorrhage

The nurse monitors the recipient for signs and symptoms of mediastinal hemorrhage and possible cardiac tamponade. Tamponade is indicated by a rise in CVP and fall in arterial pressure, decreased peripheral perfusion, decreased chest tube output, muffled heart sounds, and pulsus paradoxus. Factors that potentiate postoperative bleeding include leakage from the anastomotic sites and preexisting coagulopathy. Preoperative coagulopathy is caused by liver congestion due to right-sided heart failure. The mechanical action of CPB results in destruction of thrombocytes and may also contribute to bleeding. The nurse draws coagulation studies and replaces chest tube drainage with blood products as ordered. Treatment of coagulopathy may include the administration of fresh frozen plasma, platelets, protamine, or aquamephyton. If the coagulation report is normal and bleeding persists, the recipient returns to the operating room for exploration and hemostasis.

Dysrhythmias

Manipulation of the donor heart during surgery, as well as anesthesia and edema of the suture lines (particularly in the SA node area) may potentiate dysrhythmias. Atrial or junctional bradycardia may occur in the immediate postoperative period, requiring the use of temporary atrial pacing. Sinus rhythm usually returns within the first postoperative week, but the ECG exhibits two P waves: a donor P wave and a native P wave (Shinn, 1980) because the native SA node is preserved and innervates the atrial remnant while the donor SA node innervates the donor atria. The nurse monitors the cardiac rhythm and watches for premature ventricular contractions, tachycardia, or bradycardia. Hypokalemia caused by diuresis after surgery can also contribute to ventricular irritability. The nurse checks serum potassium frequently and makes corrections as ordered.

Renal Dysfunction

Prerenal failure may exist prior to transplant surgery due to congestive heart failure. CPB may potentiate hypotension and a decrease in renal perfusion. Cy A can also cause acute tubular necrosis (Myers, Ross, Newton, Leutscher, & Perlroth, 1984). Nursing interventions include administering dopamine to improve renal perfusion. The nurse also gives diuretics as ordered, monitors intake and output carefully, and records cyclosporine serum levels daily. Hemodialysis may be necessary to correct fluid and electrolyte imbalance.

Hypertension

Hypertension (HTN) has been seen in the early postoperative period in the recipient receiving Cy A. The mechanism of this side effect of Cy A is not clear.

Monitoring blood pressure and titrating medications to keep the blood pressure within normal ranges is an important nursing intervention.

Immediate Postoperative Complications of Combined Heart–Lung Transplantation

In addition to the complications described under heart transplantation, other unique complications may be seen in the heart-lung recipient, including respiratory insufficiency and pulmonary infection.

Respiratory Insufficiency

Heart–lung transplant recipients are at higher risk than heart transplant recipients for pulmonary problems. A major complication of heart–lung transplantation is a shock-lung-like syndrome, formerly known as reimplantation response manifested by transient pulmonary edema. This syndrome usually begins within 48 hours after surgery and continues for up to 21 days (Covner & Shinn, 1983). The exact cause is not clear. Speculation includes imperfect preservation of lungs related to ischemic injury (E. Stinson, MD, personal communication, 1989), trauma from manipulation of donor lungs during surgery, disruption of the pulmonary lymphatic system, and a drop in oncotic pressure (Covner & Shinn, 1983).

Nursing assessment focuses on the presence of dyspnea, tachypnea, and diaphoresis. Frequent auscultation of the lungs and sensorium checks are important. Optimal treatment consists of diuretics and fluid restriction to minimize the potential for pulmonary edema. When vigorous diuresis does not decrease pulmonary congestion, hemodialysis or pure ultrafiltration (PUF) is initiated. Weakness and fatigue caused by pulmonary congestion and a decrease in compliance increases the work of breathing. Reintubation is often necessary to assure adequate oxygenation and ventilation. Carefully monitoring intake and output and daily weights to maintain a negative fluid balance are important nursing interventions. Monitoring of arterial blood gases is imperative.

Pulmonary Infection

Another complication in the heart–lung recipient is the loss of a spontaneous cough reflex due to denervation of the lungs which frequently results in pulmonary infection. Nursing interventions include frequent endotracheal suction, using strict aseptic technique. After extubation, vigorous pulmonary toilet is important to prevent pulmonary infection. The nurse encourages coughing and deep breathing and assists with incentive spirometry, chest percussion therapy (CPT) and postural drainage. Bronchodilators may be added to the respiratory treatments if necessary.

Further nursing care, with nursing diagnoses, nursing interventions, and patient outcomes are listed in the nursing care plan for heart and heart–lung transplantation at the end of this chapter.

Special Considerations—Daily Care

Maintenance of Protective Isolation

Current isolation techniques for heart transplant recipients include use of a private room, handwashing with antiseptic soaps, and wearing a mask and shoe covers (optional). Protective isolation techniques for the transplant population have changed over the past 4 years as new immunosuppressants have been introduced. Complete protective isolation may be used only for heart–lung recipients at this time. Recent studies have confirmed that the intensity of protective isolation appears to have no impact on the incidence of infection and associated morbidity and mortality in the early postoperative period (Gamberg, Miller, & Lough, 1987). This reduction of isolation practice has lessened psychological effects on the recipient and family and decreased hospital costs. It adds to comfort and offers a more normal environment to the patient, staff, and visitors (Hess, Brooks-Brunn, Clark, & Joy, 1985).

After 2 or 3 postoperative days, when the recipient has stabilized, the nurse plans care for the recipient's recovery in the ICU. The nurse encourages activities of daily living (ADL) as soon as the recipient is hemodynamically stable. Most recipients are elated at this time, knowing that they have survived the procedure. The nurse also needs to encourage rest and sleep periods to promote healing and recovery from surgery. Initially, visits may be restricted to the immediate family to allow sufficient rest and to prevent spread of infections. The nurse explains the purpose of the isolation procedure and assists family members in washing their hands and putting on masks and shoe covers. The nurse is responsible for screening visits. Restrictions are that no persons with active or incubating infections (colds, flu, herpes, etc.) are allowed to enter the recipient's room.

Rejection and Infection

Refer to the nursing care plan at the end of this chapter for signs and potential symptoms of acute rejection and infection.

Occupational Therapy

Occupational therapy is initiated when the recipient is stable. Nursing interventions include encouragement of recipients to pursue or develop hobbies while confined to the hospital. To create a more pleasant environment, the family can bring in posters or pictures for walls or windows. Entering photos of the recipient's progress and documentation of his/her stay in a scrapbook will occupy time. A calendar is helpful to follow the progress of recovery.

Other examples of recipient's use of free time include watching TV or videotapes, listening to battery-operated radio/tape recorder, or doing hand-icrafts such as beadwork or puzzles.

Physical Therapy

Patients learn to do warm-up, peak, and cool-down exercises. With a denervated heart, heart rate will not increase rapidly in response to exercise. Therefore, provision of warm-up exercises allows time for circulating catecholamines to reach the heart.

Physical therapy begins after the recipient is extubated. Exercise and toning are increased as tolerated. Weights and stationary cycling are included in the exercise program. The nurse monitors vital signs and watches for signs of fatigue during this period.

Dietary Considerations

Dietary teaching may begin at this time. Transplant recipients may have low fat/low cholesterol, no-added salt diets. Food may be made by the family and brought in for the recipient with physician's orders. The nurse encourages recipients to be aware of calories and salt in the foods they eat. Prednisone will cause them to retain water, redistribute muscle/fat tissue, and increase their appetites. A dietitian will consult with family regarding safety in prepara-tion and transport of food. The following list of foods or snacks can be brought in from home:

- Peanut butter with no salt, or sugar; old-fashioned nonhydrogenated type (best place to buy is in a health food store) also, diet jams and jellies.
- Low- or no-salt crackers, melba toast.
- Sugar-free gum, dietetic hard candies, favorite teas; powdered carob may be mixed with sweetener and powdered milk for hot chocolate.
- Sugar-free sodas, moderate amounts of fresh fruit—a few pieces at a time (no fresh fruit unless peeled before being brought into room; unpeeled fruits such as oranges may carry mold in the crevices of the skin).

The nurse teaches and encourages recipients to calculate their food intake and output consistently. Because consistency is vital, the nurse may suggest that the recipients attach a piece of paper to the overbed table and write items down as they eat and drink.

Housekeeping

Housekeeping duties are performed per protocol once to twice a day by a housekeeper. All recipient-care articles—bath, basin, soap dish, urinals—need to be changed once a week. The room needs to be kept as neat and clutter-free as possible. This is the responsibility of nurses on all three shifts. No flowers or live plants are allowed in the room due to the patient's susceptibility to infection.

Immunosuppressive Protocols

Important to a speedy recovery is the regulation of acute rejection by appropriate, precise immunosuppressant therapy. Corticosteroids, Cy A, and azathioprine are routinely administered, based upon body weight for each recipient. Recently, OKT3 (a monoclonal antibody) has replaced antithymocyte globulin (ATG) as prophylaxis in the immunosuppressant protocol. Important guidelines for the administration of Cy A and OKT3 for the nurse to follow are specified in Table 5.1. At some centers adequate immunosuppression has been achieved without prophylaxis in heart transplantation. For more details of immunosuppressant therapy, refer to Chapter 2 "Immunological Aspects of Organ Transplantation."

Biopsies

Usually after 1 week, recipients will have their first biopsy to rule out acute cardiac rejection. The nurse must take special care in preparing recipients for biopsies, including the following:

- Informed consent for each biopsy and echocardiograms for all recipients. For heart–lung recipients, an additional permit may be obtained for fiberoptic bronchoscopy and bronchial lavage. A diagram of the heart biopsy forceps "(Cave's Bioptome")" may help the nurse explain the procedure to the recipient. (See Figure 5.3 for a diagram of the bioptome.)
- Discussion of biopsy procedure with recipient.
- Preoperative checklist completion.
- Preoperative medications (prophylactic antibiotics per transplant centers' protocols and a mild tranquilizer if needed).
- May be NPO.
- Anticoagulants on hold.
- Protective isolation attire.

The recipient is taken to the operating room or cardiac catheterization laboratory via gurney or wheelchair. The endomyocardial biopsy resembles a right sided cardiac catheterization and is performed under local anesthesia. The endomyocardial bioptome is inserted via the right jugular vein into the right ventricle where three specimens are taken from the right septal wall. The biopsy procedure requires 1 or 2 hours. Since the majority of recipients have acute rejection episodes, one of the most important aspects of nursing care is to emphasize to patients that rejection episodes imply adjustment of immunosuppressants, not imminent danger of death.

TABLE 5.1 Cyclosporine A and OKT3 Drug Protocols (an Example)

Name	Cyclosporine A	OKT3
Brand name Generic name	Sandimmune Cyclosporine A (Cy A)	OKT3 (Orthoclone) Muromonab-CD3
Manufacturer	Sandoz	Ortho Pharmaceutical Company

Action	Immunosuppresssant
	Prevents graft rejection
	Interferes with
	  T-lymphocyte function
		Immunosuppressant
		Prevents and reverses
		  graft rejection
		Blocks T-cell function
		Murine monoclonal
		  antibody of the
		  T3 antigen of the
		  human T cell

How supplied	100 mg/cc elixir
	4 oz. brown bottle
	Olive oil–based solution
	  or wrapped capsules in 25 mg
	  amd 100 mg doses.
		5 mg/5 cc ampule
		  stored in refrigerator
		Avoid freezing or
		  shaking vigorously.
		Filter (0.22 μm)
		  before giving.

Dosage
and route
	50–500 mg bid
	  (approx.); dependent on
	  renal and liver functions
	  as well as Cy A levels.
	Elixir diluted in 1:10
	  solution of orange juice
	  or milk
		Prophylactic dose
		  5 mg/day IV
		  (adults): In heart
		  transplant recipients
		  for 7–14 days. In
		  heart–lung trans-
		  plant recipients for
		  10 days.
		Same dose given for
		acute rejection when
		needed
		Given IV push in less
		than 1 min.

Premedication	None required	Needed for first 1–3 doses only, given every 6 hrs acetamin- ophen 650 mg po/pr Ranitidine 50–100 mg IV Benadryl® 0-50 mg Hydrocortisone 50–100 mg IV (qd before dose)

(continued)

TABLE 5.1 Cyclosporine A and OKT3 Drug Protocols (an Example, continued)

Name	Cyclosporine A	OKT3
Complications	Nephrotoxicity Hepatotoxicity Neurotoxicity (fine hand tremors, seizures) GI upset Hirsutism Gingival hyperplasia Skin changes Hypertension Lymphomas	Serum sickness (see below) Anaphylaxis (see below) Fatal severe pulmo- nary edema Aseptic meningitis syndrome Prolific infections Lymphomas Ebstein-Barr virus (EBV)–like disorders
Nursing Interventions	1. Check Cy A level daily and wait to give evening dose until new order received. 2. Notify physician if any of following symptoms occur: Increase in systolic and diastolic blood pressure Headaches Seizures Decrease in urine output Elevated hepatic or renal function tests 3. If recipient vomits within a few hours of taking dose, check with physician about repeating dose.	Notify physician if any of the following symptoms occur: Signs of serum sickness, pyrexia, chills, nausea, vomiting, diarrhea Signs of anaphylaxis or pulmonary edema. dyspnea, chest pain, wheezes Signs of aseptic meningitis, headache, neck stiffness, tremors Photophobia Neurological changes If recipient is fluid overloaded before OKT3 dose, the chances of developing pulmonary edema are increased. Watch CVP closely and auscultate lungs frequently.

(continued)

TABLE 5.1 Cyclosporine A and OKT3 Drug Protocols (an Example, continued)

Name	Cyclosporine A	OKT3
		Check weight daily. If temperature is greater than 37.8°C orally, it is recommended that acetaminophen be given before OKT3 administration.

After biopsies, nursing assessments include the following:

- Checking vital signs every hour or as ordered.
- Obtaining chest x-ray (CXR) as ordered.
- Hanging new CVP bottle and tubing (if central line remains in place) and reinforcing dressing if necessary (left internal jugular vein site is usually changed to right internal jugular vein site at time of first biopsy).
- Checking site for hematoma.
- Observing for pneumothorax, cardiac tamponade, and dysrhythmias.

After the first negative biopsy, the recipient may be transferred to a step-down unit or intermediate care area.

Recipient Teaching

Teaching the transplant recipients and their families about their drug regimens is another important nursing responsibility. The goals for the recipients before leaving the ICU include the following:

- Know the times for taking medications.
- Take all medications without supervision.
- Keep an independent record of medications.
- Know the action, dosage, and side effects of medications.

The following is an example of how to facilitate this learning:

- Place a large medication chart on the wall of the isolation room with the names, actions, dosages, and side effects of the cardiac and immunosuppressive drugs (see Table 5.2).
- Document the recipient's progress in learning medications (see Table 5.3).

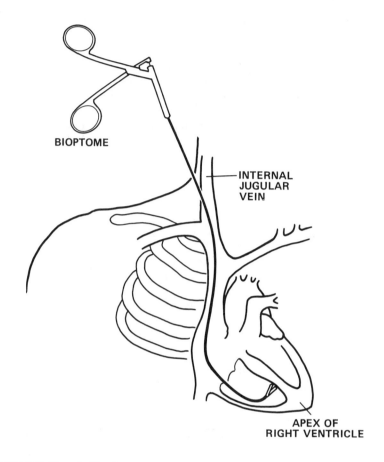

FIGURE 5.3 Cave's bioptome.

- Teach recipients to keep an accurate record of intake, output, and daily weight.
- If recipients are taking prednisone, teach urine testing for sugar and acetone and stool hemocult test.

When the patient leaves the ICU, the nurse must report on the recipient's knowledge and ability to perform the following:

- Self-medication.
- Intake and output procedure.
- Monitoring signs of rejection and infection.
- Personal hygiene and other measures to prevent infections.
- Monitoring vital signs.

TABLE 5.2 Medication Chart for Teaching of Heart and Heart–Lung Transplant Recipients (an Example)

Medication	Dosage	Action	Side effects
Dipyridamole	75 mg 4 times a day 9 am, 1 pm, 5 pm, 9 pm	Prevents platelet aggregation and the potential for atherosclerosis	Stomach irritation Dizziness Headache Flushing Skin rash Bruising
Antacid of choice	1 tsp after meals and at bedtime 9 am, 5 pm, 10 pm	Prevents ulcers and relieves heartburn by neutralizing increased gastric acids caused by prednisone and cyclosporine; Antacid acts as a calcium supplement	Constipation or diarrhea Nausea
ASA	325 mg once a day 9 am	Prevents platelet aggregation.	Bruising Bleeding GI upset
Nystatin Suspension (100,000 U/cc)	5 cc after meals and at bedtime 9 am, 5 pm, 9 pm	Protects against development of fungal mouth infections	None
Colace (100 mg)	100 mg 2 times a day as needed	Softens stool	Abdominal cramps (rare) Diarrhea
Furosemide	Varies, check medication card daily.	Diuretic necessary for the excretion of water due to the salt–retaining effects of prednisone	Loss of potassium (K+) Low blood pressure Nausea Vomiting Blurred vision Loss of hearing
Potassium chloride	30 mEq twice a day 9 am, 6 pm	Replaces potassium loss caused by diuresis	Stomach upset Stomach irritation

(continued)

TABLE 5.2 Medication Chart for Teaching of Heart and Heart–Lung Transplant Recipients (an Example, continued)

Medication	Dosage	Action	Side effects
Cyclosporine A	Varies; check medication card daily; mix with juice or milk 9 am, 6 pm	Immunosuppressant inhibits rejection of heart and lungs.	Hypertension Renal dysfunction Liver dysfunction Tremors Hirsutism Prone to infection
Azathioprine	Varies; check medication card daily 6 pm	Immunosuppressant, inhibits rejection of heart and lungs.	Decreases white blood cells Increases risk of infection GI upset Decreases platelets
Prednisone (orally)	Varies; check medication card daily.	Immunosuppressant, antiinflammatory drug, suppresses cell reactions to prevent rejection of heart and lungs; also used to treat rejection when it occurs	Diabetes mellitus Increases risk of infection Increases risk of bone fracture Increases appetite Sodium and water retention Peptic ulcers Skin rash Loss of muscle mass Redistribution of body fat (moon face) Large abdomen Mood swings—euphoria to depression
Methylprednisolone Varies (intravenously)	(given by RN)	Treatment for acute rejection May require hospitalization	Same as prednisone.
Antithymocyte globulin (ATG) (intramuscularly/ intravenously) or OKT3 (intravenously)	Varies (given by RN)	Immunosuppressant, prevents and reverses rejection of heart and lungs	Increases risk of infection Anaphylaxis

TABLE 5.3 Heart and Heart–Lung Transplant Progress Sheet (an Example)

Patient objectives	Recipient performs with assistance	Recipient performs without assistance	Nursing comments
Measure output, specific gravity, sugar, and acetone; Hematest stool Specimens: Collect urine Diet: Menu selection			

Medications:	Recognizes	Pours	Dosage	Action	Side effects
Azathioprine					
Prednisone					
Cyclosporine A					
Dipyridamole					
Antacid of choice					
ASA					
Potassium					
Furosemide					
Acetaminophen					
Nystatin					
Colace					

NURSING RESPONSIBILITIES FOR DISCHARGE PLANNING, FOLLOW-UP VISITS, AND COMPLICATIONS

Discharge Planning

Discharge planning and teaching of self-care are continued after transfer from the ICU to the step-down unit. The average hospital length of stay for a complication-free heart transplant recipient is 2 to 3 weeks; for the heart–lung recipient, about 3 to 4 weeks. Important aspects of discharge teaching include medication, nutrition, physical therapy, and prevention of infection.

Knowledge of Medication

The nurse's role is to ensure that all transplant recipients demonstrate knowledge of their medications: actions, dosages, and side effects. This is imperative because knowledge of medication is essential for the recipient's survival.

Nutrition

An individualized nutrition plan of care is introduced by a dietitian before the recipient leaves the hospital. The overall goal is the maintenance of ideal body weight. A low-cholesterol, low-sodium, and modified-fat diet is recommended (Kumar & Coulston, 1983). Target levels for serum cholesterol and triglycerides are (1) cholesterol, less than 200 mg/dl, and (2) triglycerides, less than 150 mg/dl. Studies on nutritional management of the heart transplant recipient have shown that a compromised nutritional status preoperatively may predict postoperative complications and affect rehabilitation (Frazier, Van Burren, Poindexter, & Waldenberger, 1985; Grady & Herold, 1988). These studies have further reported that long-standing heart failure contributes to muscle and adipose tissue loss, which return to normal values after heart transplantation (Grady & Herold, 1988). Dietary teaching and recommendations are essential in decreasing the risk factors associated with graft atherosclerosis and the complications of immunosuppressive therapy. Side effects of corticosteroids which may be managed by dietary intervention include diabetes mellitus as a result of gluconeogensis and decreased glucose utilization by cells, sodium and water retention, and increased calcium excretion causing osteoporosis. Nursing care includes teaching recipients to monitor urine for sugar and acetone, reduce fat and sodium intake, take calcium supplements, and exercise daily. Also, recipients should weigh themselves every day. Nurses play an important role in referring recipients with weight problems for dietary counseling and cardiac rehabilitation (Grady & Herold, 1988).

Physical Therapy

Returning to activities of daily living can be accomplished by encouraging recipients to participate in medically approved exercise programs. Physical therapy is initiated while the recipient is in the ICU setting. Exercises are gradually increased from range of motion to walking or stationary bicycle riding as tolerated. A physical therapist discusses and supervises the appropriate activity level. The recipient is taught to check his pulse and to watch for signs of fatigue, shortness of breath, and a heart rate of 130 beats per minute or greater. During exercise, increased venous return and circulating catecholamines are responsible for a gradual increase in heart rate (Stinson, Griepp, Schroeder, Dong, & Shumway, 1972). Because of this gradual response, an exercise regimen for cardiac transplant recipients must also be gradually increased in direct proportion to the response in heart rate (Stinson et al., 1972). A physical therapist or nurse will monitor and explain the reason for warm-up and cool-down exercises.

Teaching Prevention of Infection

Infections occur frequently in the immunosuppressed recipient whose natural defenses are compromised. Infections are among the major causes of mortality in the heart and heart–lung transplant group (Fragomeni & Kaye, 1988). Most infections are opportunistic and originate in the lungs. During the initial ICU period, when immunosuppressant drugs are maximized to prevent rejection, the recipient is most vulnerable to infections. Once sufficient immunosuppressive coverage is achieved, immunosuppressant drugs are gradually reduced to minimal dosages, and risk of infection lessens.

Nursing responsibilities include teaching the recipient and his/her family to identify and prevent potential infections. Recipients need to be instructed in the following before leaving the hospital:

- Check temperature daily and report any elevation above 38°C.
- Notify the physician about persistent cough, change in sputum production, shortness of breath, vomiting, diarrhea (these could indicate early signs of lung or gastrointestinal infection). Heart–lung recipients are at a higher risk for pulmonary infections. A respiratory therapist or nurse emphasizes the importance of respiratory care at home.
- Inspect skin daily and report changes; the skin may become fragile or infected due to the side effects of steroids.
- Avoid persons with infections (e.g., colds).
- Clean and dress lacerations immediately. Wound healing is decreased in patients taking steroids. Notify physician if pain, swelling, or redness is experienced.
- Request prophylactic antibiotics prior to any dental or surgical procedures to reduce the risk of bacterial endocarditis.
- Wear a face mask inside the hospital.
- Stop smoking and avoid smoky environments. Smoking will add to the risk for developing lung infection while taking immunosuppressants.
- Check with the physician before buying a pet. Animals may carry diseases that may be transmitted to humans, such as toxoplasmosis found in cat feces.

The recipient also needs to learn procedures for monitoring vital signs and other parameters before leaving the hospital, as follows:

- Check pulse at rest and during activity once daily and as needed; note and report any significant changes in rate or regularity.
- Check blood pressure daily; if taking antihypertensive medications, more frequent checks may be necessary.
- Check weight daily; call physician if gain is greater than 2 pounds per day.

- Observe for signs and symptoms of acute rejection (i.e., low blood pressure, irregular heart rate, dizziness, and fatigue).

Preparation for discharge from the hospital includes knowledge of medications, the importance of diet and exercise, the signs and symptoms of rejection, and an awareness of prevention and recognition of infections. Teaching the transplant recipient to be self-sufficient and to return to a normal lifestyle is a major nursing responsibility.

Follow-up Visits

After discharge from the initial hospitalization, recipients are seen once or twice a week in the outpatient clinic. Visits subsequently taper off, depending on the individual's health status, to one every 2 weeks, then monthly for 2 to 3 months, and finally to an annual visit. The recipient usually remains in the local area for 2 to 4 months. If the recipient lives locally, he may continue to have clinic visits two to four times per year. The clinic nurse is available for explanation and clarification of treatments. Each clinic visit includes appropriate hematology, chemistry panels, cyclosporine level, ECG, CXR, and a complete physical examination.

Heart biopsies and echocardiograms are performed frequently for all recipients after discharge from the hospital. Heart–lung recipients may also have fiberoptic bronchoscopy to monitor for lung rejection and bronchial alveolar lavage with transbronchial biopsy. If free of rejections 6 months postoperatively, checkups may be reduced to every two to four months. The annual checkup requires hospitalization and includes biopsy, echocardiogram, and cardiac catheterization with angiography for both the heart and heart–lung transplant recipient. The heart-lung recipient also requires follow-up pulmonary function tests with each visit.

The follow-up visits are an opportune time for the nurse to observe the recipient's recovery and provide further teaching and clarification. How well the recipient is coping with the treatments and how he/she is adjusting is a reflection of successful integration of teaching into a new life-style (Gunderson, 1985).

Complications of Long-Term Heart and Heart–Lung Transplantation

Acute Rejection

Rejection may occur late postoperatively and is treated according to the clinical and histologic findings. For example, if the recipient does not respond to increased oral prednisone, additional high doses of intravenous methylprednisolone are administered to control severity of acute rejection. If acute rejection continues, OKT3 or ATG may be added to the treatment.

Graft Atherosclerosis

Graft atherosclerosis is another potential concern after transplantation. Coronary artery lesions can be visible by angiography as early as 1 year after heart transplantation. The current treatment for this accelerated diffuse allograft atherosclerosis is retransplantation (Fowler & Schroeder, 1986). The pathophysiology of accelerated graft atherosclerosis is not clear at present and needs further exploration. Researchers have noted that graft atherosclerosis seems to be closely related to the frequency and severity of acute rejection episode and duration of graft survival (Fowler & Schroeder, 1986).

A silent myocardial infarction, visible on ECG, may be the first sign of advanced coronary artery disease (Hunt, 1986). The recipient does not exhibit classical signs of angina pectoris because the transplanted heart is denervated. The most reliable method of detecting and monitoring this complication is coronary angiography (Fowler & Schroeder, 1986). Angiography is performed before discharge from the hospital, to establish a baseline, and annually thereafter.

Hypertension

Arterial hypertension is frequently seen in the recipient receiving Cy A (Hunt, 1983). Hypertension often develops in the immediate postoperative period. It is difficult to control this hypertension since no standard drug regimen is consistently effective. Studies are in progress to determine the underlying cause of hypertension. Appropriate, aggressive antihypertensive and diuretic drug treatment varies for each recipient. Nursing responsibilities include monitoring of blood pressure postoperatively and teaching recipients how to take their own blood pressure before discharge.

Myocardial Fibrosis

Myocardial fibrosis has developed in some heart transplant recipients taking Cy A (Hunt, 1983). Long-term studies may identify the underlying cause. The myocardial fibrosis seems to be unrelated to rejection. Currently, the interstitial myocardial fibrosis appears to have no clinical significance.

Infection

Infectious complications are common in the immunosuppressed transplant recipient. Bacterial infections are the most frequent type seen in this population, followed by viral, fungal, and protozoan organisms (Baumgartner, 1983). Classical signs and symptoms of infection may be masked when taking chronic immunosuppressants. Nursing assessment skills are crucial in detecting and preventing infection. Mild malaise and tiredness, with a normal or slightly elevated body temperature may be the first signs of a pulmonary infection. Early diagnosis and aggressive treatment with the appropriate drug regimen are imperative.

Obliterative Bronchiolitis

A leading complication and cause for retransplantation of the heart–lung recipient is obliterative bronchiolitis (OB) (Burke et al., 1986). The pathophysiology of the obstructive and restrictive lung process is unclear. Pulmonary function tests have detected physiologic changes as early as 2 months after heart–lung transplantation (Harjula et al., 1987). There is some evidence that infections such as cytomegalovirus pneumonia may be a contributing factor to OB (Burke et al., 1986). Augmented immunosuppression appears to decrease the progression of OB (Imoto, Glanville, Baldwin, & Theodore, 1987).

The overall experience with heart–lung transplants remains limited. More experience and sophistication are needed to broaden the horizon in this area of organ transplantation.

CONCLUSION

Care of the heart and heart–lung recipient requires a multidisciplinary approach. Specialists of the health care team, such as nurses, physicians, physical therapists, dietitians, and social workers, provide expertise and have a major impact on the transplant recipient's quality of life after transplantation. Lough, Lindsey, and Shinn's (1985) study, on "Life Satisfaction Following Heart Transplantation," showed that life quality and life satisfaction were "good to very satisfactory" and that heart transplant recipients reported "good to excellent" quality of life. Quality of life after transplantation will be discussed in Chapter 13 in greater detail. The successful recovery of the recipient depends on compliance with stringent medical, nursing, dietary, and activity protocols. Nursing is a vital link between the various departments because nurses are responsible for initiating, planning, and evaluating these complex issues.

ACKNOWLEDGMENTS

We are grateful to Edward B. Stinson, MD, Professor of Cardiovascular Surgery at Stanford University Medical Center, and Vaughn A. Starnes, MD, Assistant Professor of Cardiovascular Surgery and Head of Heart/Lung Transplantation Program at Stanford University Medical Center, for their assistance and encouragement.

HEART AND HEART–LUNG TRANSPLANTATION NURSING CARE PLAN

Nursing diagnoses	Expected outcome	Nursing interventions
ALTERATION IN CARDIAC OUTPUT related to Cardiac surgery Hypothermia Hypovolemia Hemorrhage: due to heparin effect, possible preop liver dysfunction, abnormal coagulation studies, insufficient cauterization in operating room (OR).	Recipient will maintain optimum cardiac output as follows: Hemodynamic stability CVP within normal limits (wnl) Heart rate initially 110–130 beats/min Absence of dysrhythmias Normotension Fluid electrolyte balance within normal limits Adequate cerebral, renal and peripheral perfusion No rales No peripheral edema	1. Monitor BP, heart rate, respiration, temperature, CVP, chest tube drainage, per orders. 2. Watch for hypovolemia due to increased intravascular space as recipient rewarms, third-spacing, or hemorrhage. 3. Recognize signs and symptoms of cardiac tamponade. Sudden decrease in chest tube drainage; increased CVP; decreased BP; tachycardia; decreased urine output; pulses paradoxus; cold, clammy skin. 4. Optimize preload with fluids as ordered. 5. Administer inotropic/chrono-tropic agents (i.e., isoproterenol, dobutamine, dopamine) or atrial pacing to counteract bradycardia due to denervation of heart as ordered. 6. Administer vasodilator agents (i.e., nitroprusside) as ordered. 7. Adjust drugs to optimize contractility, pre- and afterload reduction as ordered. 8. Monitor and assess intake and output per routine.

(continued)

HEART AND HEART–LUNG TRANSPLANTATION NURSING CARE PLAN (continued)

Nursing diagnoses	Expected outcome	Nursing interventions
		9. Check daily weights.
		10. Assess for signs of fluid overload (i.e., pulmonary and systemic congestion).
		11. Auscultate lungs for rales, rhonchi.
		12. Check for peripheral edema. Administer fluids and diuretics as ordered.
		13. Check electrolytes as ordered.
		14. Assess level of consciousness, peripheral pulses, capillary refill.
	* * * *	
ALTERATION IN RESPIRATORY FUNCTION related to Anesthesia Endotracheal airway intubation Ineffective airway clearance	Recipient will demonstrate recovery from anesthesia Independent breathing Adequate airway clearance (i.e. effective cough). Clear chest x-ray (ABGs) within normal limits	1. While patient is intubated; monitor respiration and monitor ABGs. 2. Adjust respirator setting and acid/base balance as ordered. 3. Repeat ABGs 30 min after respirator change. 4. Auscultate lungs; listen for rales, bronchi, pericardial friction rub. 5. Administer pulmonary care as ordered. 6. Provide adequate pain control when weaning off the respirator. 7. When patient is extubated; administer O_2 as needed (via O_2 mask, nasal cannula, etc.) Encourage deep breathing, coughing, incentive spirometry every 2 hrs. 8. Utilize pillow to avoid splinting and assist with effective, productive coughing. 9. Administer pain medication as ordered.

(continued)

HEART AND HEART–LUNG TRANSPLANTATION
NURSING CARE PLAN (continued)

Nursing diagnoses	Expected outcome	Nursing interventions
		10. Draw ABGs as needed. 11. Monitor oxygen saturation. 12. Place patient in semi-Fowler's position.

FOUND IN HEART–LUNG TRANSPLANTATION ONLY

RESPIRATORY DYS-FUNCTION: related to Shock-lung-like syndrome related to ischemic lung injury, lymphatic disruption and alveolar permeability resulting in pulmonary edema
Absence of mucociliary clearance below tracheal suture line.
Pulmonary rejection
Bronchospasm
Leakage or perforation of tracheal anastomosis
Infection
Phrenic nerve paresis
Pleural effusion
Anxiety

Recipient will demonstrate:
Adequate respiratory function.
Normal CVP (6–12 mmHg)
ABGs wnl
Effective breathing pattern and rate postextubation
Oxygen saturation greater than 90%.
CXR wnl
Clear breath sounds in all lung fields.

1. Assess for signs of pulmonary edema such as distended neck veins, increased rales, color and consistency of sputum, use of accessory muscles, restlessness, deteriorating ABGs.
2. Suction as needed (prn).
3. Use strict aseptic technique; avoiding vigorous suction (use soft catheters; recipient has fresh tracheal suture line that may be irritated by vigorous suction).
4. Administer diuretics as ordered.
5. Assist with respiratory treatments as ordered (i.e., percussion, postural drainage).
6. Teach recipient how to cough effectively, because recipient does not have the sensation of "mucus" below the suture line.

(continued)

HEART AND HEART–LUNG TRANSPLANTATION NURSING CARE PLAN (continued)

Nursing diagnoses	Expected outcome	Nursing interventions
		7. Administer broncho-dilators as ordered 8. Monitor intake and output, maintain volume status "dryer" than usual. 9. Provide emotional support regarding anxiety.

* * * *

Nursing diagnoses	Expected outcome	Nursing interventions
ALTERATION IN NORMOTENSIVE STATUS as a result of Cy A therapy	Recipient will demonstrate normotension: Systolic blood pressure less than 140 mmHg Diastolic blood pressure less than 90–100 mmHg	1. Monitor blood pressure as ordered. 2. Administer anti-hypertensive as needed. 3. Observe and treat for other causes: Pain Anxiety Tremors Nausea/vomiting Vasoconstriction with decreased renal perfusion *Note:* Prolonged hypertensive state will increase myocardial workload and increase O_2 consumption.

* * * *

Nursing diagnoses	Expected outcome	Nursing interventions
ALTERED IMMUNO-LOGICAL RESPONSE causing potential acute rejection episodes	Recipient will be adequately immunosuppressed as exhibited by heart biopsies without rejection. Absence of signs and symptoms of rejection: No fever No weakness No fatigue No dysrhythmias (PACs, PVCs)	1. Administer daily immunosuppressants as ordered. 2. Observe and report changes in hemodynamics, (i.e., dysrhythmias, hypotension, weakness, cardiac failure). 3. Explain to recipient that rejection will occur and is treatable with adjustment of immunosuppresants.

(continued)

HEART AND HEART–LUNG TRANSPLANTATION
NURSING CARE PLAN (continued)

Nursing diagnoses	Expected outcome	Nursing interventions
	No hypotension No congestive heart failure <div align="center">* * * *</div>	4. Provide emotional support.

POTENTIAL FOR INFECTION related to
  Immunosuppression
  Invasive lines
  Altered nutri-
  tional state
	Recipient will be free of
	infection with:
	  Lungs clear to auscul-
	  tation
	  No fever
	  No drainage from
	  incisional sites
	  All cultures negative
		1. Maintain protective
		   isolation as indicated.
		2. Monitor temperature.
		3. Auscultate lungs,
		   check sputum for
		   color and consistency.
		4. Check incision sites
		   for redness, swelling,
		   tenderness, pain, exudate.
		5. Check mouth for oral lesions.
		6. Administer antibiotics
		   as ordered.
		7. Change sterile dressing once
		   a day as needed.
		8. Change IV bags/bottles
		   tubings per protocol.
		9. Obtain blood, sputum,
		   and urine cultures as ordered.
		10. Consult with dietitan
		   to provide optimal
		   dietary support.
		11. Encourage adequate
		   caloric intake to
		   promote healing (i.e.,
		   nutritional snacks,
		   vitamin supplements).
		12. Organize nursing care
		   to facilitate maximal
		   intake at mealtime.

	<div align="center">* * * *</div>	

POTENTIAL SYSTEMS DYSFUNCTION related
to immunosuppressive
therapy:
  Renal status
  Hepatic status
  Neurological
  status
	Recipient will exhibit
	normal kidney, liver and
	neurological function:
	  Creatinine and BUN wnl.
	  Urine output 100 cc/hr.
	  Liver enzymes wnl
	  No jaundice
	  Neurological assess-
	  ment wnl
		1. Monitor and record kidney
		   and liver lab data (BUN,
		   creatinine, bilirubin,
		   liver enzymes).
		2. Draw cyclosporine level
		   every day or as ordered.
		3. Assess recipient for
		   headaches, tremors, and
		   seizure activity.

(continued)

HEART AND HEART–LUNG TRANSPLANTATION
NURSING CARE PLAN (continued)

Nursing diagnoses	Expected outcome	Nursing interventions
	Recipient alert, oriented to time and place, moving all extremities equally.	
	* * * *	
ALTERATION IN MOBILITY related to Side effects of Corticosteroids Denervated heart Decreased nutritional status.	Recipient will demonstrate a progressive increase in exercise tolerance.	1. Assess readiness to begin physical therapy. 2. Assess degree of muscle wasting due to corticosteroids or preoperative nutritional state. 3. Assist in physical therapy,(i.e., passive/active range of motion, weights, bicycle). 4. If recipient is in rejection, withhold physical therapy. 5. Monitor vital signs before, during, and after exercise.
	* * * *	
ALTERED SKIN INTEGRITY related to Immunosuppression, Nutritional status, Impaired mobility	Recipient will be free of skin breakdown.	1. Assess and document condition of skin and mucous membranes every 8 hrs. 2. Turn and position recipient every 2 hrs. 3. Explain and stress importance of early ambulation, hygiene, nutrition, and hydration to promote healing. 4. Use preventive measures to avoid skin breakdown because recipients are slow to heal due to side effects of corticosteroids.
	* * * *	

(continued)

HEART AND HEART–LUNG TRANSPLANTATION NURSING CARE PLAN (continued)

Nursing diagnoses	Expected outcome	Nursing interventions
POTENTIAL COM-PLICATIONS RELATED TO ENDOMYOCARDIAL BIOPSY	Recipient will be free of complications. No bleeding at site of biopsy No cardiac tamponade No dysrhythmias No pneumothorax	1. Assess and monitor vital signs. 2. Check pressure dressing for bleeding swelling, etc. 3. Obtain CXR if needed 4. Monitor for signs and symptoms of cardiac tamponade/pneumothorax: Increased dyspnea Increased respiration Increased restlessness, Confusion tachycardia Hypotension Pulsus paradoxus. Change in skin color

FOUND IN HEART–LUNG TRANSPLANTATION ONLY

POTENTIAL COM-PLICATIONS REL-ATED TO BRONCHIAL LAVAGE AND CLOSED LUNG BIOPSY related to Residuals of anesthesia and inability to breathe adequately Inability to clear secretions Onset of pulmonary edema due to trauma of procedure	Requires no respiratory support	1. Assess and monitor respiratory status. 2. Maintain airway with adequate respirator settings, suctioning as needed. 3. Watch for: Tracheal bleeding, Pulmonary edema, Pneumo/hemothorax 4. Wean from respirator as tolerated.

*   *   *   *

ALTERED PSYCHO-SOCIAL status related to Potential anxiety Depersonalization Potential dependency Potential isolation Fear of rejection Body image changes Altered life-style	Recipient will be free of anxiety. Recipient will begin to adjust appropriately to changes in life-style. Recipient will perform ADLs.	1. Assess recipient for anxiety, fear of the unknown. 2. While in ICU setting, reduce unnecessary stimuli. 3. Assure consistency in recip-ient care routine and allow for scheduled periods of rest.

(continued)

HEART AND HEART–LUNG TRANSPLANTATION NURSING CARE PLAN (continued)

Nursing diagnoses	Expected outcome	Nursing interventions
		4. Encourage family and staff to communicate with recipient through verbal and tactile stimuli.
		5. Explain procedures and rationale
		6. Allow choices in care; encourage ADLs as much as possible.
		7. Individualize environment (i.e., pictures, posters, hobbies).
		8. Contact other resources prn (i.e., social worker, pastoral care, occupational therapy).
		9. Reassure recipient that rejection is expected in the first months after transplantation and that it is treatable.
		10. Teach recipient about side effects of immunosuppressants, i.e., mood swings, redistribution of body fat ("moonface"), hirsutism, etc.
		11. Set priorities and goals with recipient and family.
	* * * *	
KNOWLEDGE DEFICIT related to transplantation		1. Establish specific plan of teaching utilizing appropriate resources.
		2. Record and communicate recipient's progress on teaching flow sheet.
		3. Reinforce teaching throughout hospital stay in following areas:

(continued)

HEART AND HEART–LUNG TRANSPLANTATION
NURSING CARE PLAN (continued)

Nursing diagnoses	Expected outcome	Nursing interventions
		Medication Activities, exercises Diet Recognition of changes that require notification of physician and nurse Signs and symptoms of infection Signs and symptoms of rejection.

REFERENCES

American Council on Transplantation (1990). UNOS 1990 Statistics. Available from Act, 700 N. Fairfax Street, Alexandria, VA 22314.

Baumgartner, W. A. (1983). Infection in cardiac transplantation. *The Journal of Heart Transplantation, 3*(1), 75–79.

Burke, C. M., Glanville, A. R., Macoviak, J. A., O'Connell, B. M., Tazelaar, H. D., Baldwin, J. C., Jamieson, S. W., & Theodore, J. (1986). The spectrum of cytomegalovirus infection following human heart-lung transplantation. *The Journal of Heart Transplantation, 5*(4), 267–272.

Covner, A. L., & Shinn, J. A. (1983). Cardiopulmonary transplantation: Initial experience. *Heart and Lung, 12*(2), 131–135.

Dawkins, K. D., Oldershaw, P. J., Billingham, M. E., Hunt, S. A., Oyer, P. E., Jamieson, S. W., Popp, R. L., Stinson, E. B., & Shumway, N. E. (1984). Changes in diastolic function as a noninvasive marker for cardiac allograft rejection. *The Journal of Heart Transplantation, 3*(4), 286–294.

Fowler, M. B., & Schroeder, J. S. (1986). Current status of cardiac transplantation. *Modern Concepts of Cardiovascular Disease, 55*(8), 37–41.

Frazier, O. H., Van Burren, C. T., Poindexter, S. H., & Waldenberger, F. (1985). Nutritional management of the heart transplant recipient. *The Journal of Heart Transplantation, 4*(4), 450–451.

Funk, M. (1986). Transplantation: Postoperative care during the acute period. *Critical Care Nurse, 6*(2), 27–44.

Gamberg, P., Miller, J. L., & Lough, M. E. (1987). Impact of protection isolation on the incidence of infection after heart transplantation. *The Journal of Heart Transplantation, 6*(3), 147–149.

Grady, K. L. (1985). Development of a cardiac transplantation program: Role of the clinical nurse specialist. *Heart and Lung, 14*(5), 490–494.

Grady, K. L., & Herold L. S., (1988). Comparison of nutritional status in patients before and after heart transplantation. *The Journal of Heart Transplantation, 7*(2), 123–127.

Gunderson, L. (1985). Teaching the transplant recipient. *The Journal of Heart Transplantation, 4*(2), 226–227.

Hammer, C., Reichenspurner, H., Ertel, W., Lersch, C., Plahl, M., Brendel, W., Reichart, B., Uberfuhr, P., Welz, A., Kemkes, B. M., Rebel, B., Funccius, W., & Gokel, M. (1984). Cytological and immunologic monitoring of cyclosporine treated human heart recipients. *The Journal of Heart Transplantation, 3*(3), 228–231.

Harjula, A. L. J., Baldwin, J. C., Glanville, A. R., Tanzelaar, H., Oyer, P. E., Stinson, E. B., & Shumway, N. E. (1987). Human leukocyte antigen compatibility in heart-lung transplantation. *The Journal of Heart Transplantation, 6*(3), 162–165.

Haverich, A., Kemnitz, J., Fieguth, H. G., Wahlers, Th., Schäfers, H. J., Hermann, G., Schröder, H. J., Wonigeit, K., Maisch, B., Gratz, K. F., & Borst, H. G. (1987). Noninvasive parameters for detection of cardiac allograft transplantation. *Journal of Clinical Transplantation, 1*(3), 151–158.

Hess, N., Brooks-Brunn, J. A., Clark, D., & Joy, K. (1985). Complete isolation: Is it necessary? *The Journal of Heart Transplantation, 4*(4), 458–459.

Hess, N., Brooks–Brunn, J. A., Clark, D., & Joy, K. (1985).Complete isolation: Is it necessary? *The Journal of Heart Transplantation, 4*(4), 458–459.

Hunt, S. A. (1983). Complications of heart transplantation. *The Journal of Heart Transplantation, 3*(1), 70–74.

Hunt, S. (1986). *Outpatient care of the Stanford cardiac transplant patient: The cyclosporine era, Unpublished manuscript.*

Imoto, E. M., Glanville, A. R., Baldwin, J. C., & Theodore, J. (1987). Kidney function in heart-lung transplant recipients: The effect of low dosage cyclosporine therapy. *The Journal of Heart Transplantation, 6*(4), 204–211.

Jamieson, S. W., Billingham, M., Oyer, P. E., Stinson, E., Baldwin, J., & Shumway, N. E. (1984). Heart transplantation of end-stage ischemic heart disease: The Stanford experience. *The Journal of Heart Transplantations, 3*(3), 224–227.

Kriett, J.M., & Kaye, M.P., (1990). The Registry of the International Society for Heart Transplantation: Seventh Official Report - 1990. *The Journal of Heart Transplantation, 9*, (4), 323–330.

Kumar, M. R., & Coulston, A. M., (1983). Nutritional management of the cardiac transplant patient. *Journal of the American Dietary Association, 83*, 463–465.

Lekander, B.J. (1988). Preventing complications for the Heart and Lung Transplant Recipient. *Dimensions of Critical Care Nursing, 7* (1), 18–26.

Lough, M. E., Lindsey, A. M., & Shinn, J. A. (1985). Life satisfaction following heart transplantation. *The Journal of Heart Transplantation, 4*(4), 446–449.

Lough, M.E., Williams, B.A. (1985). Stanford University Medical Center Cardiovascular Intensive Care Unit Nursing Care of the Transplant Candidate, Donor, and Heart or Heart-Lung Recipient Self-Learning Module. Unpublished Manuscript.

Mersch, J. (1985). End-stage cardiac disease: Cardiomyopathy. In M.K. Douglas, & J.A. Shinn. (Eds.), *Advances in cardiovascular nursing* (pp. 117–139). Rockville, MD: Aspen Systems Corporation.

Myers, B. D., Ross, J., Newton, L., Leutscher, J., & Perlroth, M. (1984). Cyclosporine associated chronic nephropathy. *New England Journal of Medicine, 311*(11), 699–705.

O'Connell, J. B., & Gunnar, R. M. (1982). Dilated-congestive cardiomyopathy: Prognostic features and therapy. *The Journal of Heart Transplantation, 2*(1), 7–17.

Oyer, P. E., Stinson, E. B., Jamieson, S. W., Hunt, S. A., Perlroth, M., Billingham, M.,

& Shumway, N. E. (1983). Cyclosporine in cardiac transplantation: A 2½ year follow-up. *Transplantation Proceedings, 15*(4) (Suppl. 1), 2546–2552.

Reitz, B. A., Pennock, J. L., & Shumway, N. E. (1981). Simplified operative method for heart and lung transplantation. *Journal of Surgical Heart Research, 31*, 1–5.

Reitz, B. A., Stinson, E. B., Oyer, P. E., Jamieson, S. W., & Shumway, N. E. (1982). Heart-lung transplantation: Development and case histories. *Primary Cardiology,* 45–63.

Sandiford, D. M. (1976). Cardiac transplantation: Eight years experience. *Heart and Lung, 5*(4), 566–570.

Shinn, J. A. (1980). *Cardiac transplantation and the artificial heart.* New York: Appleton-Century-Crofts.

Shinn, J. A. (1985). New issues in cardiac transplantation. In M. K. Douglas & J. A. Shinn (Eds.), *Advances in cardiovascular nursing* (pp. 185–195). Rockville, MD: Aspen Systems Corporation.

Stinson, E. B., Griepp, R. B., Schroeder, J. S., Dong, E., Jr., & Shumway, N. E. (1972). Hemodynamic observation one and two years after transplantation in man. *Circulation, 45*, 1183–1193.

CHAPTER **6**

LUNG TRANSPLANTATION

Bernice Coleman
Johanna Salamandra

The feasibility of lung transplantation was demonstrated in 1948 by Metras (1950) when the first canine transplant was performed in France. In 1963, the first human lung transplant was performed in the United States by Hardy (Hardy, Webb, Dalton, & Walker, 1963). Between 1963 and 1978, further attempts at human lung transplant met with dismal results. Only 2 of 40 patients survived more than 1 month (Malen & Boychuck, 1989); the longest survival was 10 months following single lung transplant (Veith, Montefusco, Kamholz,& Mollenkopf, 1983). Disruption of the airway anastomosis, infection, and rejection were found to be the most common causes of death in these early cases, with poor donor and recipient selection as contributing factors. The use of steroids in the pre- and postoperative periods and interruption of the recipient's bronchial artery blood supply to the transplanted donor bronchus were found to diminish the healing capacity of the airway anastomoses (Lima et al., 1981; Schreinemaker et al., 1990). High doses of immunosuppressive drugs, such as prednisone and azathioprine, were necessary to prevent rejection but greatly predisposed these patients to life-threatening infections.

It was not until the introduction of more effective and selective immunosuppression, such as cyclosporine A (Cy A), and the implementation of techniques designed to improve airway healing (Dubois, Choiniere & Cooper 1984) that the first successful single lung transplant was performed in 1983 by the Toronto Lung Transplant Group. In 1986, this group reported survival of up to 44 months for 8 of 11 patients (Toronto Lung Group, 1986). Double lung transplant was later attempted with long-term success in 1986 by the same group (Cooper et al., 1989).

Ever-improving surgical techniques and better immunosuppression have greatly increased survival and decreased morbidity and mortality in this patient population. Subsequently, successes demonstrated by the Toronto Lung Transplant Group have been reproduced elsewhere, leading to the proliferation of lung transplant programs worldwide. As of 1990 the International Society for Heart Transplantation (ISHT) received data from 58 centers documenting 157 single lung and 48 double lung procedures (Kriett & Kaye, 1990). These statistics do not include all international centers.

The special needs of these patients often present a challenge to nurses caring for them. This chapter will cover indications for single and double lung transplantation, recipient evaluation and selection, donor selection and management, organ procurement and preservation, preoperative recipient preparation, surgical technique, nursing care of the lung transplant recipient, immunosuppression, long-term and follow-up care, and future trends.

INDICATIONS

Indications for lung transplantation are ever changing and expanding. Today a much broader array of end-stage lung diseases is being successfully treated through lung transplantation. As well, single lung transplants are being performed for diseases previously thought to require the more difficult double lung or heart–lung transplant. Double lung transplant now often replaces heart–lung transplant, sparing the patient potential cardiac complications and providing scarce donor organs for both a lung and a heart recipient.

Pulmonary fibrosis is a common indication for single lung transplant (Toronto Lung Transplant Group, 1988). Due to the decreased compliance and increased pulmonary vascular resistance in the native lung, the allograft receives preferential shunting of both blood flow and ventilation. This matched shift in ventilation and perfusion from the diseased native lung to the "normal" transplanted lung makes end-stage fibrosis ideally suited for single lung transplant.

Although previously indicated for double lung or combined heart–lung transplant, disease processes such as emphysema of any cause (including alpha-1- antitrypsin deficiency), primary pulmonary hypertension, Eisenmenger's syndrome with correctable lesions, and lymphangiomyomatosis have been most recently and successfully treated with single lung transplant.

The most common indications for double lung transplant are disease states, such as cystic fibrosis and bronchiectasis, that produce copious amounts of pulmonary secretions and chronic bilateral pulmonary sepsis. Any of the aforementioned disease processes may require double lung transplant if they also present with pulmonary sepsis. Single or double lung transplant, may be contraindicated in otherwise acceptable candidates if irreversible right- and/or left-sided heart failure is present; heart–lung transplantation may be required.

RECIPIENT EVALUATION AND SELECTION

Although many patients suffer from end-stage pulmonary disease, the key to successful lung transplantation is appropriate screening and selection of recipients and donors. The goals of the recipient evaluation process include the following:

- To determine transplant suitability.
- To rule out extrapulmonary disease and potential contraindications.
- To assess the overall medical and psychosocial condition of the patient.
- To allow the patient and family the opportunity to become acquainted with the transplant process and team members.
- To determine the appropriate medical, surgical, nursing, and psychosocial plan of care.

The typical lung transplant candidate is oxygen-dependent, with severely limited exercise tolerance and life expectancy. (See Table 6.1.) These patients must also possess a strong desire and commitment to undergo the necessary evaluation, transplant, and rehabilitation.

TABLE 6.1 Lung Recipient Selection

INCLUSION CRITERIA
Age <60 years
Limited life expectancy (< 6–24 months)
Unresponsiveness to other treatment.
Severely limited exercise tolerance
Oxygen dependent.
Adequate support system.

EXCLUSION CRITERIA
History of recent malignancy
History of smoking
Overt right- and/or left-sided heart failure
Severe coexisting extrapulmonary disease/disorder
High-dose steroid dependence
Ventilator dependence
Severe malnutrition
History of severe psychiatric disorder

Review of the patient's past medical history, as well as initial interviews and examinations by the transplant surgeon and pulmonologist, is necessary to identify appropriate candidates. Following initial acceptance, an extensive evaluation is conducted (see Table 6.2). The patient's condition is often tenuous due to the effects of the disease; therefore, hospitalization may be required during evaluation.

Complete pulmonary testing is conducted to determine the extent of the disease state and to provide a basis for pretransplant therapy, testing, and decision making. Right ventricular ejection fraction and pulmonary artery pressures are measured in an attempt to predict the need for cardiopulmonary bypass at the time of transplant. In addition, the presence of hematologic, renal, hepatic, immunologic, and other metabolic abnormalities is determined by laboratory assessment and may prompt further investigative studies.

Consultation and study results are reviewed at lung transplant team conferences to determine the patient's suitability for transplantation. Essential lung transplant team members include the thoracic surgeon, transplant pulmonologist, transplant coordinator, cardiologist, psychiatrist, clinical nurse specialist, social worker, nutritionist, and other necessary consultants. Results of studies and the decision regarding transplant are promptly communicated to the patient and referring physician.

Once a patient is accepted for lung transplantation, a pretransplant plan of care is established that may include the following:

- Participation in ongoing pulmonary rehabilitation, education, and counseling programs.
- Recommendations for adjustments of medications/treatments.
- Follow-up testing and transplant clinic visits.
- Logistical arrangements for patient to remain within 2 hours of the medical center.
- Donation of autologous or donor-directed blood.

DONOR SELECTION AND MANAGEMENT

Shortage of suitable donor lung allografts is the primary obstacle to lung transplantation. Conditions in an organ donor that may preclude lung donation are aspiration, prolonged intubation predisposing to pneumonitis, pulmonary contusion, and neurogenic pulmonary edema. These conditions are frequently associated with head injury and brain death. Lung recipients may therefore wait longer for transplantation than do other solid organ recipients. The criteria for lung donor selection may differ from center to center (see Table 6.3).

TABLE 6.2 Evaluation Process for Lung Transplantation

Review of past medical history

Pulmonary studies
   Chest x-ray
   Complete pulmonary function testing
   Exercise testing
   Arterial blood gas analysis
   Ventilation/perfusion scan
   Chest CT scan

Cardiovascular studies
   Electrocardiogram
   Echocardiogram/Doppler study
   Radionuclide ventriculogram with resting wall motion
   Cardiac catheterization (right and/or left|)
   Duplex scan of legs

Multidisciplinary assessment
   Cardiothoracic surgery
   Pulmonology
   Cardiology
   Psychiatry
   Nursing
   Social service
   Infectious disease
   Nutrition

Laboratory assessment
   Hematology studies
   Chemistry panels
   Immunologic profile
   Coagulation studies
   Metabolic studies
   Disease-specific assays
   Creatinine clearance

Infectious screening
   Laboratory serological testing
   Skin testing for anergy
   Cultures (sputum or bronchoalveolar larvage [BAL] and urine)
   Dental clearance

In order to optimize the number of usable donor lung allografts for transplantation, all donor management must include close monitoring and meticulous pulmonary care. (See Table 6.4) Monitoring hemodynamics, chest x-rays, blood gas analysis, and breath sounds will help to minimize the occurrence of pulmonary edema and signal early problems. The following information is needed to determine the quality of donor lung allografts:

- Present and past medical history.
- Recent serial chest radiographs.
- Sputum Gram's stains and/or cultures.
- Results of hyperoxygenation testing:(arterial blood gas on FIO_2 of 100% and PEEP of 5 cm.

Recipient/donor matching is based on ABO blood compatibility and size. To determine the appropriate-size allograft, the transplant team matches height and weight as well as the following chest and radiographic lung field measurements:

- Transverse diameter (side to side at dome of diaphragm).
- Longitudinal size (from apex of lung to top of diaphragm on the right and left sides).
- Circumferential chest wall dimension (at the fourth to fifth intercostal space).

A discrepancy between donor and recipient lung size may be preferred, depending on the disease process and the procedure to be performed. Usually, a larger donor single lung allograft is used to normalize lung capacity in restrictive lung diseases such as pulmonary fibrosis. Single or double lung allografts for obstructive lung disease should match or be slightly smaller than the recipient's own. Appropriate size matching is important because

TABLE 6.3 Lung Donor Criteria

Brain Death
Age < 50 years
Clear chest x-ray
PaO2 greater 300 torr with ventilatory settings of FIO2 100% and PEEP
   5.0 cm × 10 min
No airway sepsis
No history of presence of bilateral pulmonary disease or injury
No significant smoking history
No history of malignancy
ABO compatibility
Appropriate size matching

TABLE 6.4 Lung Donor Management

Check arterial blood gases every 3–4 hr and maintain adequate oxygenation with ventilatory settings of FIO_2 40–50% and PEEP 5.0 cm.

Maintain vigorous pulmonary toilette.

Maintain central venous pressure <10.0 mmHg; keep IV fluids to a minimum.

Monitor chest x-ray and measure size of chest.

Monitor peak inspiratory pressures.

Send endotracheal sputum analysis for stat Gram's stain and culture with sensitivity.

Notify recipient center of changes immediately.

Prepare for intraoperative flexible fiberoptic bronchoscopy.

---

oversized lungs may cause cardiac compression and/or atelectasis; undersized lungs may result in residual pleural air space, predisposing the recipient to pleural effusion and empyema.

ORGAN PROCUREMENT AND PRESERVATION

Inspection of the donor lungs by the organ retrieval team is done first through flexible bronchoscopy. The donor airways should be free of obstruction or purulence. Bronchial washings are sent for Gram's stain and culture. The condition of the donor graft is reported back to the transplant center before recipient surgery proceeds.

The donor pneumonectomy is performed through a median sternotomy. An adequate double lung donor specimen consists of both lungs, the distal trachea, the main pulmonary artery, and a cuff of left atrium containing the four pulmonary veins. In single lung transplant, each lung may be used for a different recipient. In this case, two donor lung grafts are created by separating the bronchi at the carina, the pulmonary arteries at the bifurcation of the main pulmonary artery, and obtaining a left atrial cuff for each lung containing the respective pulmonary veins. With each of these techniques, a suitable donor graft can also be obtained for heart transplant.

Two methods of donor lung preservation most frequently used are (1) immersion of the partially inflated lung in 4°C Euro-Collins or other solution, and (2) pulmonary artery flush with 4°C Euro-Collins or other solution followed by immersion as above. The donor trachea/bronchus is stapled prior to immersion to prevent flooding of the airways. Both techniques are followed by cold storage for transport (Starkey et al., 1986, Toronto Lung

Transplant Group, 1988). When using the latter technique, prostaglandin E_1 (PGE$_1$) is injected directly into the pulmonary artery just prior to cross-clamping the aorta and starting cardioplegia. PGE$_1$ dilates the pulmonary vascular bed, thus enhancing uniform distribution of perfusate (Zenati et al., 1989). Using these preservation techniques, satisfactory function can be restored after average cold ischemic times of 4 to 6 hours, which is measured from aortic cross-clamp in the donor until release of pulmonary artery clamp in the recipient.

Preoperative Recipient Preparation

Coordination and cooperation of many professionals is necessary for the successful completion of any solid-organ transplant. Restrictions of ischemic time and the unpredictable nature of organ donation lead most programs to require their recipients to live within 2 hours of the transplant center to allow enough time for preoperative and intraoperative preparation prior to beginning surgery.

Preoperative preparations are done stat and include the following:

- Informed consent.
- Chest x-ray.
- Laboratory studies (hematology and coagulation studies, chemistry panels, blood bank screening and preparation, immunology tests, and urinalysis).
- 12-lead ECG.
- Medical clearance.
- Administration of preoperative antibiotics and immunosuppression.

The patient is transferred to the operating suite for final preparations such as placement of pulmonary artery and radial artery lines.

Timing of anesthetic induction depends upon the condition of the patient, the estimated time of organ retrieval (including travel time from the donor hospital), and the time required for surgical preparation of the recipient prior to placement and anastomosis of the donor organ. The patient is shaved, prepped, and draped in the usual fashion according to the surgical approach intended.

SURGICAL TECHNIQUE

Single lung transplant without anticipated cardiopulmonary bypass (CPB) is performed through a standard posterolateral thoracotomy. From this approach, if the patient fails to tolerate single lung ventilation, femoral venoarterial bypass is initiated. CPB is generally required in patients with greatly elevated pulmonary artery pressures and/or low right ventricular ejection fractions, as in primary pulmonary hypertension. In these patients, single lung transplant is performed on the right side through mediastinotomy. Other factors may infuence the choice of sides, such as past thoracotomies or pleurodesis, perfusion flow, and/or pleural scarring or thickening.

The surgical approach and technique for double lung transplant continues to evolve. Traditionally, double lung transplant has been done via mediastinotomy with use of CPB (Cooper et al., 1989). Utilizing this approach, anastomoses with the donor allograft are performed at the right and left mainstem bronchi, the main pulmonary artery, and the left atrium of the recipient. CPB is required with this technique. More recently, successful double lung transplant has been performed without the use of CPB, significantly reducing bleeding and other bypass-associated risk factors (Pasque et al., 1990). This technique is commonly referred to as bilateral sequential–single lung transplant and requires a transverse, transthoracic incision at the level of the fourth or fifth intercostal space. After the incision is made, the operation proceeds much the same as a single lung transplant, with the surgeon completing the anastomoses of one lung and the respective bronchus, pulmonary artery, and pulmonary veins contained within the left atrial cuff while the patient is ventilated via the contralateral lung. Ventilation is then shifted to the newly transplanted lung, and the same anastomoses are performed on the opposite side.

In all of the above procedures, the bronchial anastomosis is performed first, followed by anastomoses of the pulmonary arteries and then the left atrium and donor cuff. Upon completion of all anastomoses, the bronchial blocker and vascular clamps are removed simultaneously.

The final stage of lung transplant involves wrapping the bronchial anastomosis with a pedicle flap of omentum to provide revascularization of the site. This omentopexy also acts to contain potential contamination and air leak should the anastomosis fail. The pedicle flap of omentum is excised via laparotomy and tunneled through a small defect created in the diaphragm. It is brought posterior to the airway anastomoses, which are then wrapped circumferentially. After ensuring hemostasis, a flexible bronchoscopy is performed to assess the interior integrity of the bronchial anastomoses. (See Figures 6.1 and 6.2.)

NURSING CARE OF THE LUNG TRANSPLANT RECIPIENT

The nurse can expect the recipient to arrive in the intensive care unit (ICU) with an endotracheal tube, pulmonary artery catheter, radial artery catheter, peripheral intravenous lines, chest tubes, pulse oximeter, and Foley catheter. The patient may also require vasoactive medications to improve cardiac contractility. Care is directed toward optimizing gas exchange, improving

DOUBLE-LUNG TRANSPLANT

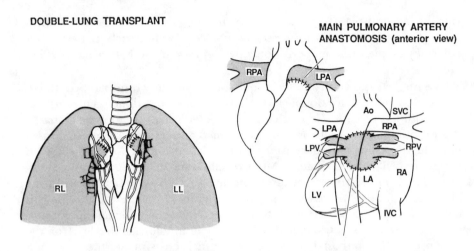

MAIN PULMONARY ARTERY
ANASTOMOSIS (anterior view)

(1) MAINSTEM BRONCHIAL ANASTOMOSES
WITH OMENTAL WRAP (anterior view)

(3) LEFT ATRIAL CUFF ANASTOMOSIS
(posterior view)

FIGURE 6.1 The three sites of anastomoses for double lung transplantation are (1) mainstem bronchial with omental wrap, (2) main pulmonary artery, and (3) left atrial cuff containing the four pulmonary veins. Drawing by Bayard Colyear, medical illustrator.

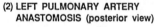

(2) LEFT PULMONARY ARTERY
ANASTOMOSIS (posterior view)

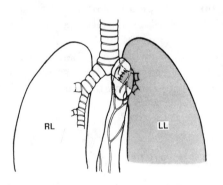

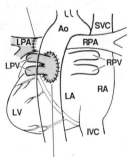

(1) LEFT MAINSTEM BRONCHIAL ANASTOMOSIS
WITH OMENTAL WRAP (anterior view)

(3) LEFT ATRIAL CUFF ANASTOMOSIS
(posterior view)

FIGURE 6.2 The three sites of anastomoses for left single lung transplantation are (1) left mainstem bronchial with omental wrap, (2) left pulmonary artery, and (3) left atrial cuff containing the two left pulmonary veins. Drawing by Bayard Colyear, medical illustrator.

contractility, stabilizing cardiac and pulmonary hemodynamics, monitoring secretions, observing for bleeding, and promoting adequate urine output.

The average ICU length of stay is 3 to 6 days. Total hospital length of stay may average 21 days.

Lung transplant patients provide a challenge to nurses caring for them throughout their hospitalization. The major concerns for nursing management of these patients are a clear understanding of the physiology of the transplanted lung; alteration in gas exchange, cardiac output, and fluid balance; immunosuppression; rejection; and infection. (See the nursing care plan at the end of this chapter.)

Physiology of the Transplanted Lung

Clinical management of lung transplant patients in the perioperative phase is based on a working knowledge of resultant physiologic changes in the lung. Common changes are central denervation of the organ(s), altered ventilation and perfusion patterns, impaired lymphatic drainage, altered rate and rhythm of respirations, and impaired secretion clearance. Additionally, spontaneous deep cough reflex is lost distal to the airway anastomosis. Recognizing and understanding these substantial, yet manageable physiologic changes is cardinal for planning the nursing care of lung transplant patients.

Normally, smooth muscles found in airways and blood vessels throughout the pulmonary circuit are innervated by both sympathetic and parasympathetic nerve fibers (Richardson, 1979). Stimulation via these autonomic pathways results in either excitory or inhibitory responses on airway diameter, pulmonary vasculature, and glandular activity such as mucus production and, to some extent, cilia movement (Guyton, 1986; Murray, 1986). Although less clearly documented, there exists anatomic and physiologic evidence that receptors such as pulmonary stretch fibers (Clark & Von Euler, 1972) and irritant receptors (Widdicombe & Sterling, 1970), in conjunction with autonomic nervous system innervation, contribute to the dynamic process of breathing.

The question then arises: How does the act of breathing and the process of adequate gas exchange continue after single or double lung transplant? The definitive answer is unclear; however, it is thought that two mechanisms are responsible. The first involves the role of the phrenic nerves in the act of breathing. During the surgical procedure, care is taken to prevent injury to the phrenic nerves, which innervate both hemidiaphragms. This central innervation causes flattening of the diaphragm, pulling down the lower surfaces of the lung to facilitate inspiration. At the same time, the intercostal muscles of inspiration raise the ribs and the sternum to increase the anterior and posterior diameters of the chest by 20% (Guyton, 1986). Upon expiration, the diaphragm relaxes passively while active contraction of the expiratory muscles pull downward upon the lower ribs. Another theory is that chemoreceptors continue to impact on inspiratory and expiratory muscles in regulating the depth and rate of breathing. Serum carbon dioxide (CO_2) levels act directly on the medulla, while circulating oxygen (O_2) levels impact indirectly by way of the chemoreceptors in the carotid bodies and aortic arch to regulate serum gas levels (Guyton, 1986).

The lung receives blood supply from both the pulmonary and bronchial circulations. The pulmonary circulation receives all of the cardiac output and provides perfusion to the lungs. The bronchial circulation, on the other hand, receives only 1% to 2% of the cardiac output and perfuses the tracheal and bronchial structures. Communication of both circulations occurs at the junction of the bronchus and alveoli. The significance of this communication is best demonstrated when a pulmonary artery embolism occurs and the distal perfusion is preserved, albeit to a lesser extent, via the bronchial arteries.

As a result of lung transplantation, the bronchial blood supply is lost in the transplanted lung. Early approaches to connecting the airways utilized the tracheal anastomosis, which often resulted in necrosis and dehiscence of the suture line (Veith et al., 1983). Concerns over this complication, sparked attempts at revascularization utilizing omental or other highly vascular tissue to wrap the bronchus or trachea (Cooper et al., 1989; Dubois et al., 1984). In view of better perfusion to the distal segment by the pulmonary circulation, bronchial anastomoses (in conjunction with omental wrap) are now preferred over tracheal anastomosis (Pasque et al., 1990). With this technique, should one anastomosis fail, the patient can still be adequately ventilated, allowing time for emergency measures such as single lung retransplant.

Following transplantation, the combination of the underlying disease process, the degree of intrapulmonary shunting, and amount of interstitial lung water will contribute to the ventilation and perfusion patterns. Close monitoring of daily chest x-rays and periodic perfusion scans provide clinical data regarding the ventilation and perfusion matching in the transplanted lung.

Thoracotomy and removal of the diseased lung disrupts the native lymphatic system. This change impedes the usual drainage pattern of lung water, causing the wet chest x-ray patterns often seen in the early postoperative period (Morrison & Ostrow, 1989). During this time, drainage of lung water occurs by way of the pleural lymphatic system. Usually the donor and recipient lymphatic systems coalesce within 21 to 60 days (LeKander, 1988). Patients may require diuretics to facilitate the loss of lung water.

Secretion clearance is of concern in these patients. Denervation of the transplanted lung causes a change in cilia movement and mucus production. Normally, the epithelial lining of the lower airways has 200 cilia per cell beating 10 to 20 times per second, moving a layer of mucus about 1.0 cm/min toward the upper airways (Guyton, 1986). It is postulated that after transplant there is a change in the rate of cilia movement, and mucus production becomes tenacious. Such changes contribute to the clinical problem associated with secretion clearance. To compound matters, the cough reflex is obliterated in patients with tracheal anastomosis, incidental to the denervation of the donor allograft below the suture line. These areas are new foci for research, and very little literature is now available.

Alteration of Gas Exchange

Alteration in gas exchange is of primary concern. The loss of lymphatic drainage, ischemic time of the donor organ, and impaired secretion clearance may all contribute to poor ventilation and oxygenation. Care must be taken not to inoculate the lower airways when suctioning. The immunosuppressive state predisposes patients to infection. The patient must cough and breathe deeply to expectorate secretions and prevent atelectasis. Positioning and early, progressive exercising will help to mobilize secretions. The presence of crepitus with air leak in the chest tube water seal and/or a significant difference between inspired and expired tidal volumes in the mechanically ventilated patient signals possible airway anastomosis failure. These findings warrant immediate notification of the physician. Hypercapnea is also frequently noted in the postoperative period and is most prevalent in patients with severe preoperative chronic obstructive pulmonary disease (COPD) with CO_2 retention. This occurrence may be related to abnormality in central CO_2 responsiveness and generally normalizes during the ensuing weeks after transplantation.

Alteration of Cardiac Output

Alteration in cardiac output, specifically right ventricular function, is of particular concern in this population. Patients requiring CBP, as discussed above, may experience transient right ventricular dysfunction. Right ventricular function improves significantly after lung transplantation due to afterload reduction. Hypotension should be avoided, as such episodes can lead to ischemia and subsequent stricture or dehiscence of the airway anastomosis.

Alteration in Fluid Balance

Alteration in fluid balance is an important clinical issue, especially in the early postoperative period. The goal is to establish euvolemia to prevent pulmonary edema and promote adequate ventilation and oxygenation. Patients must be weighed daily. This is essential to accurate dosing of medications and provides validation of the intake and output.

Immunosuppression in Lung Transplant Recipient

The goal of immunotherapy is to strike a balance between adequate immunosuppression and maintenance of competent host defenses. This is important because infectious complications following lung transplant are the leading cause of death in this population.

Typically, Cy A and azathioprine are used preoperatively for immunosuppressive induction. These drugs are continued postoperatively in conjunction with a 2-week course of monoclonal (such as OKT3) or polyclonal (such as ALG, RATG) antibody therapy. Steroid use is avoided within the first 2 weeks following transplant to encourage adequate healing of the airway anastomosis. Regardless, usual treatment for rejection episodes is 3 days of pulsed dose methylprednisolone. A moderately high-dose oral steroid is introduced upon completion of monoclonal or polyclonal antibody therapy. The dose of oral steroids is titrated to lower maintenance doses over the ensuing weeks.

OKT3 is usually started on the first postoperative day and given daily thereafter for 10 to 14 days. This monoclonal antibody is specific for the T3 (CD3) complex located on the human T lymphocyte (Cosimi, 1987). Because more often than not the drug is given to an immunocompetent patient with normal CD3 values, a varying clinical response occurs with administration of the first and, sometimes, second doses. Patients may exhibit signs and symptoms of oxygen desaturation, restlessness, meningismus, fever, rigor, impaired gas exchange, and pulmonary edema. In order to prevent pulmonary edema, the patient should be euvolemic prior to first dose administration. The use of adjunctive medications such as methylprednisolone, diphenhydramine HC1, H2 blockers, and acetaminophen for premedication may help decrease the severity of first and second dose reaction.

Potential for Rejection

A diagnosis of rejection in lung transplant patients is based on the combination of clinical presentation, chest x-ray, and histologic findings. It is not unusual for these patients to experience a mild episode of rejection within the first 2 weeks following transplant. These early episodes are most often characterized by oxygen desaturation, decreased exercise tolerance and/or dyspnea, general malaise, and elevated temperature (Toronto Lung Transplant Group, 1988), with radiograph findings of hilar flare and/or new infiltrates (Morrison & Ostrow, 1989). However, episodes of allograft rejection in the later posttransplant period may not be apparent radiographically, and monitoring of pulmonary function tests for air flow obstruction may be beneficial.

In order to differentiate rejection from infection (which may have a similar presentation), the timing of onset of symptoms must be considered. The first episode of rejection generally does not occur before the fifth to seventh day postoperatively, whereas infection may occur at any time. A diagnostic bronchoscopy is performed to obtain bronchoalveolar lavage and transbronchial biopsy (Higenbottam, Steward, Penketh, & Wallwork, 1988). In rejection, histologic tissue examination demonstrates lymphocytic peribronchial infiltration and perivascular cuffing (Halasz et al., 1973). Identification of infectious agents may offer a further explanation as to the cause of developing symptomatology. Finally, empirical diagnosis is made on the basis of response to a pulse dose of methylprednisolone, with worsening of radiographic findings and oxygen requirements in infectious states and rapid amelioration of all findings in rejection (Toronto Lung Transplant Group, 1988). In single lung transplant, nuclear perfusion scanning may be useful in demonstrating reduced flow to the transplanted lung during rejection (Herman et al., 1989).

Potential for rejection can be diminished with proper monitoring and observation. Patient/family teaching is extremely important to decrease anxiety and provide a basis for early detection and treatment. The patient must be well versed in the proper administration of medication, the rationale and importance of these medications and regimens, and when and how to call the transplant team after discharge. Close monitoring of serum Cy A levels, chemistries, and hematologies is necessary to provide accurate dosing of medications and prevent complications. Nurses need to be particularly sensitive to the patient's vague somatic complaints, as these may be the first sign of rejection.

Potential for Infection

Clinical presentation of infection is similar to that of rejection. The patient with respiratory infection additionally presents with leukocytosis, change in sputum production and character, and positive cultures. Prompt identification and treatment of the causative organism is critical. Adjunctive therapy may include oxygen administration and adjustment of the immunosuppressive regimen. Potential for donor-transmitted infections is higher in the lung transplant population. Cultures of donor sputum are generally unavailable at the time of transplant. Donor-acquired bacterial and fungal infections may require treatment retrospectively. Cytomegalovirus (CMV) may be transmitted to serologically negative recipients from positive donors with devastating results. CMV pneumonitis may cause irreversible graft dysfunction in addition to other serious sequelae. Debate rages with regard to the practicality and effectiveness of donor/recipient CMV matching. However, CMV prophylaxis is recommended when matching is deferred (Emmanuel, 1990).

Nurses must be ever mindful of the potential for infection in this therapeutically immunosuppressed patient population. During hospitalization, most centers utilize some type of isolation technique to protect recipients from nosocomial infection. Strict hand washing is the most important and effective defense against this threat. Early detection and notification of any sign of infection and/or subtle somatic symptoms are key to effective treatment.

Other essential nursing care aspects that demand special attention are progressive ambulation, oxygen weaning and pulmonary rehabilitation, relief

NURSING CARE PLAN FOR LUNG TRANSPLANTATION RECIPIENT

Nursing Diagnosis	Expected Outcome	Nursing Interventions

ALTERATION IN GAS EXCHANGE secondary to
   Altered mucocillary
     clearance
   Increased alveolar
     capillary permeability
   Fluid overload
   Altered lymphatic drainage
	Optimal gas exchange and maintenance of respiratory muscle strength	<u>Intubated Patient</u>
		1. Document respiratory setting and keep pleural pressures low.
		2. Monitor for:
		   Air leak in drainage systems and the presence of crepitus on chest wall, neck, arm, and abdomen. Desaturation effects associated with positioning and activity.
		3. Maintain aseptic suctioning techniques.
		<u>Extubated Patient</u>
		1. Instruct/reinforce triflow usage.
		2. Initiate pulmonary rehabilitation prescription while monitoring for desaturation states.

*   *   *   *

Nursing Diagnosis	Expected Outcome	Nursing Interventions

POTENTIAL ALTERATION IN CARDIAC OUTPUT secondary to
   Right or left ventricular dysfunction
   Cardioplegia and cold ischemia
   Elevation in afterload
   Bleeding from vascular anastomosis or pleural surface (secondary to cardiopulmonary bypass heparinization and subsequent coagulopathy) or adhesions from previous surgeries.
	Optimal cardiac function and tissue perfusion	1. Monitor cardiac hemodynamics
		2. Monitor pulmonary pressure, left and right.
		3. Treat hypertension or volume overload with appropriate therapy.
		4. Watch for signs and symptoms of tamponade
		5. Monitor coagulation.

*   *   *   *

(continued)

NURSING CARE PLAN FOR LUNG TRANSPLANTATION RECIPIENT (continued)

Nursing Diagnosis	Expected Outcome	Nursing Interventions
ALTERATION IN FLUID BALANCE secondary to Intake > output Decreased serum oncotic pressure	Patient weight remains within 3–5 lbs of dry weight.	1. Weigh patient every day. 2. Monitor intake and output. 3. Monitor cardiac hemo-dynamics for early signs of right or left ventricular failure. 4. Auscultate chest for pulmon-ary status at the beginning and end of shift and as needed. 5. Assess for pedal edema and periorbital edema. 6. Monitor renal function and electrolyte balance. 7. Administer immunosuppres-sive drugs fluids and diuretics as ordered.
* * * *		
POTENTIAL FOR ALLOGRAFT REJECTION secondary to Immune response Donor HLA	Absence of signs and symptoms of rejection	1. Administer immunosup-pressants and monitor serum levels of drugs and other laboratory tests. Azathioprine (white blood cells (WBC). Cy A (serum level and renal function) OKT3–CD3 levels (or ALG, RATG levels) 2. Monitor for clinical signs of rejection: Observe for elevated temp-erature, fatigue, short-ness of breath, anor-exia, and hypoxemia at rest or with exertion. Be alert to subjective somatic complaints. Provide rationale for bronchoscopy, trans-bronchial biopsy, and broncho alveolar lavage. Teach the patient signs and symptoms of rejection and when to call the physician.

(continued)

NURSING CARE PLAN FOR LUNG TRANSPLANTATION RECIPIENT (continued)

Nursing Diagnosis	Expected Outcome	Nursing Interventions
POTENTIAL FOR INFECTION secondary to Immunosuppression.	No evidence of nosocomial infection	1. Monitor isolation procedures. 2. Suction using aseptic techniques. 3. Culture sputum, urine, and blood as ordered for bacterial and fungal infection. 4. Monitor results of cultures from both recipient and donor to assure that antibiotic coverage is appropriate. 5. Monitor clinical parameters such as WBC with differential, temperature, and serum levels of antibiotics.

LONG-TERM AND FOLLOW-UP CARE

After discharge the patient returns to the transplant clinic for follow-up visits with the transplant pulmonologist. The frequency of clinic visits is dictated by the patient's condition. Graft function is monitored by chest x-ray, spirometry, and physical examination. Changes in any of these may signal rejection or infection and warrant further assessment with arterial blood gas analysis. Differential diagnosis is established by performing flexible fiberoptic bronchoscopy with bronchoalveolar lavage and transbronchial biopsy. Treatment of rejection and infection is described above. Histology of transbronchial biopsy specimens is monitored closely for signs of bronchiolitis obliterans. This uncommon potential posttransplant complication is thought to be the result and manifestation of chronic rejection and may necessitate retransplantation   (Burke et al., 1984; Higenbottam et al., 1988).

Along with pulmonary function, patient's chemistries, hematologies, and drug levels are monitored closely, as with other solid-organ transplant recipients receiving immunosuppression therapy. Pulmonary rehabilitation, which includes progressive ambulation and extremity strengthening several times a week, begins soon after surgery and continues for a period of approximtely 3 months after transplant. Exercise studies are performed periodically during the first year following transplant and then yearly.

Due to chronic immunosuppression and changes in mucociliary clearing capabilities, lung transplant patients are especially susceptible to a wide variety of respiratory infections, including *Pneumocystis carinii* pneumonia. Prophylaxis can be achieved through use of oral trimethoprim and sulfamethoxazole or monthly treatments with nebulized pentamidine. Patients are immunized, postoperatively, against influenza and are taught to be vigilant with regard to exposure to communicable infections.

FUTURE TRENDS

Although lung transplantation has been established as an effective treatment modality for select patients with end-stage lung disease (Stevens, Raffin, & Baldwin, 1989), the future will depend upon increased donor availability, and improved preservation techniques (Cooper et al., 1989; Toronto Lung Group, 1986). In addition, improved immunosuppression, and development of more effective means of detecting rejection are needed.

ACKNOWLEDGEMENT

The authors would like to acknowledge Dr. Paul Waters, Director, and Dr. David Ross, Medical Director, Lung Transplantation, Cedars-Sinai Medical Center, for their support and review of the manuscript.

REFERENCES

Burke, M., Theodore, J., Dawkins, K., Yousen, S., Blank, N., Billingham, M., Kessel, A., Jamieson, S., Oya, P., Baldwin, J., Stinson, E., Shumway, N. & Robin, E. (1984). Posttransplant obliterative bronchiolitis and other late lung sequelae in human heart transplantation. *Chest, 88*, 824–829.

Clark, F., & Von Euler, C. (1972). On the regulation of the depth and rate of breathing. *Journal of Physiology, 222*, 267–295.

Cooper, J., Patterson, A., Grossman, R., Maurer, J., & the Toronto Lung Group. (1989). Double-lung transplant for advanced chronic obstructive lung disease. *American Review of Respiratory Diseases, 139*, 303–307.

Cosimi, A. (1987). Clinical development of orthoclone OKT3. *Transplant Proceedings, 19*, 7-16.

Dubos, P., Choiniere, L., & Cooper, J. (1984). Bronchial omentopexy in canine lung allotransplantation. *Annals of Thoracic Surgery, 38*, 211–214.

Emmanuel, D. (1990). Treatment of cytomegalovirus disease. *Seminars in Hematology, 27*, 22–27.

Green, A., & Claibourne, C. (1989). A nursing challenge: Cytomegalovirus in the transplant recipient. *Focus on Critical Care, 16*, 349–354.

Guyton, A. (1986). Respiration. A. Guyton (Ed.) *Textbook of medical physiology* (7th ed. pp. 466–479). Philadelphia: W. B. Saunders.

Halasz, N., Catanzaro, A., Trummer, M., Tisi, G., Saltzstein, S., & Moser, K. (1973). Transplantation of the lung: Correlation of physiologic immunology and histologic findings. *Journal of Thoracic Cardiovascular Surgery, 66*, 581–587.

Hardy, J., Webb, W., Dalton, M., & Walker, G . (1963). Lung transplantation in man. *Journal of the American Medical Association, 186*, 1065, 1070.

Herman, S., Rappaport, D., Weisbrod, G., Olscamp, G., Pattersen, A., Cooper, J., & the Toronto Lung Group. (1989). Single-lung transplantation imaging features. *Radiology, 170*, 89-93.

Higenbottam, T., Stewart, S., Penketh, A., & Wallwork, J. (1988). Transbronchial lung biopsy for the diagnosis of rejection in heart-lung transplant patients. *Transplantation, 46*, 532–539.

Kriett, J. M., & Kaye, M. P. (1990). The registry of the International Society of Heart Transplantation: Seventh official report—1990. *The Journal of Heart Transplantation, 9*(4), 323–330.

LeKander, B. (1988). Preventing complications for the heart and lung transplant recipient. *Dimensions in Critical Care Nursing, 7*, 18–27.

Lima, O., Cooper, D., Peters, W., Ayaba, H., Townsend, E., Luke, S., & Goldberg, M. (1981). Effects of methylprednisolone and azathioprine on bronchial healing following lung autotransplantation. *Journal of Thoracic Cardiovascular Surgery, 82*, 211–215.

Malen, J., & Boychuck, J. (1989). Nursing perspective on lung transplantation. *Critical Care Clinics of North America, 1*, 707–727.

Metras, H. (1950). Note preliminaire sur la graffe. Totale du pouman chez le chien. *French Academie Science, 3*, 1176–1177.

Morrison, N., & Ostrow, D. (1989). Evaluating pulmonary infiltrates in immunocompromised patients. *Journal of Respiratory Disease, 10*, 37–51.

Murray, J. (1986). Lymphatic and nervous system. In J. Murray (Ed.), *The normal lung* (pp. 61–82). Philadelphia: W. B. Saunders.

Pasque, M., Cooper, J., Kaiser, L., Haydock, D., Triantafillon, A., & Trulock, E. (1990). Improved technique for bilateral lung transplantation: Rationale and initial clinical experience. *Annals of Thoracic Surgery, 49B*, 785–791.

Richardson, J. (1979). Nerve supply to the lungs. *American Review of Respiratory Disease, 119*, 784–802.

Schreinemaker, H., Weder, W., Miyoshi, S., Harper, B., Shimokawa, S., Egan, T., McKnight, R., & Corper, J. (1990). Direct revascularization of bronchial arteries for lung transplantation: An anatomical study. *Annals of Thoracic Surgery, 49*, 41–54.

Starkey, T., Sakakibara, N., Hagberg., R., Tazelaar, H., Baldwin, J., & Jamieson, S. (1986). Successful six hour cardiopulmonary preservation with simple hypothermic crystalloid flush. *Journal of Heart Transplantation*, 291–297.

Stevens, J., Raffin, T., & Baldwin, J. (1989). The status of transplantation of the human lung. *Surgery, Gynecology and Obstetrics, 169*, 179–185.

The Toronto Lung Group. (1986). Lung tansplantation for pulmonary fibrosis. *New England Journal of Medicine, 314*, 1140-1145.

The Toronto Lung Transplant Group. (1988). Experience with single-lung transplantation for pulmonary fibrosis. *Journal of the American Medical Association, 259,* 2258–2262.

Vieth, F., Montefusco, C., Kamholz, S., & Mollenkopf, F. (1983). Lung transplantation. *Heart Transplantation, 2,* 155–164.

Widdicombe, J., & Sterling, G. (1970). The autonomic nervous system and breathing. *Archives of Internal Medicine, 126,* 311–329

Zenati, M., Dawling, R., Aritage, J., Kormos, R., Dummen, J., Hardesty, R., & Griffith, B. (1989). Organ procurement for pulmonary transplantation. *Annals of Thoracic Surgery, 48,* 882–886.

CHAPTER 7

LIVER TRANSPLANTATION

Vicki L. Fioravanti

The first successful human orthotopic liver transplant was performed in March 1963 by Thomas E. Starzl, MD, with limited clinical trials continuing through the 1970s (Starzl et al., 1982). With the advent of a new immunosuppressive drug in 1980, cyclosporine A, and refined surgical technique, the number of patients undergoing liver replacement has increased dramatically. Worldwide, approximately 1,000 patients per year undergo liver transplantation with 85% of adult recipients returning to active productive lives (Sebesin & Williams, 1987). This chapter will discuss the indications for liver transplantation, the evaluation process, and the nursing implications of caring for a patient undergoing liver replacement.

INDICATIONS FOR LIVER TRANSPLANTATION

Patients who are referred for liver transplantation suffer from various types of end-stage liver disease that may be due to a chronic illness with a long protracted course, or to an acute illness such as fulminant hepatic failure. All other accepted means of medical management have been exhausted and liver replacement is the only hope for long-term survival.

In adults, the leading indication for transplantation is cirrhosis (Gordon et al., 1987). This may be due to a variety of causes including, but not limited to, chronic active hepatitis, primary and secondary biliary cirrhosis, Laennec's (alcoholic) cirrhosis or postnecrotic cirrhosis (cirrhosis secondary to viral, autoimmune, or cryptogenic mechanisms). See Table 7.1 for a complete list of indications for transplantation.

TABLE 7.1 Indications for Liver Transplantation

Cirrhosis
  Chronic active hepatitis
  Primary biliary cirrhosis
  Secondary biliary cirrhosis
  Laennec's cirrhosis

Metabolic diseases
  Wilson's disease
  Alpha-1-antitrypsin deficiency
  Hemochromatosis

Sclerosing cholangitis

Vascular disorders
  Budd-Chiari syndrome.
  Veno-occlusive disease

Fulminant disease
  Viral
  Drug induced
  Hepatitis B

THE EVALUATION PROCESS

The evaluation period is a necessary and crucial phase of the transplant process. The medical staff must judge the suitability, urgency, and degree of risk for each patient. It is also a time for preoperative teaching of both the patient and family members.

Each transplant program develops its own evaluation protocol; however, the goals are the same for each. The first major goal is to determine and/or confirm the specific pathologic process and to determine the severity of hepatic illness. This is accomplished by reviewing the patient's past medical history and any procedures, pathology, and laboratory studies performed by the referring institution and supplementing these studies as necessary.

The second goal is to correct any metabolic abnormalities. The patient suffering from hepatic encephalopathy may require adjustment of medications or diet. Because the liver synthesizes fibrinogen and pro-thrombin (essential for blood clotting) and is responsible for vitamin K storage, patients with end-stage liver disease may require vitamin K replacement and/or transfusions of fresh frozen plasma to prevent hemorrhage. Patients with end-stage liver disease develop massive ascites due to obstruction of flow in the vena cava or portal vein, disturbance in electrolyte balance, or depletion of plasma proteins necessitating diuretic therapy and often intravenous salt-poor albumin. This type of medical management requires close observation of the patient's body weight, electrolyte profile, and renal function.

The third goal of the evaluation process is to determine suitability for transplantation, both physically and psychologically. Abdominal ultrasound is performed to identify the hepatic vessels and their patency along with abdominal computer-aided tomography (CT) scan for calculation of liver volume. Various other laboratory and radiologic studies are performed, and appropriate consultations are obtained. The consultants may include anesthesiologists, cardiologists, pulmonologists, endocrinologists, and nutritionists.

With the rapid development and refinement of liver transplantation, the list of absolute contraindications to transplantation has gradually decreased, and many variables are now considered relative contraindications. Table 7.2 lists contraindications for liver transplantation.

In addition to the physical evaluation, social and psychological evaluations are also performed. A transplant social worker assesses the patient's and family's ability to cope with transplantation. Potential candidates may also be referred for psychiatic evaluation if indicated. With the exception of those patients with liver disease secondary to alcohol abuse, psychiatric referrals are often made on a case-by-case basis. Such referrals are usually required for patients with Laennec's (alcoholic) cirrhosis as well as commitment to an alcohol rehabilitation program.

Preoperative teaching of patients and families is initiated during the evaluation process. Frequently, patients are given so much information during the evaluation that it is extremely difficult for them to remember it all (especially if patients have any degree of encephalopathy). Therefore, the information must be reinforced repeatedly during the waiting period.

TABLE 7.2   Contraindications for Liver Transplantation

Absolute
  Extrahepatic malignancy
  Sepsis outside the hepatobiliary system
  Multisystem disease that would preclude surgery or sharply reduce potential for
    long-term survival
  Active use of hepatotoxic drugs
  HIV-antibody-positive serology

Relative
  History of alcohol abuse or active alcohol abuse
  Portal vein thrombosis
  Hepatitis B surface antigen positivity
  Age greater than 60 years
  Advanced chronic renal disease
  Prior portacaval shunting procedure
  Prior complex hepatobiliary surgery

Patients are taught what to expect during the immediate postoperative period and long-term. If possible, they tour the intensive care unit (ICU) to familiarize themselves with the unit and meet some of the nurses who may be caring for them after surgery. They are also given the opportunity to meet other transplant patients who are in the recovery phase.

Various medications and potential posttransplant complications are discussed in detail with the entire family. This includes the need for long-term immunosuppressive therapy and its adverse effects, potential surgical complications, possibility of rejection, and long-term outlook. Questions and expression of concerns are encouraged and addressed appropriately.

The information obtained during the pretransplant evaluation is compiled by the hepatologist and presented to the entire transplant team at a weekly conference. (See Table 7.3 for evaluation protocol.) This conference is usually attended by transplant surgeons, hepatologists, nurse coordinators, social workers, dietitians, psychiatrists, financial counselors, and any interested nursing staff. A patient may be accepted or rejected for liver transplantation based on the information available. The results of the evaluation and the decision reached at the transplant conference are then forwarded to the referring physician. Patients who are accepted as candidates are placed on the transplant list to await a suitable organ donor.

TABLE 7.3   Liver Transplantation Evaluation Protocol

1. History and physical examination with particular attention to the gastrointestinal system.
2. Consultations:
   Gastroenterologist, transplant coordinator, transplant surgeon, anesthesiologist, cardiologist, psychiatrist (when indicated), social worker, dietitian, dentist, and hospital finance representative.
3. Diagnostic tests:
   ECG, chest x-ray, portal vein sonogram and Doppler, CT scan of abdomen. Further testing as indicated, e.g., CT scan of head, EEG, flexible sigmoidoscopy/colonoscopy, upper gastrointestinal endoscopy, pulmonary function studies, angiography, echocardiogram, magnetic resonance imaging, liver biopsy, nuclear medicine scan, bone densitometry
4. Laboratory tests:
   Liver function studies, chemistry and hematologic screens, coagulation factors, renal workup, blood cultures, urine, sputum and blood typing with antibody screen.
5. Optional tests as indicated: abdominal paracentesis, skin tests.

Note: If test results are abnormal, further tests/procedures may be necessary.

THE RECIPIENT OPERATION

A bilateral subcostal or midline incision with right chest extension is used most commonly to provide maximum surgical exposure (Makowka et al., 1988) (see Figure 7.1). The native hepatectomy can be the most difficult phase of transplantation. Previous abdominal surgeries, coagulopathy, and the presence of portal hypertension can make this a tedious procedure with high potential for hemorrhage.

The liver hilum is carefully dissected, and the hepatic artery, portal vein, and supra- and infrahepatic vena cava are clamped, in that order, and the liver is removed. Clamping of the vena cava can cause acidosis, bleeding, swelling of the intestines, and renal congestion. In adults and selected pediatric recipients, many of these problems have been avoided by the use of veno-venous bypass (Shaw, Martin, & Marquez, 1984). Large-bore cannulae are inserted into the axillary and femoral veins. Blood is drained from the infrahepatic vena cava through a nonheparinized biopump and returned to the heart via the axillary vein, thereby decompressing the intestinal tract and kidneys. This also makes anesthetic management of the patient easier secondary to maintenance of good cardiac output (Makowka et al., 1988).

The donor liver is inspected in the operating room and prepared for implantation. The supra- and infrahepatic vena cava are anastomosed, followed by the portal vein, thereby establishing blood flow to the graft. Finally the hepatic artery is anastomosed, followed by biliary reconstruction.

There are two types of biliary reconstruction that may be performed. When the bile duct is of suitable size (and not damaged by the recipient's disease), a duct-to-duct anastomosis (choledochocholedochostomy) is performed. A T-tube is placed to prevent strictures at the anastomotic site and brought out through the skin. An alternative method for biliary reconstruction is a Roux-

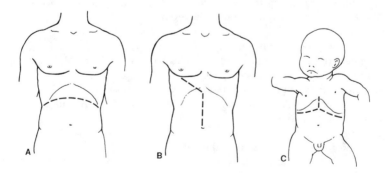

FIGURE 7.1 **Three types of incisions used in liver transplantation: (A) bilateral subcostal incision, (B) midline incision with right chest extension, and (C) bilateral subcostal incision with midline extension (Mercedes Benz incision). Drawing by Bayard Colyear, medical illustrator.**

en-Y choledochojejunostomy. The donor bile duct is connected to a Roux limb devised of proximal jejunum (Figure 7.2).

Finally, three Jackson-Pratt drains are placed in the abdomen and the incision is closed. The entire surgical procedure may last from 8 to 24 hours with an average of 12 hours.

POSTOPERATIVE NURSING CARE IN THE ICU

Immediately following liver transplantation, the patient is admitted to the ICU. A variety of invasive tubes and lines are necessary to support both functions for a period of time. An endotracheal tube, orally placed, is connected to a ventilator for respiratory support. A nasogastric tube is placed and connected to intermittent low suction. Hemodynamic monitoring is accomplished via arterial and central venous pressure lines. A Swan-Ganz catheter may be used to monitor pulmonary artery and pulmonary capillary wedge pressures. An arterial line is usually placed in one of the upper extremities; central venous pressure lines may be placed in external jugular or subclavian sites. Multiple peripheral venous catheters are placed in other areas of the upper extremities for volume support and emergency access.

The large abdominal incision is usually closed with staples and covered with a sterile gauze dressing. Jackson-Pratt drains are placed in the peritoneum

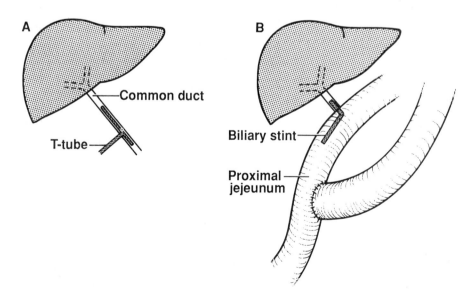

FIGURE 7.2 Two types of biliary reconstruction used in liver transplantation: (A) end-to-end choledochocholedochostomy, and (B) Roux-en-Y choledocho-jejunostomy. Drawing by Bayard Colyear, medical illustrator.

and under the liver intraoperatively (Makowka et al., 1988). Two drains are placed on the right side; one is placed on the left side. These drains are attached to bulb suction. If an end-to-end biliary reconstruction is performed, the T-tube is connected to an external bile bag. A urinary drainage catheter is connected to an hourly gravity collection system.

One hour is usually required to admit the patient, receive the report and perform preliminary nursing assessments. Laboratory studies, consisting of an electrolyte panel, clotting studies, and liver function tests (i.e, SGOT, SGPT, GGT, bilirubin, etc.) are performed every 4 to 6 hours. Arterial blood gases are performed frequently also.

Immunosuppressive therapy may be initiated perioperatively. The patient is usually given methylprednisolone after revascularization of the liver, and it is continued as a single daily dose. Cyclosporine A (Cy A) is given intravenously during the early postoperative period, usually in divided doses (either bid or tid). Once gastrointestinal motility has been established, a daily oral dose in two divided doses is started, overlapping with the intravenous dose. Daily trough levels are monitored, the intravenous dose weaned, and the oral dose adjusted to assure adequate blood levels (Gugenheim, Samuel, Saliba, Castaina, & Bismuth, 1988).

During the first 24 hours after liver transplantation, there are several important nursing diagnoses: potential for infection, alteration in pulmonary and cardiovascular function.

Potential for Infection

Infection is a major postoperative threat to the immunosuppressed patient. The patient is not placed in isolation following surgery; however, patients presenting preoperatively with active hepatitis may be isolated. Usually, only good handwashing is enforced, and sterile technique is utilized for all procedures.

Common sites for infection are the liver, bile ducts, T-tube site, surgical incision, invasive lines, drainage tubes, urinary tract, and lungs. Prophylactic coverage with broad-spectrum antibiotics is often begun preoperatively and is continued for 48 to 72 hours to prevent opportunistic infections. In addition, respiratory treatments with aerosolized pentamidine may be initiated for prophylaxis against (*Pneumocystitis carinii*) pneumonia. Prophylaxis usually continues throughout the hospital stay. At the time of discharge, prophylactic therapy may be changed to trimethoprim/sulfa, single strength, daily. The transplanted patient is vulnerable to wound infections from bacteria such as *Pseudomonas*, and *Escherichia coli*, or fungi such as *Aspergillus* species. Fungal infections in the mouth or peritoneum and systemic bacterial and viral infections may also occur (Kusne et al., 1988).

Continuous nursing assessment for signs of infection is very important. Vital signs are monitored frequently in the ICU and regularly on the general nursing unit. The mucous membranes of the mouth are inspected daily, and prophylactic nystatin may be used following oral care four times a day. Viral (cytomegalovirus, Epstein-Barr virus) and bacterial blood cultures are obtained for all fevers greater than 38.5°C, as well as urine, sputum, wound, and drainage tube cultures. Fever is investigated aggressively and thoroughly. Skin integrity is maintained by lotions, repositioning, and massaging of bony prominences. As early as the second postoperative day, most patients are out of bed, and sitting in a chair. As soon as possible, physical therapists and occupational therapists are consulted to begin range-of-motion and strengthening exercises.

Incisions and invasive lines are inspected frequently for inflammation or infection. The abdominal dressing is removed the second or third postoperative day, and the incision is exposed to air to promote healing. All invasive line dressings are changed daily. The sites are cleansed according to each hospital's standards of care, and a sterile occlusive dressing is applied. The Jackson-Pratt bulbs and biliary drainage bag are emptied every 2 to 4 hours. Insertion sites are cleansed every shift and new dressings applied. Urinary catheter care is provided every 4 to 8 hours.

Alteration in Pulmonary Function

Stasis of pulmonary secretions that may lead to respiratory complications is prevalent secondary to prolonged anesthesia, the large abdominal incision, immobility, and atelectasis. The patient's pulmonary status is evaluated frequently following ICU admission. As the patient regains consciousness, adjustments in the FIO_2, tidal volume, rate, and positive end-expiratory pressure (PEEP) are based on arterial blood gas analysis. Extubation is usually accomplished within 24 to 48 hours.

Even a limited degree of atelectasis can lead to pneumonia in the immunosuppressed patient. Aggressive pulmonary toilet is instituted immediately postoperatively. While intubated, the patient is suctioned every 2 hours and prn. Once extubation is accomplished, and throughout the postoperative period, incentive spirometry and coughing/deep breathing exercises are instituted. Vigorous chest physiotherapy and postural drainage are performed. Early ambulation and aggressive pulmonary toilet are keys to prevention of respiratory complications in the liver recipient.

Alteration in Cardiovascular Function

Alteration in cardiac output can be life threatening. The primary focus of care is adequate perfusion of body organs, especially the transplanted liver. Nursing assessment of tissue perfusion is made by evaluation of capillary refill, color of mucous membranes and extremities, and the presence of peripheral pulses. Normothermia is maintained with warming blankets and heat lamps to prevent vasoconstriction and decreased perfusion of the transplanted liver.

Continuous assessment of the patient's hemodynamic status is necessary. Surgical hemorrhage most frequently occurs within the first 48 hours postoperatively. Hypotension, decreasing hematocrit, evidence of frank blood or an increase in the amount of blood-tinged sanguinous fluid in the Jackson-Pratt drains, or expanding abdominal girth may all be indicative of hemorrhage. If hypotension is not corrected with volume replacement (crystalloids and blood products), temporary vasopressor support with dopamine or dobutamine may be required until surgical intervention can be accomplished.

Hypertension is commonly seen immediately after transplant and throughout the postoperative period. It usually resolves by 6 months postoperatively. The exact etiology is unclear, but it is thought to be secondary to steroid or Cy A therapy (Dindzans, Schade, & Van Thiel, 1988). It is treated with drug therapy that may include one or more drugs. Hypertension must be brought under control for prevention of intracranial hemorrhage, seizures, and renal complications.

Fluid and Electrolyte Disturbances

The balancing of fluid and electrolytes is a postoperative problem that may be difficult to solve. Hypokalemia and hyperkalemia may be seen after surgery due to the expanded extra-cellular fluid volume. Hypokalemia can occur early in the postoperative period when potassium is drawn back into the well-functioning transplanted liver. Hyperkalemia can occur from graft necrosis causing the release of potassium from the liver cells. Therefore, additional potassium is rarely added to intravenous solutions. Later in the postoperative period, hyperkalemia may occur secondary to cyclosporine-induced nephrotoxicity. This is treated with sodium polystyrene sulfonate, given either orally or rectally, and adjustments in the Cy A therapy.

Potential for Renal Dysfunction

Patients may experience kidney dysfunction after liver transplantation. Strict intake and output is evaluated hourly in the ICU. In addition, patients are weighed daily, and abdominal girths may be obtained. Blood urea nitrogen,(BUN) and serum creatinine levels are monitored daily to assess renal function. Patients with poor kidney function at time of transplantation may be unable to tolerate conventional doses of Cy A. Therefore, the dose of Cy A may be sharply reduced or withheld altogether, and an antilymphocyte-antibody preparation may be given instead. OKT3 monoclonal antibody and Minnesota antilymphocyte globulin are the most frequently used preparations. On occasion, hemodialysis may be instituted until the kidneys recover.

If no unusual postoperative complications occur, the patient is usually transferred to the general nursing unit on the third or fourth postoperative day.

NURSING CARE ON THE GENERAL NURSING UNIT

Before transfer from the ICU, the majority of intravenous lines, monitoring devices, etc. have been removed. The patient usually still has a peripheral intravenous line, subclavian catheter, T-tube with biliary drainage bag, Jackson-Pratt drains and, occasionally, a nasogastric tube. The patient is excited and pleased to be "going to the floor," as this is indicative of a giant leap forward in the recovery process.

Four major diagnoses are important for the nurse caring for the recovering liver transplant patient: (a) potential infection related to altered immune response, (b) potential rejection of the transplanted liver related to physiologic processes, (c) potential surgical complications related to biliary and arterial obstruction, and (d) knowledge deficit regarding drug therapy and altered life-style. Each goal will be examined separately. For further explanations of nursing interventions, see the liver transplation nursing care plan at the end of this chapter.

Infection

For the liver transplant patient, infection is one of the most worrisome postoperative complications, even more so than rejection. As a final measure, rejection can be treated with retransplantation, but infection in the immunosuppressed patient can be lethal.

The nurse continuously assesses the patient for signs and symptoms of infection. Vital signs are taken every 4 hours, and temperature elevations are reported to the physician. As in the ICU, fevers are aggressively evaluated with cultures from peripheral blood, subclavian lines, and any drains or catheters that remain, as well as throat, urine, and sputum cultures. The specimens are sent for viral and bacterial cultures. Chest x-rays are obtained, and if the fever is accompanied by headache, lumbar puncture is performed. Frequently, the patient is begun on broad-spectrum antibiotic coverage until the culture results are available.

Approximately 20% of liver transplant recipients develop pulmonary difficulties; therefore, the prevention of respiratory complications continues after the patient is transferred from the ICU (Wood, Shaw, & Starzl, 1985). With a large abdominal incision, the patient is reluctant to cough, deep-breathe, and ambulate. Incentive spirometry is used, and ambulation is aggressively enforced. Each shift the nurse evaluates for rales, rhonchi, and other adventitious sounds by auscultating the patient's lung fields. Any change in respiratory status is reported to the physician.

The nurse observes all incision sites every shift for signs of redness, swelling, or purulent drainage. The veno-venous bypass sites in the groin and axillae should not be overlooked. Because of the number of lymphatic vessels in the area of the axillary and saphenous veins, lymphoceles may occur. The lymphoceles eventually resolve; however, percutaneous drainage is often necessary.

Good oral hygiene is encouraged, and the mouth is inspected every shift. Patients may be placed on nystatin oral suspension for prophylaxis against oral candidiasis. Patients may also be placed on prophylactic acyclovir to prevent herpes infections, and as mentioned earlier, aerosolized pentamidine may be used to prevent *pneumocystis carinii* pneumonia. If renal function is adequate, the patient may take trimethoprim/sulfa upon discharge. With increased serum creatinine levels, the patient may continue to receive pentamidine treatments on an outpatient basis.

Rejection

Rejection of the transplanted liver can occur at any time during the postoperative period. Laboratory studies consisting of complete blood count, electrolyte panel, BUN, serum creatinine, and liver function studies (bilirubin-total and direct-SGOT, SGPT, alkaline phosphatase, and gamma-GTP) are performed frequently. In addition, cyclosporine trough levels are obtained daily. Frequently, rejection will manifest itself by a slight rise in the serum transaminase and may be accompanied by a low grade fever and a feeling of general malaise.

Abdominal ultrasound or cholangiogram may be performed to differentiate rejection from other possible problems such as vascular or biliary complications. Definitive diagnosis of rejection is made by percutaneous liver biopsy.

Liver biopsy, although a relatively safe procedure, is not without potential complications, including intraperitoneal hemorrhage, pneumothorax, hemothorax, intrahepatic or subcapsular hematoma, and bacteremia. The procedure is performed in the patient's room or treatment room. Using sterile technique, a local anesthetic is given, and using a Menghini-type needle, a small piece of tissue is obtained and sent to the pathology department for microscopic examination.

After the liver biopsy, the nurse observes the patient for signs of respiratory distress or severe abdominal pain. Vital signs are monitored frequently and hemoglobin and hematocrit readings are obtained 6 hours postprocedure. (See Table 7.4.)

Initial treatment for rejection frequently consists of giving a "pulse" of high-dose steroids, usually 1 g of methylprednisolone or hydrocortisone sodium succinate as a one-time drug (Nery et al., 1988). With a large dose, the

TABLE 7.4 Example of Postoperative Liver Biopsy Orders

1. Vital signs:
    q 15 minutes x 4, then
    q 30 minutes x 4, then
    q 60 minutes x 3, then
    q 4 hours until morning.

2. Hemoglobin and hematocrit in 6 hrs.

3. Contact Dr._____ for change in vital signs:
    Systolic blood pressure <100 mmHg
    Pulse >120 bpm
    Severe abdominal pain
    Decreased hemoglobin or hematocrit
    Acute respiratory distress

4. Patient to lie on right side with pressure dressing applied to biopsy
   site for 2 hrs. Patient may then lie supine with head elevated 30° × 4 hrs.

5. Resume pre-liver-biopsy diet orders.

---

drug should be given as an intravenous infusion in 50 cc of 5% dextrose over 30 to 40 minutes. Following the steroid pulse, the patient may be given a "taper" or "recycle" of steroids. The following is an example of a steroid (prednisone) recycle for adults:

Day 1: 200 mg (50 mg q6h)
Day 2: 160 mg (40 mg q6h)
Day 3: 120 mg (30 mg q6h)
Day 4: 80 mg (40 mg q12h)
Day 5: 40 mg (20 mg q12h)
(Thereafter: Baseline: 20 mg qd)

Recalcitrant rejection is usually treated with an antilymphocyte preparation, usually OKT3, a monoclonal antibody. The usual dose of OKT3, is 5 mg given intravenously once daily for a total of 10 to 14 days (Nery et al., 1988). Drug side effects include fever, malaise, nausea, headaches, and arthralgias. Premedication with steroids and antihistamines are given for the first several days of therapy, when these side effects are most common.

The first rejection episode is an extremely anxious time for the patient. Even though patients are taught preoperatively to expect at least one episode of rejection, they are still surprised and frightened when it occurs. They need the nurses' support and reassurance during this time. The nurse encourages the patient to express fears and concerns and to verbalize questions. All procedures, drugs, and test results are explained carefully and at a level appropriate for that particular patient. Rejection does not automatically indicate retransplantation, but when rejection does not respond to medical therapy, the patient must be prepared for that possibility.

Technical Complications

Technical complications after liver transplantation stem from the vascular and biliary anastomoses. Vascular complications include thrombosis and stenosis of the portal vein and hepatic artery thrombosis. Two types of biliary complications appear in the liver transplant patient: bile leaks and biliary tract obstruction (Koneru et al., 1988).

Vascular Problems

Portal Vein Thrombosis Although rarely seen (Wozney, Zajko, Bron, & Starzl, 1986), portal vein thrombosis early in the postoperative period has life-threatening consequences (Lerut et al., 1987). It usually results in severe graft dysfunction, and in patients with preexisting esophageal varices, bleeding may occur. Diagnosis is made with angiography, and emergency portal vein thrombectomy is indicated (Koneru et al., 1988).

Hepatic Artery Thrombosis Hepatic artery thrombosis is the second most common serious surgical complication (after hemorrhage) following liver transplantation (Koneru et al., 1988). Clinical manifestations range from septic shock due to massive hepatic necrosis to being essentially asymptomatic. For patients who develop massive necrosis, the only chance for survival is emergency retransplantation.

Because the intrahepatic biliary tree is supplied by branches of the hepatic artery, the biliary system is also at risk when hepatic artery thrombosis occurs. Frequently, the patient will present with a clinical picture of biliary sepsis. Diagnosis of hepatic artery thrombosis is made by Doppler ultrasound and/or angiography. Once acute systemic sepsis is controlled, patients face the potential complications of intrahepatic biliary strictures and recurrent cholangitis necessitating chronic antibiotic therapy.

Biliary Tract Problems

Bile Leak Nurses caring for liver transplant patients should be alert to signs and symptoms that may indicate complications of the biliary tract. With a choledochocholedochostomy reconstruction, bile leaks can occur at the anastomosis site or at the point of exit of the T-tube from the common hepatic duct (Koneru et al., 1988). Clinical manifestations of bile leaks may include one or more of the following: fever, abdominal pain, bilious drainage, leukocytosis, and rising serum bilirubin, alkaline phosphatase, and gamma-GTP. Diagnosis is confirmed by T-tube cholangiogram, and the only treatment is surgical intervention.

Those patients whose biliary reconstruction was a choledochojejunostomy are subject to bile leak at the biliary-enteric anastomosis. Unfortunately, there is no easy access to the biliary tree via T-tube. The diagnosis of bile leak is made on the basis of clinical manifestations and percutaneous transhepatic cholangiogram such as those mentioned in the preceeding paragraph (Zajko, Zemel et al., 1988).

Bile leaks may also occur late in the postoperative course in the patient with a T-tube. The T-tube is usually left in place until 3 to 6 months after surgery, at which time it is removed in the physician's office. On occasion, removal of the tube can create a small leak at the insertion site. Again, this is manifested by severe abdominal pain and fever. The patient is immediately readmitted to the hospital for surgical repair.

Obstruction Biliary tract obstruction is a complication that may occur later in the postoperative period (Koneru et al., 1988). The patient may present with acute bacterial cholangitis (fever, chills, abdominal pain, jaundice), recurrent episodes of low-grade fever, or a gradual increase in serum transaminase with no associated symptoms. Diagnosis is made by ultrasonography and cholangiogram. The obstruction is usually secondary to an anastomotic narrowing, multiple intrahepatic strictures (usually associated with hepatic artery thrombosis), or obstruction due to a T-tube or internal stent (Koneru et al., 1988). In the case of obstruction from the tube, the tube is simply removed. Obstruction due to strictures at the anastomosis is treated with percutaneous balloon dilatation (Zajko, Campbell et al., 1988).

Discharge Teaching

Discharge planning and teaching begins when the patient arrives from the ICU. Prior to release from the hospital, a patient must be able to name each medication, take the proper dose, and state the frequency, purpose, and side effects for each drug. In addition, each patient is given a teaching tool in booklet form that reviews the signs and symptoms of rejection and infection, medications, wound care, and follow-up clinic visits. The staff nurse and transplant coordinator review the booklet with the patient. The patient's family is encouraged to review it and ask questions.

LIVER TRANSPLANTATION NURSING CARE PLAN

Nursing Diagnoses	Expected Outcome	Nursing Interventions
POTENTIAL FOR INFECTION secondary to immune response	Patient will remain afebrile.	1. Inspect all drainage tube and invasive line sites each shift for signs of infection. 2. Collect specimens from drainage tubes using sterile technique. 3. Assess mouth each shift for white patches, which may be indicative of oral candidiasis. 4. Assess breath sounds each shift for rales, rhonchi. 5. Encourage coughing and deep breathing, incentive spirometry. 6. Monitor vital signs every 4 hr. 7. Enforce universal precautions and good handwashing techniques.
	* * * *	
POTENTIAL FOR REJECTION of transplant secondary to patient's immune response.	Patient will not reject transplanted liver.	1. Monitor liver function studies (bilirubin, SGOT, SGPT, AP, GGTP) frequently. 2. Assess bile for color, quantity, consistency each shift. 3. If no T-tube, monitor stool color for presence of bile. 4. Monitor vital signs.
	* * * *	
ALTERATIONS IN NUTRITION secondary to increased caloric needs.	Patient will receive adequate nutrition to meet caloric needs.	1. Administer TPN/ nasogastric tube feedings as ordered. 2. Perform calorie counts. 3. Encourage family to bring foods from home. 4. Seek dietary consultation
	* * * *	

(continued)

LIVER TRANSPLANTATION NURSING CARE PLAN
(continued)

Nursing Diagnoses	Expected Outcome	Nursing Interventions
KNOWLEDGE DEFICIT of health care maintenance after discharge	Patient will demonstrate knowledge of health care maintenance. Patient will demonstrate wound care and care of T-tube. Patient will verbalize appropriate reporting mechanisms for any difficulties that may occur.	1. Begin discharge teaching based on patient's motivation to learn. 2. Teach patient and family about medication administration, signs and symptoms of infection, rejection and wound care.

The patient assumes responsibility for self-care. Frequently, patients may attempt to make their spouses primarily responsible for their care. This is not acceptable and should be discouraged because a major goal in transplantation is to return the patient to a self-sufficient and active life.

Because of the high incidence of hypertension following liver transplantation, all patients learn to take their own blood pressure, and they learn the parameters for which they should call the physician or nurse. A self-use digital sphygmomanometer is appropriate for patient use, and patients are therefore not dependent on others to take their blood pressure.

During the first postoperative year, immunosuppressive therapy is maintained at relatively high levels, placing the patient at increased risk for various types of infections. Therefore, patients are taught to report immediately such signs and symptoms of infection as diarrhea, vomiting, shortness of breath, cough, fever above 38.5°C, and flulike symptoms. Although patients should not view themselves as fragile, they should not become complacent and overlook any potential problems. Symptoms should be aggressively evaluated, and appropriate therapy should be instituted.

After discharge, patients are usually seen in the transplant center twice weekly. Complete blood chemistries are obtained, including cyclosporine trough levels. The physician examines patients for any late complications and makes necessary adjustments in their medical regimens.

LONG-TERM FOLLOW-UP

As patients continue to do well, the frequency of laboratory tests is decreased. However, because the possibility of rejection remains, the patient's liver function is usually evaluated at least every 6 weeks. Late rejection episodes are treated with immunosuppressive dosages similar to those administered in the early postoperative period.

Patients are encouraged to return to work as soon as they are physically able. Limited restrictions are placed on physical activity during the first year (no contact sports, water skiing, etc.). Return to a normal life-style is an important goal for patients who have had liver transplantation.

Patients undergo a more extensive evaluation on a yearly basis. A complete physical examination is performed, as well as biochemical studies, and the transplanted organ is evaluated by ultrasonography. Although adjustments in immunosuppressive therapy are made throughout the follow-up period, many of the physical side effects of drug therapy can only be appreciated on a "face-to-face" basis. The follow-up visit allows the transplant team to make further adjustments in medications if indicated.

REFERENCES

Dindzans, V., Schade, R., & Van Thiel, D. H. (1988). Medical problems before and after transplantation. *GI Clinics of North America. 17,* 19–31.

Gordon, R. D., Iwatsuki, S., Esquivel, C. O., Makowka, L., Todo, S., Tzakis, A., Marsh, J. W., & Starzl, T. E. (1987). Progress in liver transplantation. *Advances in Surgery, 21,* 49–64.

Gugenheim, J., Samuel, D., Saliba, F., Castaina, D., & Bismuth, H. (1988). Use of cyclosporine A in combination with low dose corticosteroids and azathioprine in liver transplant. *Transplantation Proceedings, 20,* 366–368.

Koneru, B., Tzakis, A. G., Bowman, J., Cassavilla, A., Zajko, A., Starzl, T. E., & Ho, M. (1988). Postoperative surgical complications. *GI Clinics of North America, 17,* 71–92.

Kusne, S., Dummer, J. S., Singh, N., Makowka, L., Esquivel, C., Starzl, T. E., & Ho, M. (1988). Fungal infections after liver transplantation. *Transplantation Proceedings, 20,* 650–651.

Lerut, J., Tzakis, A. G., Bron, K., Gordon, R. D., Iwatsuki, S., Esquivel, C., Makowka, L., Todo, S., & Starzl, T. E. (1987). Complications of venous reconstruction in human orthotopic liver transplantation. *Annals of Surgery, 205,* 404–415.

Makowka, L., Steiber, A., Sher, L., Kahn, D., Mieles, L., Bowman, J., & Starzl, T. E. (1988). Surgical technique for orthotopic liver transplantation. *GI Clinics of North America, 17,* 33–51.

Nery, J., Klintmalm, G., Olson, L., Neely, S., Rippert, L., Gonwa, T., & Husber, B. (1988). Incidence and outcome of acute rejection in liver transplantation. *Transplantation Proceedings, 20,* 375–377.

Sebesin, S. M., & Williams, J. W. (1987). Status of liver transplantation. *Hospital Practice, 22,* 75–86.

Shaw, B. W., Jr., Martin, D. J.,& Marquez, J. M. (1984). Venous bypass in clinical liver transplantation. *Annals of Surgery, 200,* 524–534.

Starzl, T. E., Iwatsuki, S., Van Thiel, D. H., Gartner, J., Zitelli, B., Malatack, J., Schade, R., Shaw, B., Hakala, T., Rosenthal, J., & Porter, K. (1982). Evolution of liver transplantation. *Hepatology, 2,* 614–636.

Wood, R. P., Shaw, B. H., Jr., & Starzl, T. E. (1985). Extrahepatic complications of liver transplantation. *Seminars in Liver Disease, 5,* 377–384.

Wozney, P., Zajko, A. B., Bron, K., & Starzl, T. E. (1986). Vascular complications after liver transplantation. *American Journal of Radiology, 147,* 657–663.

Zajko, A. B., Campbell, W. L., Bron, K. M., Schade, R., Koneru, B., & Van Thiel, D. H. (1988). Diagnostic and interventional radiology in liver transplantation. *GI Clinics of North America, 17,* 105–143.

Zajko, A. B., Zemel, G., Skolnick, M. L., Bron, K. M., Campbell, W. L., Iwatsuki, S., & Starzl, T. E. (1988). Percutaneous transhepatic cholangiogram rather than ultrasound as a screening test for postoperative biliary complications in liver transplant patients. *Transplantation Proceedings, 20,* 678–681.

CHAPTER **8**

BONE MARROW TRANSPLANTATION

Carol S. Viele
Catherine M. Cebulski

The past three decades of cancer research in the area of bone marrow transplant have made long-term survival a reality for patients diagnosed with an immune deficiency disease (specifically acute and chronic leukemia) and aplastic anemia. There has also been limited success in using bone marrow transplantation for treatment of solid tumors.

However, bone marrow transplantation remains experimental, and indications for treatment are continually changing. Under the best of circumstances, bone marrow transplantation is a high-risk procedure with a mortality rate of 30% to 40% due to transplant-related complications or recurrent malignancies. Thus, transplantation is inappropriate when other modalities offer a chance of cure at a lower risk (Blume & Petz, 1983). Many considerations, including disease, age, current health status of the patient, and the availability of a histocompatible donor (Blume & Petz, 1983) have to be addressed when offering bone marrow transplant as a treatment option. Another consideration is that of expense resulting from lengthy hospitalization with complex care and necessary follow-up care after discharge.

Some of the most significant advances that have made bone marrow transplant a treatment option for patients have been the development of human leukocyte antigen (HLA) typing, techniques to harvest platelets and store blood products, and the development of second- and third-generation antibiotics, antiviral and antifungal drugs (Blume & Petz, 1983). It is because of these developments that patients have been able to sustain long periods of immunosuppression after transplantation.

Bone marrow transplantation is offering hope to patients who otherwise would have died, just 10 years ago, for lack of appropriate and supportive therapy. The future of bone marrow transplantation is exciting to researchers, who now look for ways to combat graft-versus-host disease (GVHD), veno-occlusive disease, and interstitial pneumonia. This chapter will focus on some of these posttreatment complications and related nursing care and also provide a complete overview of bone marrow transplant as a viable alternative for patients with malignant and nonmalignant hematologic disorders.

THE HISTORY OF BONE MARROW TRANSPLANTATION

During 1891, the first attempt to use bone marrow therapeutically was documented when Brown-Sequard and his colleagues administered bone marrow by mouth for nutritional purposes to patients with anemia secondary to leukemia. Later therapeutic attempts involved intermedullary and intravenous infusions of living marrow to patients suffering from anemia from various causes (Freedman, 1988).

Not much interest was generated in bone marrow transplantation until the 1940s, when World War II ended with the use of the first atomic bomb. For the first time, scientists saw the effects of exposure to ionizing radiation on human beings. This experience was the driving force behind bone marrow transplant experimentation.

In 1948, it was found that if the spleen of a mouse was protected by lead shielding from ionizing radiation, the mouse would survive (Blume & Petz, 1983). This piece of information was especially important because shielding other organs was found to be much less effective. Shortly afterward, it was discovered that lethally irradiated mice or guinea pigs could be protected by intraperitoneal injections of autologous bone marrow cells after radiation (Blume & Petz, 1983).

Over time, attempts were made to perform bone marrow transplant in humans, but most failed because the experiments were done on terminally ill patients. In the 1950s and 1960s, there were a few successful grafts, but many people died of GVHD, which is an attack of the donor's marrow against the tissue of the host patient. Other complications occurred secondary to the inability to select compatible donors, the unavailability of adequate platelet and white blood cell (WBC) transfusions, the absence of methods to prevent infections, and the lack of potent antibiotics to treat infections (Freedman, 1988).

Much research has taken place over the past 30 years, and it was in the early 1970s that human histocompatibility typing made it possible to match the recipient's tissue type with that of the donor's marrow (Freedman, 1988). Advances in blood product support have made it possible for patients to sustain long periods of aplasia when the patient's bone marrow is still unable to make WBCs, red blood cells (RBCs), and platelets. The ability to store blood products for long periods of time and advancement of techniques using selected donors for platelet and WBC infusions have increased the number of blood products available.

It was the discovery of HLA typing that changed the course of bone marrow transplantation. The first report of successful marrow transplant between HLA-identical siblings came from a group in Minneapolis headed by Dr. Robert Good (Blume & Petz, 1983).

To date, there have been over 10,000 bone marrow transplants performed (Corcoran-Buchsel & Ford, 1988; Ford & Ballard, 1988). New centers are opening yearly around the world. This trend will continue as advances in research make bone marrow transplantation a treatment option for long-term survival and cure.

WHO CAN BE TREATED USING BONE MARROW TRANSPLANTATION?

The first successful bone marrow transplants were in children and young adults with either partial or complete bone marrow failure. Patients with an immune deficiency disease and aplastic anemia can benefit greatly from an allogeneic bone marrow transplant. In an allogeneic transplant, the donor can be a brother or sister who is HLA-identical and mixed lymphocyte culture (MLC)–compatible. Only one in four siblings have genetic matchings similar enough to donate marrow successfully. At present, national statistics show that patients with the diagnosis of aplastic anemia have an 80% chance of long-term survival if they have received no prior blood transfusions and a 40% to 50% chance of survival if they have been previously supported with blood products (Bozdech, 1986.)

For young patients with chronic myelogenous leukemia in stable chronic phase, there is an 80% chance of survival without recurrence of disease. For patients with acute myelogenous leukemia in first remission, current results with subsequent remission show an overall survival of 30% (Bozdech, 1986). Patients with acute lymphoblastic leukemia in second or subsequent remission have an overall survival of 30%, whereas patients with lymphoma or Hodgkin's disease who are refractory to standard therapy have a long-term disease-free survival rate of 30% to 40% (Bozdech, 1986).

Currently, three types of bone marrow transplants are being performed: autologous (using the patient's own bone marrow), allogeneic (using a sibling's marrow), and synergeneic (using a twin's bone marrow).

The type of bone marrow used is dependent on the disease being treated and the results of the histocompatibility typing (Freedman, 1988). Presently, there are over 2,500 allogeneic and more than 1,000 autologous transplants performed every year (Corcoran-Buchsel, 1986; Ford & Ballard, 1988). Autologous transplants are performed only for malignant diseases, and patients are usually in a state of remission when marrow is collected. The bone marrow is then stored until it is needed.

The most common source of bone marrow is allogeneic. The donor can be a brother or sister but under some circumstances may be unrelated. The major difference between allogeneic bone marrow transplant and autologous transplant is the greater chance of relapse with autologous bone marrow, since there may still be undetected malignant cells present when the bone marrow is harvested and reinfused. Patients who undergo allogeneic transplant have a greater chance of long-term survival but a higher risk of mortality because of the potential for GVHD and interstitial pneumonitis. Hospital stays tend to be longer for patients with allogeneic transplants secondary to posttransplant complications and longer periods of aplasia.

Patients who undergo synergeneic transplant have a high chance of long-term survival because this type of transplant eliminates the problems of graft rejection and GVHD (Freedman, 1988). However, they run a greater risk of leukemic relapse; it is thought that mild GVHD serves to reduce the risk of relapse in patients who have undergone allogeneic transplantation.

Patients who are unable to donate their own bone marrow and who do not have a matched sibling may opt for an unrelated transplant (a donor who has identical tissue typing and is screened from a national donor registry) or a mismatched transplant (the donor being a mother or father who is not completely HLA-matched). However, both kinds of transplants have the greatest risk of mortality because of graft rejection.

Bone marrow transplantation for other types of cancer is considered experimental, and there are no clear indications concerning when and if it should be performed. Patients with cancers other than leukemias, lymphomas, and aplastic anemias, are considered on an individual basis, preferably within the guidelines of an approved research protocol.

Once a decision is made for bone marrow transplantation, routine preadmission visits are scheduled with the departments of radiation therapy, oral medicine, physical therapy, and psychiatry. Patients are scheduled for an electrocardiogram (ECG), cardiac scan, and pulmonary function tests.

Once all of these tests are completed, an informed-consent conference is scheduled. Because bone marrow transplantation may be a research therapy and can cause many potentially serious complications, it is necessary for health professionals to disclose all relevant information regarding the treatment process before the treatment begins (Carney, 1987). In the case of bone marrow transplantation, the physician is legally responsible for informing the patient and obtaining consent (Murchinson, Nicholos, & Hanson, 1982). Other health care workers who are present during the informed consent process include the primary nurse and social worker. After the bone marrow process has begun, it will be their job to support and reinforce the information disclosed at the informed-consent conference.

During the informed consent process, each aspect of the treatment is discussed including benefits and risks. Patients are asked to sign appropriate consent forms prior to receiving treatment. Patients and family members are free to ask questions and seek clarification of treatment plans from both a medical and a nursing perspective.

Prior to hospitalization, patients will have an indwelling central line placed. Long-term access is crucial for the infusion of hyperalimentation, antibiotics, and blood products and for frequent blood sampling (Hickman & Buckner, 1979).

BONE MARROW TRANSPLANT DONORS

Donor Selection

The basis for selection of the most appropriate donor begins with an understanding of the HLA that are analyzed during tissue typing. HLA tissue typing is essential in predicting GVHD and marrow graft rejection, either of which may prove crucial to the clinical course of the bone marrow transplant recipient (Ruggiero, 1988).

Histocompatibility is determined by two tests, HLA typing and the MLC. HLA typing can identify antigens at only 4 of the 5 known genetic loci (A, B, C, and DR) that can be found on the surface of peripheral blood lymphocytes (Ruggiero, 1988). The HLA-D locus is determined by the MLC. This test requires mixing lymphocytes from the potential donor with those of the recipient in a culture medium for 5 to 6 days. A nonreactive MLC signals compatibility.

The goal of histocompatibility testing is to find the closest match so that the likelihood of graft rejection or GVHD is reduced (Ruggiero, 1988). Although donors may have identical HLA typing and be MLC-nonreactive, they may have different ABO blood types.

Although ABO antigens do not appear to be disease targets of GVHD, ABO incompatibility between donor and recipient may present unique clinical problems (Ruggiero, 1988). Major incompatibility between donor and recipient exists in approximately 10% to 15% of HLA-matched pairs and 15% to 20% of HLA-mismatched combinations (Bensinger et al., 1987). ABO-incompatible transplants carry the risk of a hemolytic transfusion reaction at the time of marrow infusions (Bensinger et al., 1987). Steps to prevent this from occurring include plasma exchange or RBC depletion before infusion of the marrow. These techniques, however, could prevent engraftment and account for delays in platelet and RBC transfusion independence (Bensinger et al., 1987).

Donor Evaluation

Bone marrow withdrawal or harvesting is a minor surgical procedure with no significant risk to the donor. However, it is performed under general or spinal anesthesia in order to minimize the pain of multiple bone marrow aspirations, which are required to withdraw a suitable amount of bone marrow. Nevertheless, donors who are allogeneic (brothers, sisters, parents) or twins must be in reasonably good health. Prior to the procedure, a complete history, physical examination, ECG, and laboratory tests for hepatitis, human immunodeficiency virus (HIV) antibody, syphilis, ABO and Rh groups, and cytomegalovirus (CMV) antibody status are performed.

Multiple factors influence the extent of preparation that a donor receives prior to bone marrow transplant. These factors include accessibility of the donor and the current relationship of the donor with the recipient and family (Ruggiero, 1988).

Physicians not only look at the physical findings in donor selection but also evaluate the donor's perceptions and attitudes toward the transplant process. They identify any distortions in donor conceptualization of the procedure, assess the donor's pretransplant relationship with the marrow recipient, evaluate the support systems available to the donor, and assess the degree of potential disruption to the donor's life-style. Adequate preparation of the donor should follow the standard of obtaining informed consent (Ruggiero, 1988).

Recent advances in bone marrow transplant have made it a viable treatment option for many, but what about those patients who do not have a matched donor and are not candidates for an autologous transplant in which they donate their own marrow?

In Western Europe and North America, the average size of families (2– children) restricts the number of patients with an HLA-identical sibling donor to approximately one third of the total number requiring allogeneic bone marrow transplant (Hows et al., 1986). Approximately 12,000 individuals annually are predicted to be candidates for transplantation from a national donor pool (Gale, 1986).

Who are the volunteers who make up a donor registry? Volunteers are solicited by organized donation drives sponsored by nonprofit agencies, or in some centers blood donors are asked if preliminary HLA typing can be performed on their blood and entered into the donor registry for possible marrow donation.

When a patient has no other option but accessing volunteer donors from the national registry, a computer search identifies all donors whose HLA-A and B antigens are identical to that of the patient's. The donors are then HLA-DR-typed. Once a match is confirmed, the donor blood is used for MLC testing (McCullough et al., 1986).

At present, the process for identifying a well-matched unrelated donor is both costly and time-consuming. The chances of finding a donor are 1 in

20,000 or better. The median time taken to select an unmatched donor is 4 months, and there is no guarantee that the volunteer will be willing or able to donate at the time the marrow is needed (McCullough et al., 1986).

It should be noted that the survival of patients after receiving marrow from an HLA-identical donor is superior to that of patients receiving transplants from two or more HLA-mismatched donors. The incidence of GVHD is much higher in patients who have partially matched donors (McCullough et al., 1986). However, the one advantage of using partially matched family donors rather than volunteer donors is that transplant is less likely to be delayed by a prolonged search for a suitable donor, and in the end, the patient may have a greater chance of long-term survival if transplanted in remission (Hows et al., 1986).

Experimental studies have shown some success in manipulating bone marrow to allow partially matched brothers, sisters, and parents to donate marrow. However, the incidence of complications following transplantation, particularly GVHD, remains very high. Some patients may also be eligible for autologous/purged bone marrow transplantation, in which the marrow is treated in vitro with a drug called 4HC that destroys any remaining malignant cells.

BONE MARROW DONATION PROCEDURE

After the donor evaluation process is completed, arrangements are made for 2 pints of blood to be withdrawn from the donor and stored, to be returned to him/her at the time the marrow is withdrawn. This prevents the patient from becoming anemic after the procedure.

Usually, the donor is admitted to the hospital the morning of the procedure and taken directly to the operating room (OR). Approximately 2 hours is required to withdraw 1 L of bone marrow from the posterior iliac crest. It takes approximately 100 aspirations to yield the appropriate amount of stem cells because only 5 to 10 cc can be withdrawn with each aspiration. The donor will only have two to three puncture sites on each side of the iliac crest because with each aspiration the needle is redirected to various marrow spaces. One liter of marrow constitutes approximately 10% to 15% of the body's bone marrow. This bone marrow is replaced by the body within 4 to 6 weeks, so there is no significant adverse risk to the donor. Specifically, there is no increased risk of infection or susceptibility to infection since the remainder of the marrow is more than adequate to protect the donor.

Patients usually require narcotics to control pain in the first 12 to 24 hours after the procedure. They describe the pain as a dull ache and are encouraged to ambulate as tolerated after returning to the floor. The patient will be transfused with the blood they donated prior to the procedure and given a prescription for iron pills to take for 1 month following the harvest to assure complete recovery of RBC production. They are generally discharged from the hospital the day after the procedure.

The donor is asked to return for a follow-up exam 1 week after the procedure. At this time, the donor's hematocrit level and the aspiration sites are checked. Donors may still experience soreness at the aspiration sites, but they are able to resume their regular activity level and should not require any additional follow-up care.

Although the risks of marrow donation are considered minimal, the potential for complications exists. The International Bone Marrow Transplant Registry and Seattle's Fred Hutchinson Cancer Center transplant team analyzed major complications of marrow harvesting in 3,290 donor episodes and found a complication incidence of 0.27%. No deaths or permanent sequelae were reported (Ruggiero, 1988). The Seattle team reviewed minor complications and found that fewer than 1% of donors experienced prolonged pain. This pain may relate to hematomas developing at aspiration sites, swelling of soft tissue, or the donor's pain tolerance and anxiety associated with the procedure. Postharvest fever of unknown etiology was reported in approximately 10% of patients but resolved without complication and often without the use of antibiotic therapy (Ruggiero, 1988). The same study also reported six life-threatening complications, three associated with anesthesia (Ruggiero, 1988).

Implantation of Bone Marrow

When a sufficient amount of bone marrow is collected in the OR, the marrow is filtered through a fine screen to remove any pieces of bone or fat cells. If the patient is undergoing an autologous transplant, the bone marrow is preserved and stored until it is needed.

With allogeneic transplantation, the donor's marrow is infused into the patient within 1 to 2 hours after the aspiration procedure is completed. The bone marrow is brought up in plastic bags and infused through the patient's central line. The procedure for infusions follows that of a normal red cell transfusion with one exception: Filter tubing should not be used because it would prevent stem cells, which are essential for engraftment, from passing through the filter. With the infusion of bone marrow, patients may develop allergic reactions, including hives, chills, and tachycardia. Therefore, patients are premedicated with acetaminophen and diphenhydramine. Depending on the volume of bone marrow, the infusion is given over a 2- to 4-hour period.

Experts still do not understand the exact body mechanism controlling the migration of stem cells to the bone marrow cavities, but physicians begin to detect signs of engraftment within 1 to 2 weeks after transplantation.

COMPLICATIONS OF BONE MARROW TRANSPLANTATION

Many complications are associated with bone marrow transplantation. Each of them will be covered in detail so that nursing care can subsequently be discussed.

Infection

One of the great nursing challenges in caring for bone marrow transplant patients is the prevention and early detection of infection. According to Ford and Ballard (1988), virtually all lines of defense in the host are disrupted simultaneously with a prolonged state of neutropenia. This disruption can, in effect, have lethal consequences. Infection can be caused by a wide variety of pathogens, including bacteria, fungi, and viruses as well as those organisms categorized as opportunistic. During this suppressed period, a number of anti-infectious agents must be administered simultaneously to protect the host against infection. Managing the patient receiving these medications can be a significant nursing challenge in this patient population. Risk factors for developing infection have been identified and are listed in Table 8.1. For treatment of infection in this patient population, combination therapy is often utilized.

Organisms commonly seen after bone marrow transplantation are gram-negative pathogens, gram-positive pathogens, and fungi. A list of specific organisms is found in Table 8.2.

Therapy for gram-negative organisms requires a broad-spectrum anti-pseudomonal penicillin (e.g., piperacillin or ticarcillin) and an aminoglycoside (e.g., tobramycin or amikacin). An international study is currently underway to compare two treatment alternatives for bacterial infection: use of

---

TABLE 8.1   Risk Factors for Infection in Bone Marrow Transplant Patients

1. Prolonged neutropenia
2. Graft versus host disease
3. Older age
4. Hematologic malignancy
5. Relapsed disease state
6. Extensive antibiotic use
7. Higher radiation dose
8. Colonization with organisms early after transplant

Note: From "Acute Complications after Bone Marrow Transplantation" by R. Ford and B. Ballard, 1988, *Seminars in Oncology Nursing*, 4(1). Copyright 1988 by Grune and Stratton, Incorp. Reprinted by permission.

the single agent ceftazidime, a cephalosporin, versus combination therapy of piperacillin and tobramycin. Preliminary data by Linker (1988) show no difference in effective antibacterial coverage between the two arms of the study. Monotherapy, the use of one antibiotic agent, may be the future treatment in these patients.

Other types of organisms that have demonstrated significant morbidity in the transplant population are the gram-positive organisms. Treatment of gram-positive organisms requires the use of combined antibacterials. The usual therapy in some centers is cefotaxime, a third-generation cephalosporin, and vancomycin. Vancomycin is chosen in the transplant setting for its activity against *Staphylococcus epidermidis*, an organism resistant to routine antibacterial coverage. Patients with indwelling central lines frequently culture this organism. As mentioned above, the transplant patient requires an indwelling central line for medication administration. Vancomycin is the only intravenous preparation that has shown sensitivity and good cell kill. Burnett and McDonald (1987) identified resistance by *S. epidermidis* to most antibacterials but noted that, fortunately, rapid clinical deterioration of the patient does not usually occur with this organism. The usual therapy for treatment of this infection is vancomycin 1 gm every 24 hours or 500 mg every 12 hours, depending on renal function. If a patient has a multilumen catheter, drug delivery is rotated among lumens to assure drug presence in each lumen to eradicate the organism. Another organism in the gram-positive group that is increasing in frequency is *Corynebacterium* CDC-JK. It is a highly resistant organism, and the only available therapy is vancomycin and ciprofloxacin.

Fungal organisms are the second most frequently found pathogens in bone marrow transplant patients. Fungal infections usually occur during the first

TABLE 8.2 Organisms Prevalent Post Bone–Marrow Transplantation

Gram-negative bacteria	Gram-positive bacteria	Fungi
Escherichia coli	Staphylococcus aureus	Candida albicans
Klebsiella pneumoniae	Staphylococcus epidermis	Candida tropicalis
Enterobacter	Staphylococcus viridans	Aspergillus species
Serratia marcescens	Corynebacterium CDC-JK	
Proteus mirabilis	Streptococcus pneumoniae	
Pseudomonas aeruginosa	Enterococci	

Note: Data in Column 1 are from *Infection in the granulocytopenic host.* Paper presented at University of California, San Francisco. Reprinted by permission.

Note: Data in Column 2 are from "Approaching controversies in antibacterial management of cancer patients by P. Pizzo, J. Commers, D. Cotton, J. Gress, J. Harthorn, J. Hiemenz, D. Longo, D. Marshall, and K. Robichaud. 1984, *American Journal of Medicine, 76*, p. 436–449. Copyright 1984 by Technical Publishing New York, Division of Dun-Donnelley Publishing Corp. Company of Dun and Bradstreet Corporation. Reprinted by permission.

month after transplant, according to Pizzo and Schimpff (1983) and De Gregorio, Lee, Linker, Jacobs, and Ries (1982). Therapy for fungal infections has involved the early use of amphotericin B. Administration of amphotericin B has major implications for nursing because nurses must manage the side effects of this agent, which include fevers, chills, rigors, dypsnea, and hyper- or hypotension. The nurse must provide the correct medication to allow the patient to receive the amphotericin with minimal toxicity and must monitor for toxicity while administering the drug. Prior to each dose, BUN and creatinine should be evaluated. Amphotericin also interferes with the reabsorption of magnesium and potassium from the renal tubules; therefore, nurses should monitor these levels prior to infusing the dose. If the patient's potassium level is below normal, 3.0 to 5.0 mEq/L, potassium replacement should be given prior to the amphotericin infusion to prevent cardiac arrhythmias.

In addition to bacteria and fungi, viral infection is common in bone marrow transplant recipients. The viruses and their median duration of onset are presented in Table 8.3. Pizzo et al. (1986) noted that herpes simplex may occur in the oropharynx during the first 2 weeks after transplant. Pizzo et al. and Schryber, Lacasse, and Barton-Burke (1987) described patients who had had previous infections or were seropositive and therefore were at increased risk of reactivating the infection. Bennett and Brachman (1985) state that these infections are seldom life-threatening but may have a major impact on patient well-being and compliance with oral medication or nutrition. Acyclovir is used prophylactically in all bone marrow transplant patients to prevent reactivation of the herpes simplex virus. The prophylactic dosage of acyclovir is 5 mg/kg every 8 hours, given intravenously. The dose is adjusted on the basis of renal function. Acyclovir had been documented as effective not only prophylactically but also in established infections as measured by pain reduction, healing, and viral shedding (Bennett & Brachman, 1985).

Herpes zoster poses a threat to patients from days 100 through 365. According to Corcoran-Buchsel (1986), after documentation of positive herpes zoster culture or symptom assessment, this infection is treated with acyclovir. The dosage for treating varicella zoster is 10 mg/kg, intravenously,

TABLE 8.3 Viruses Prevalent Post–Bone Marrow Transplantation

Occurrence	Organism
1st month	Herpes simplex virus
2nd–3rd month	Herpes simplex virus
	Herpes zoster/varicella virus
	Cytomegalovirus
3rd month and later	Herpes zoster virus

every 8 hours for 21 doses (7 days). The frequency of zoster infection is directly related to the degree of prolonged immunosuppression. Corcoran-Buchsel (1986) noted that patients without GVHD became infected with herpes zoster less than 50% of the time; however, in patients with chronic GVHD, the frequency rate of infection rose to greater than 75%. When caring for a patient with varicella zoster, strict isolation procedures must be maintained. With disseminated zoster, the virus becomes airborne, and nurses who have not had chickenpox or those whose titers are not known should not provide direct care to these patients.

CMV is usually a pulmonary complication that McGlave (1985) reports can occur during the second through the third month after transplant. CMV infection during this time may be the result of either reactivation of endogenous virus or a primary infection (Burnett & McDonald, 1987). The mortality rate for patients in whom CMV has been diagnosed may be as high as 90% in allogeneic and autologous transplant patients (Burnett & McDonald, 1987; Wingard et al., 1988). Wingard et al. reported the frequency of interstitial pneumonitis caused by CMV after autologous bone marrow transplant at 14%. Synergeneic transplant patients experienced a rate of 15%, while the rate in allogeneic recipients of bone marrow transplants was 43%. Therapy for CMV pneumonitis is under investigation. The agents currently approved are DHPG, or Ganciclovir® (an analog of acyclovir), and an anti-CMV immunoglobulin. Patients are routinely tested before transplant to determine their CMV status. All patients who are CMV-negative should receive CMV-negative blood products in an effort to prevent the transmission of the virus via the blood and the occurrence of CMV pneumonia.

In patients who are severely immunosuppressed, the major opportunistic pathogen has been *Pneumocystis carinii*, which is categorized as a protozoan. By definition, an opportunistic organism is one that is found within the hospital normally but takes advantage of the immune-suppressed state and becomes pathogenic. *P. carinii* is most often found in the lung and, as one would expect when the individual is immunosuppressed, it results in pneumonia. This pathogen has been almost totally prevented in transplant patients because they receive prophylaxis with trimethoprim–sulfamethoxazole on a regular schedule. The schedule is institution-dependent. For patients who have a sulfa allergy, inhaled pentamidine, recently approved by the FDA, is given on a monthly basis. These prophylactic medications have prevented patients from developing potentially life-threatening complications.

The nursing implications for the prevention and detection of infection are significant, and the management is complex. The infection may grow from an insignificant problem to a life-threatening situation within a few hours. The nurse plays an integral role in monitoring, assessing, and instituting therapy for infectious complications. Table 8.4 presents a list of prophylactic measures against infection.

Mucositis

As noted earlier, there are many complications associated with transplantation. One of the initial problems encountered by the patient is gastrointestinal distress. The patient will usually develop mucositis within 5 to 7 days of starting the high-dose chemotherapy preparative regimen. Oral mucositis is a universal side effect of high-dose chemotherapeutic regimens. The oral mucosa are extremely susceptible to damage by these agents because of the rapid turnover of cells in this tissue, resulting in a painful, denuded mucosa. The remaining area of the gastrointestinal tract may be involved to a lesser degree. The combination of chemotherapy and radiation promotes the occurrence of severe mucositis. If each treatment were given singly, the toxicity would not be as significant. Frequently, severe mucositis involving the oropharynx requires narcotic analgesia for appropriate pain relief.

Nausea and vomiting can be a major problem, beginning with the initial day of chemotherapy and possibly persisting for 3 to 4 weeks posttransplant. Appropriate antiemetic therapy should be instituted by the nurse to prevent or curtail the nausea and vomiting as much as possible.

Diarrhea may result from the preparative regimen but does not usually commence until 1 week after therapy has begun. Diarrhea should also be treated as early as possible. In addition, diarrhea may be a sign of GVHD. GVHD should be suspected if the diarrhea continues 10 to 14 days after transplant. Nurses play a major role in assessing and intervening to decrease the complications of

TABLE 8.4 Prophylactic Measures Against Infection

Protective isolation
Laminar air flow rooms
HEPA filtration
Prophylactic systemic antibiotics
Trimethoprim–sulfamethoxazole
Acyclovir
Oral non-absorbable antibiotics
Passive immunization with antibodies (gamma globulin)
Blood screening for CMV
Granulocyte transfusions (rarely used)
Nutrition (low bacteria, no fresh fruits or vegetables)
Sterile diet
Avoid damage to body barriers
Care with any venipuncture
Care with bone marrow aspiration
Routine mouth care
Routine perirectal care
Attention to proper housekeeping procedures

Note: Data from Ford & Ballard, 1988, and Pizzo & Schimpff, 1983.

the preparative regimen. Table 8.5 lists the common clinical manifestations of mucositis. Table 8.6 presents a grading system utilized at the University of California, San Francisco for gastrointestinal toxicity.

Nursing interventions for treatment of gastrointestinal toxicities are numerous. Interventions for nausea and vomiting associated with the preparative regimen should occur in a timely fashion. The nurse can intervene through the use of antiemetics and by decreasing the frequency of patient stimulation during chemotherapy. While there is no prophylaxis for mucositis, treatment should be directed toward supportive care. Oral hygiene regimens should be instituted at the onset of therapy and maintained during the entire transplant process. Among the numerous regimens available for mouth care, the Medical Center at the University of California has chosen a simple regimen of salt and baking soda rinses. If the salt proves to be too irritating, 1 tsp of baking soda in 1 pt of warm water, at least four times a day, is used. An oral assessment guide may provide a useful tool for nurses on the unit (Eilers, Berger, & Petersen, 1988). Ongoing nutritional assessment is also needed and can be provided by nursing and dietary staff. When the nurse believes a patient is no longer able to tolerate his/her diet, appropriate interventions are a calorie count and dietary consultation. Hyperalimentation is used frequently in this population to provide the calories needed during this stressful period. Appropriate nursing assessment, along with intake and output, daily weight, and laboratory assessments, can assist the health care team in delivering adequate nutrition. Nursing input in the management of gastrointestinal toxicities provides a significant contribution to patient outcome.

Veno-Occlusive Disease

Veno-occlusive disease is another major complication associated with bone marrow transplantation. This complication is thought to arise from the

TABLE 8.5 Common Clinical Findings of Mucositis

Site	Findings
Oropharyngeal	Profuse, watery-to-thick ropy mucus; severe pain; bleeding; infection; potential airway obstruction
Esophageal	Dysphagia, bleeding, infection
Gastric	Anorexia, emesis, bleeding, infections
Intestinal	Watery diarrhea, cramping pain, ulcerations, infections.

Note: From "Acute Complications after Bone Marrow Transplantation" by R. Ford and B. Ballard, 1988, *Seminars in Oncology Nursing,* 4(1), p. 16. Copyright 1988 by Grune & Stratton. Reprinted by permission.

conditioning regimens. It is, by definition, a nonthrombotic obliteration of the small intrahepatic veins by loose connective tissue (Rollins, 1986). The incidence of hepatic veno-occlusive disease is approximately 20%, with a mortality ranging from 7% to 75% (Ford, McClain & Cunningham, 1983; Rio et al., 1986; Rollins, 1986). The clinical manifestations of hepatic veno-occlusive disease are the appearance of jaundice, an enlarged liver and/or right upper quadrant pain, and ascites or unexplained weight gain occurring within 4 to 5 weeks after the marrow graft (Rollins, 1986). The clinical symptomatology may also include encephalopathy and abnormal liver function tests (Ford et al., 1983).

Risk factors associated with the development of veno-occlusive disease are hepatitis prior to transplantation, a diagnosis of acute nonlymphoblastic leukemia or chronic myelogenous leukemia (as opposed to acute lymphoblastic leukemia or aplastic anemia), and increased age (Ford et al., 1983). The treatment for veno-occlusive disease is supportive care (Ford et al., 1983). There is no known prophylaxis as yet for veno-occlusive disease. Treatment is aimed at maintaining intravascular volume and renal perfusion and minimizing accumulation of extravascular fluid. The use of blood products has also been recommended to keep the hematocrit above 35% (Ford & Ballard, 1988). Patients considered for transplantation should have normal liver function tests for at least 2 weeks prior to admission.

Nursing interventions in the treatment of veno-occlusive disease include accurate intake and output, daily weights, and abdominal girths every shift. The nurse should be aware of patient fluid and electrolyte status along with changes in liver function tests. The nurse should also monitor for any change in mental status as an indicator of encephalopathy. It is through accurate patient assessment that initial signs of veno-occlusive disease can be

TABLE 8.6 Grading System Utilized at UCSF for Gastrointestinal Toxicity (an Example)

Site	0	1	2	3	4
Oro-pharynx	None	Pain, erythema	>Pain, erythema, no oral intake, parenteral narcotics	Grade 2 with deep ulceration (30% surface involved)	Intubation
Gastro-intestinal	None	Mild pain or diarrhea not requiring therapy	Pain or diarrhea requiring therapy	Mild peritoneal findings	peritonitis or perforation

identified. It is important to remember that the goal in treating veno-occlus-ive disease is supportive care, as there is currently no effective therapy (Schryber et al., 1987).

Pulmonary Complications

Pulmonary complications after transplantation can occur at any time. The incidence is as high as 70% (Corcoran-Buchsel, 1986). They can occur during administration of the preparative regimen, wherein the mucositis may become so severe that the patient requires intubation as a method to protect the airway while the mucositis heals. Other pulmonary complications include interstitial pneumonia, CMV, *Pneumocystis carinii* pneumonia (PCP), and idiopathic pneumonia.

Interstitial pneumonia is a frequent complication, occurring in about 40% of allogeneic transplants and 14% of autologous bone marrow transplants (McGuire & Almgren, 1987; Wingard et al., 1988). The etiology of interstitial pneumonia is related to several factors including total body irradiation, GVHD, methotrexate immunosuppression, and increasing age (McGuire & Almgren, 1987).

Clinical manifestations of interstitial pneumonia include fever, dry cough, dyspnea, nasal flaring, tachypnea with rates of 40 to 60 per minute and rales (Ford & Ballard, 1988). Chest x-rays show diffuse infiltrates, and arterial blood gases demonstrate hypoxia (Ford & Ballard, 1988). A diagnosis may be difficult; bronchoscopy with lavage is usually attempted. If no diagnosis can be made, patients may be taken to the OR for open lung biopsy. Open lung biopsy can have significant morbidity in a thrombocytopenic patient, and it yields an accurate diagnosis only part of the time.

CMV is the most common infectious cause of interstitial pneumonia, occurring in about 45% to 50% of all transplant patients (Ford & Ballard, 1988). The mortality rate for CMV pneumonia has been reported to be between 13% and 90% (McGuire & Almgren, 1987). The incidence of CMV pneumonia has been reported to be significantly less in autologous transplantation than in allogeneic transplantation, ranging from 11% to 42% (Wingard et al., 1988). The risk factors associated with CMV pneumonia include previous CMV infection (patients who are seropositive to CMV), GVHD, age greater than 30 years, and exposure to the virus through blood products (Ford & Ballard, 1988).

The diagnosis of CMV pneumonia is made after bronchoalveolar lavage during bronchoscopy and an attempt to culture the lavage and evaluate for inclusion bodies. Inclusion bodies indicate the presence of the virus within the cell, as determined by microscopic evaluation. As noted previously, the current therapy for CMV pneumonia is treatment with Ganciclovir or anti-CMV immune globulin.

As mentioned in the section on infection, PCP can be a frequent occurrence in this patient population. PCP is not a significant problem for transplant patients unless individuals are allergic to trimethoprim–sulfamethoxazole. Trimethoprim–sulfamethoxazole is administered twice per week to prevent PCP. Patients who are allergic to trimethoprim–sulfamethoxazole receive aerosolized pentamidine once a month as prophylaxis.

Idiopathic pneumonia presents as adult respiratory distress syndrome and is diagnosed when no infectious organisms are found with bronchoscopy or open lung biopsy (Ford & Ballard, 1988; Wingard et al., 1988). The idiopathic pneumonias are thought to represent treatment toxicity (Ford & Ballard, 1988; Wingard et al., 1988). Yet there may also be unidentified pathogens accounting for some cases of idiopathic pneumonia.

Nursing interventions for patients with pulmonary complications include accurate respiratory assessment and teaching the patients signs and symptoms of pneumonia. The types of pneumonias discussed above may occur before transplant or as long as 100 days after transplant. Inpatient and outpatient nursing staffs, therefore, must be aware of this serious complication.

Renal Complications/Bladder Toxicity

Renal complications of transplants are the result of the administration of nephrotoxic therapy in the form of antibiotics, cyclosporine (Cy A), and chemotherapy. The etiology of renal failure for bone marrow transplantation is found in Table 8.7. Therapy for renal disease requires continuing evaluation of fluid and electrolyte balance. It may also require adjustment of nephrotoxic agents such as antibiotics and Cy A to continue treating both infectious complications and GVHD.

An important nursing intervention for patients with impaired kidney function is continuous assessment. Assessment parameters include intake and output, specific gravity, abdominal girths, and daily weights.

Bladder toxicity is a direct result of treatment with high-dose cyclophosphamide (Cytoxan®) preparation. Schryber et al. (1987) state that toxic metabolites of this drug are irritating to the transitional epithelium of the ureters and bladder, resulting in hemorrhage from the affected uroepithelium. Hemorrhagic cystitis may occur during therapy or may be delayed, usually occurring within 6 weeks of drug administration. The major sign is hematuria.

Nursing interventions for patients treated with high-dose cyclophosphamide include accurate monitoring for hematuria. Prior to the institution of a cyclophosphamide regimen, a three-way Foley catheter should be inserted to deliver 1 L/hr of isotonic fluid continuously during the days that the patient receives cyclophosphamide, continuing for 24 hours after therapy. The rationale for continuing the irrigation for 24 hours after therapy is the prolonged half-life of cyclophosphamide. The catheter may then be removed and urine output evaluated during the remainder of the hospitalization.

Cardiac Complications

Cardiac damage is a rare occurrence in bone marrow transplantation; estimates are that it occurrs in less than 5% of patients. Cardiac damage occurs as a direct result of combination chemotherapy and total body irradiation. All patients should have echocardiograms prior to institution of the preparatory regimen and ECGs should be completed prior to administration of cardiotoxic therapy. There is currently no real therapy for severe (Grade 4) cardiotoxicity. The mortality rate associated with this infrequent toxicity is 95%. Table 8.8 presents a grading system utilized at the Medical Center at the University of California for evaluation of cardiovascular function. Nursing assessment should include recording lying and standing blood pressures to evaluate for postural hypotension, checking for edema, and assessment of neck veins for jugular venous distention.

Graft Versus Host Disease

GVHD is a serious complication of allogeneic transplant. Ford and Ballard (1988) defined GVHD as "the consequence of the reaction initiated by a graft of immunologically competent lymphocytes introduced into a host that con-

TABLE 8.7 Etiology of Renal Failure in Bone Marrow Transplants (Prerenal conditions)

Hypovolemia
  Dehydration
  Third-space fluid
  Veno-occulusive disease
  Hemorrhage
Impaired circulation of blood volume
  Septic shock
  Congestive heart failure
  Cardiotoxic effects
  Renovascular constriction
  Pressor drugs
  Acute tubular necrosis
  Nephrotoxic drugs
  Prolonged ischemia
Tumor lysis syndrome
  Massive tumor lysis
Postrenal obstruction
  Hemorrhagic cystitis

Note From "Acute Complications after Bone Marrow Transplantation" by R. Ford and B. Ballard, 1988 *Seminars in Oncology Nursing,* 4(1), p. 20. Copyright 1988 by Grune & Stratton.. Reprinted by permission.

fronts the graft with a histocompatibility difference yet is unable to mount a similar immunological attack against the intrusive donor lymphoid system" (p. 17). GVHD occurs in 20% to 80% of all allogeneic transplants (Champlin & Gale, 1984; Ford & Ballard, 1988; Parker & Cohen, 1983). The organs affected by GVHD are the skin, gastrointestinal tract, and liver. Ford and Ballard (1988) identified patients at highest risk for GVHD as those over the age of 30, those with an opposite-sex donor, and those who are not perfectly matched with their donors.

The clinical onset of GVHD may occur as early as 7 days after transplant, with the median duration of onset at day 25 (Ford & Ballard, 1988; Parker & Cohen, 1983). The patient may experience symptoms in any one or all three body systems. Skin GVHD usually begins as a generalized maculopapular rash on the trunk, palms, soles and ears, which may progress to generalized erythroderma with possible desquamation of skin (Ford & Ballard, 1988).

Liver GVHD is characterized by increases in serum bilirubin, serum transaminases, and alkaline phosphatase (McDonald, Shulman, Sullivan, &

TABLE 8.8 Grading System for Cardiovascular Toxicity

Parameters	0	1	2	3	4
Arrhythmias	None	Asymptomatic, transient	Asymptomatic, requires therapy	Symptomatic, requires therapy	Asystole, ventricular tachycardia, ventricular fibrillation, emergency cardioversion
Ischemia	None	ECG negative	ECG negative	Reversible ECG changes	Documented infarction
Function	Normal	Asymptomatic but evidence of decreased left ventricular function	Symptomatic, requiring therapy but transient	Symptomatic, requiring therapy and irreversible	Hemodynamic instability, need hemodynamic monitoring

Spencer, 1986; McGuire & Almgren, 1987). Patients may complain of right upper quadrant pain and demonstrate hepatomegaly on abdominal examination (Ford & Ballard, 1988). As the disease progresses, jaundice may occur.

Gastrointestinal GVHD is characterized by secretory diarrhea and abdominal pain (McGuire & Almgren, 1987; Tutschka, 1987). It usually presents as green, watery diarrhea that may ultimately become hemorrhagic, associated with progressive and severe denudation of the gastrointestinal mucosa (Ford & Ballard, 1988; Tutschka, 1987). The patient's usual symptoms are abdominal cramping prior to a loose stool, as well as anorexia, nausea, and vomiting (Ford & Ballard, 1988). If untreated, patients may experience several liters of diarrhea within a 24-hour period (Ford & Ballard, 1988).

Diagnosis of GVHD is usually confirmed through a biopsy of the affected system. The system most easily accessed for diagnosis, with the least risk, is the skin. A skin biopsy may be obtained by a dermatologist with relatively few complications. If necessary, a gastrointestinal biopsy may be obtained during endoscopy after appropriate platelet transfusion. The risk-to-benefit ratio must always be identified when considering invasive procedures in the transplant population.

Prophylaxis for acute GVHD varies from center to center. Many institutions use more than one agent for prophylaxis. The most common agent utilized is Cy A (Klemm, 1985). Cy A may be used as a single agent or in combination with methotrexate (Ford & Ballard, 1988). Cy A may also be used in combination with early aggressive corticosteroids (Ford & Ballard, 1988; Ruutu, Volin, & Elonen, 1988). The prophylaxis is directed at the prevention or limitation of GVHD. The aim of prophylactic therapy is to remove or inactivate T lymphocytes that are responsible for the attack and to reduce the number of microorganisms that may aggravate the response (Ford & Ballard, 1988). Monoclonal antibodies and T-cell depleted marrows have also been used for prophylaxis or prevention of GVHD. Therapy used for acute GVHD, should prophylaxis not be effective, includes increasing doses of Cy A, high-dose corticosteroids, azathioprine, antithymocyte globulin, and monoclonal antibodies (Ford & Ballard, 1988; Tutschka, 1987; Ruutu et al., 1988).

Nursing interventions for the management of GVHD include scrupulous nursing assessment to detect early signs and symptoms. This assessment should include inspection of the patient's skin, with particular attention to palms, soles, ears, and trunk. Ford and Ballard (1988) also recommend strict measuring of input and output, hematesting of urine, guaiac of all stools, and monitoring of liver function tests. Nurses must also be knowledgeable about the side effects of the prescribed agents to answer patient questions accurately and reduce patient anxiety.

Chronic GVHD usually occurs 100 days after transplantation and occurs in approximately 30% of all bone marrow transplant patients (McGuire & Almgren, 1987). Most patients who develop chronic GVHD have had acute GVHD. Twenty percent of patients who may not have had acute GVHD develop chronic GVHD. Chronic GVHD may attack any organ, with 90% of patients having extensive disease of the skin, liver, eyes, mouth, esophagus, and joints (McGuire & Almgren, 1987; Tutschka, 1987). Chronic GVHD has often been described as a syndrome of disordered immunity displaying clinical features strongly resembling autoimmune diseases (Tutschka, 1987). Limited disease restricted to the skin, with or without liver involvement, is usually not treated. Extensive disease must always be treated to prevent life-threatening infection and disabling contractures (McGuire & Almgren, 1987). About 25% of patients with extensive chronic GVHD will die from infection (McGuire & Almgren, 1987).

Therapy for chronic GVHD may or may not include Cy A. Steroids are commonly used (McGuire & Almgren, 1987). Other agents that may be utilized to treat chronic GVHD are azathioprine, antithymocyte globulin, and cyclophosphamide. As the disease improves, therapy is tapered and eventually discontinued.

The patient should be given specific instructions regarding notification of the nurse or physician when nausea, vomiting, diarrhea, or abdominal or joint pain occur after discharge from the hospital. Nurses provide the patient with information for all agents prescribed to treat chronic GVHD. These patients are very anxious, and anxiety-reducing measures, including teaching, are an important part of nursing intervention.

In summary, the complications of bone marrow transplantation described in this chapter do not occur in all patients, but nurses must be aware of the major complications that can arise. Nurses play a significant role in the assessment and management of these severely ill patients. It can be a frustrating and yet rewarding experience to provide care for these incredibly complex and challenging patients.

PSYCHOLOGICAL ISSUES

The psychological issues related to bone marrow transplantation are complex and varied. In 1976, Brown and Kelly described eight psychosocial stages of bone marrow transplantation. The initial stage was found to be informed consent, but Brown and Kelly doubted that real informed consent could ever be obtained. The first stage actually begins with the initial greeting of the patient during the informed-consent conference. During the first conference, the nurse can assess the patient's level of understanding and establish rapport with the patient and family. Stage 2 appears to occur during evaluation and planning. At this time coping skills may be assessed by the team (Wolcott, Fawzy, & Wellisch, 1986). These coping responses are influenced by the natural course of the disease as well as the specific therapeutic regimens. They are (a) peaks and valleys, (b) descending plateaus, (c) downward slopes, and

(d) gradual slants (Martocchio, 1985). Knowledge of coping responses can help the nurse plan her care appropriately.

Stage 3 encompasses the conditioning regimen that Brown and Kelly (1976) characterized as "the point of no return." During this stage, patients become more concerned about death and dying. Brown and Kelly state that the patient's typical personality features intensify in response to psychological stress. Nurses should be aware of this information and allow more time for verbalization and institute supportive measures for the patient.

Stage 4 occurs on the day of transplantation. Brown and Kelly (1976) found Stage 4 to be a psychologically undramatic event; yet that has not been the experience of these authors. Most patients have reported a multitude of feelings: The allogeneic patients report feelings of gratitude, while the autologous patients report having concern over their potential for engraftment. Both transplant recipients experience a wealth of emotions on this day. Families also have heightened emotional experiences on this day, too.

Stage 5 (the pre-engraftment phase) is characterized by patients' having expectations that may or may not be met. Patients may experience greater difficulty coping with isolation procedures. Also, patients exhibit less emotional expression (Brown & Kelly, 1976). The nursing staff must realize that this is a time of great physical symptomatology and provide support by decreasing the symptoms and allowing the patient to verbalize as needed. Quiet time should be provided. It is important for the nurse to provide support to the family during this time of decreased patient coping.

Stage 6, a time of possible GVHD in allogeneic patients, is characterized by anger and severe depression on the part of the patient, family fatigue and discouragement, and donor guilt if GVHD develops. The autologous patient awaits patiently or impatiently for engraftment. The patient also experiences anger, depression, and discouragement if the projected time line of recovery of cell counts is not met. During this stage, patients may develop many of the complications described previously in the chapter. Nurses can help patients by performing frequent physical assessments and intervening to assist the patient through this stressful time.

Stage 7 occurs during the preparation for discharge, which Brown & Kelly (1976) found was characterized by ambivalence about leaving the hospital and concern about reestablishing typical daily activities. Nurses can assist patients during this stage by performing discharge teaching, promoting independence, and allowing the family to play an active role in patient care.

According to Brown & Kelly (1976), Stage 8 (adaptation out of the hospital) has not been fully studied. Wolcott, Wellisch, Fawzy, and Landsverk (1986) have completed a study of bone marrow recipient survivors. They found that recipients manifested low levels of psychological symptoms when they were not in extraordinarily stressful circumstances. Their self-rated current role functioning indicated somewhat more impairment than reported by a historically healthy community sample. Wolcott, Wellisch, Fawzy, and Landsverk found a lack of correlation between the date of bone marrow transplant and the recipient's level of adaptation; that is, time alone will not necessarily improve the recipient's adaptation response. The health status they found is clearly related to psychosocial measures of adaptation in bone marrow transplant recipients, so poor health status in recipients may be an indication of poor psychosocial adaptation. Knowledge of the psychological stages of transplantation will assist the nurse in developing an effective care plan to assist patients with the major psychosocial issues.

Psychological issues related to being a bone marrow donor must also be considered (Folsom & Popkin, 1987). Because of minimal morbidity and lack of long-term physical sequelae, little emphasis has been placed on screening donors psychologically. Folsom and Popkin reported recipient feelings of resentment toward the donor because the gift is "unrepayable." Folsom and Popkin also reported that donors struggle with a sense of tremendous responsibility for the outcome of the transplant and express inappropriate feelings of guilt when GVHD occurs. Wolcott, Wellisch, Fawzy, and Landsverk (1987) state that donor preparation should be emphasized as a critical step during the pretransplant workup. During this preparation, nurses must involve the donor in discussions and explanations. The donor must feel like an integral part of the transplantation process. The donor should not be the forgotten individual.

In conclusion, psychological issues related to bone marrow transplantation are important to nurses. The stages described provide for appropriate assessment opportunities and detailed intervention by the nursing staff. If appropriate nursing interventions are provided, this patient population will receive the high-quality psychosocial care that is so richly deserved.

CLINICAL MANAGEMENT

The clinical management of a bone marrow transplant patient is a multi-faceted procedure. The procedure begins with the destruction of the host's bone marrow prior to the actual transplant. This process is termed ablative and is usually accomplished with combined modality therapy, including total body radiation and chemotherapy for the allogeneic transplant. In the autologous transplant, chemotherapeutic agents take the place of total body irradiation. The preparative regimen usually takes 7 days. The patient is admitted 1 week prior to transplantation, which is termed Day –7, as are all days prior to the actual day of transplantation. He/she receives 2 days of high-dose chemotherapy followed by 3 days of fractionated total body irradiation. On day 0, the patient undergoes transplantation. In most regimens the patient has 1 to 2 days of rest when no therapy is given. This allows the patient to be ready for the transplant and provides the body time to metabolize and excrete the chemotherapy. In autologous transplants, patients receive chemotherapy on days –7, –6, –5, –4, and –3; and on days –2 and –1, they rest to clear the chemotherapy from their systems. Because of the large number of preparative regimens currently in use, this chapter will not provide information on them. The reader is referred to his/her institution's protocols for information on individual preparative regimens.

Isolation Procedures

While consideration must be given to isolation precautions when managing a patient undergoing a bone marrow transplant, controversies surrounding these procedures exist. The actual procedures usually reflect the personal preferences of the medical staff. This chapter will discuss the most common types of isolation utilized.

Laminar air flow is the most extreme form of isolation, providing for a total protective environment. The process includes high-efficiency particulate air (HEPA) filtration with horizontal or vertical laminar air flow; sterile or low-organism-content food; frequent disinfection of walls, floors and other environmental surfaces; sterile linen and drinking water; toilet water disinfection; use of sterile booties, gowns, caps, and gloves for personnel and visitors entering the room; and elaborate protective garb when patients leave the room (Bennett & Brachman, 1985). In an attempt to sterilize the patient's gastrointestinal tract, oral nonabsorbable antibiotics and/or systemic antimicrobials are usually given (Petersen et al., 1987). Topical antimicrobials may also be used to suppress normal skin flora (Storb et al., 1983). This type of isolation is extremely expensive and time-consuming and may have negative psychological effects on patients due to the severe limitation of physical human contact. Petersen et al. (1987) retrospectively reviewed 99 patients at the Fred Hutchinson Cancer Research Center, where patients were randomized to either laminar air flow rooms or conventional rooms. They found no statistically significant difference in mortality rates between the two groups of patients. Storb et al. found that laminar air flow rooms decrease the incidence of GVHD in the aplastic anemia transplant population. The etiology of this is unclear; however, it is thought to be related to the absence of total body irradiation in the preparative regimen (Petersen et al., 1987). In deciding on isolation procedures in any unit, the economic factors as well as institutional needs must be considered.

Other types of isolation procedures include protective isolation (reverse isolation) or neutropenic precautions. In reverse, or protective, isolation, the patient is placed in a single room equipped with an HEPA filtration system. This system filters air at the 0.3-μ level, with positive pressure to hallway, decreasing the incidence of contamination from within the unit. Anyone entering the room must wear a gown, gloves, and mask. Handwashing with an antibacterial agent, whether povidone-iodine scrub or chlorhexidine, is required. In addition, patients are not permitted to drink or bathe in tap water; sterile water is used for drinking and bathing. Dietary restrictions are in place: no fresh fruits or vegetables. Upon leaving the room, patients wear gowns, caps, masks, gloves, and booties. These patients are also given oral nonabsorbable antibiotics. This type of isolation is usually an easier adjustment for the patient than the completely sterile environment of laminar air flow.

Neutropenic precautions are implemented at the authors' transplant center. The precautions include a single room equipped with an HEPA filter and positive pressure relative to the hallway. Handwashing with povidone-iodine or chlorhexidine prior to touching the patient is mandatory. Masks are utilized only for sterile or invasive procedures. Gowns and caps are worn for invasive procedures. Fresh fruits and vegetables are not allowed. Upon leaving their rooms, patients wear masks. Oral, nonabsorbable antibiotics are prescribed for the patients. This type of isolation is the easiest to tolerate by both the patient and the nursing staff.

As noted previously, the use of isolation is not consistent among transplant programs. Many questions remain unanswered. They are based on a multitude of factors that the center must consider before implementing their specific procedures. What is known is that the principles of asepsis remain the single most effective method of preventing infection.

Nursing Care Plan

The nursing care plan for a bone marrow transplant patient is complex. There are a multitude of organ systems that may be affected. The nursing care plan at the end of this chapter is designed to include all possible organ system toxicities for a patient. It should be obvious to the reader that not every patient will have all toxicities, but any patient may develop multiple problems.

THE DISCHARGE PROCESS

Criteria for Discharge

Patients are discharged from the hospital when their bone marrow has engrafted and their absolute neutrophil count is at least 500 units. Many patients may not have an appetite prior to going home, but they should be able to drink fluids and tolerate solid food. Also, patients should be instructed about the care of their indwelling catheters at home since they will require multiple platelet and blood transfusions and close monitoring of their blood counts for several months after discharge (Bozdech, 1986).

Follow-Up after Discharge

Close monitoring and follow-up of bone marrow transplant patients in the outpatient setting are imperative to the overall success of treatment. Patients are followed weekly for several months after transplant. During clinic visits, blood tests, chest x-rays, and bone marrow biopsies are required as part of routine care.

Patients continue to be immunosuppressed for at least 1 year after treatment and require blood and platelet transfusions. Patients who have had an autologous transplant will require blood components for approximately 3 to 6 months and will not regain complete B- and T-cell function for at least 6 months. Patients who have had an allogeneic transplant will require blood component support for a shorter period of time (approximately 1–3 months) but will not regain complete B- and T-cell function for at least 1 year. Patients who receive allogeneic bone marrow transplant will be closely monitored for signs and symptoms of GVHD. Medications are also reevaluated with every visit.

Many times, patients are not prepared for the impact that multiple clinic visits and long-term side effects such as GVHD will have on their life-styles. It is at this point that outpatient nurses play a key role in identifying physical problems and providing the patient with the psychosocial support they need through their recovery phase.

The readmission rate for posttransplant complications after initial discharge is 20% at the Medical Center at the University of California. The primary cause of readmission is fever associated with sepsis and GVHD. GVHD is a major cause of morbidity and occurs in almost 30% of long-term survivors (Corcoran-Buchsel, 1986).

Patient Discharge Teaching

Comprehensive discharge teaching is essential prior to patients' leaving the hospital. Patients often express fears of leaving the hospital and need reassurance that they can return to their normal life-styles provided they follow certain guidelines.

Patients will continue to be susceptible to infections for at least 1 year after bone marrow transplantation. It is important that they are well informed of the signs and symptoms of infection prior to discharge.

Patients are instructed to take their temperature once a day or whenever they are experiencing any signs of infection. If they have a fever of 38.5°C, they should call the physician.

The following illustrations include possible signs of infection that patients may experience after discharge and ways they can prevent infection. Also included with this discharge information are activities to resume and ways to cope with the psychosocial impact bone marrow transplant can have on one's life-style and quality of life.

Sample Discharge Instructions for Patients[1]

Signs of Infection

- Temperature elevation. Take your temperature once a day and whenever you have symptoms. Call your physician or the clinic if you have a fever of 38.5°C.
- Chills and sweats. A shaking chill is a medical emergency. Call immediately.
- Cold symptoms such as headache, nasal congestion, runny nose, sore throat, cough, earaches.
- Burning or pain on urination.
- Vaginal itching or drainage.
- Rectal pain or painful inflamed hemorrhoids.
- Diarrhea.
- Skin problems such as blisters, sores, rashes, reddening, swelling at catheter site or along tunnel area, drainage from site.
- Sore throat or mouth, difficulty swallowing.
- Shortness of breath, pain with breathing.
- Sinus tenderness or pain.

Prevention of infection

- Avoid crowds and peak-hour activities such as sports events, movie theaters, classes, church, stores.
- Wear a mask when outside your home. You may take your mask off outdoors if you are not close to people and it is not too windy. Wash your hands before touching your Hickman catheter, your face, your mouth or your food. Wash after being in public places and after handling other people's clothing or personal items.
- Avoid kissing loved ones on the mouth if they have mouth or lip sores.
- Do not share eating utensils or toothbrushes.
- Avoid contact with plants and soil. No gardening or farming.
- Avoid construction sites where soil may be disturbed.
- Avoid walking in the woods.
- Avoid contact with pets (handling, licking, kissing). (If possible, send pets away or keep them outside. Do not clean cages or litter boxes. Wash hands after contact with any animals.)
- Avoid areas where animals have been or are kept (i.e., farm, zoo).
- Avoid contact with people who are ill. Wear a mask at home if you believe that your children might have been exposed to a viral illness

[1]Reprinted with permission of M.J. Bozdech, MD, Director Bone Marrow Tranplant Program, University of California, San Francisco, 1986–1989.

such as measles, mumps, or chickenpox. Inform your physician of the exposure. Call if you or your children have been exposed to chickenpox.

- Do not swim with your central line catheter or immerse it in water when taking a bath.
- Do not take rectal temperatures, rectal medications or enemas.
- NO SMOKING. Smoking increases lung problems and increases the risk of infection.

With every clinic visit, you will have your blood drawn to monitor your complete blood count (CBC) and platelet count. The signs of low platelet count are petechiae, easy bruising, mouth bleeding, blood blisters, nosebleeds, rectal bleeding, blood in urine or stools, or black stools. (If you are on an iron supplement, your stools may be black.) The following are signs of low red cell count: fatigue, pale skin, weakness, dizziness and fainting, shortness of breath, headache, and palpitations.

All blood products you have received have been irradiated while in the hospital. You will continue to need irradiated blood after discharge. (This measure is to prevent GVHD.)

Food

- No fresh fruits or vegetables unless well washed at home.
- Eat a well balanced diet; your first year is not the time for weight-reduction diets.
- You may eat or take out food from reputable food chains. Be sure the restaurant is clean. Do not eat salads or other raw foods.
- Do not eat Mexican food that contains raw vegetables or lettuce. Chinese food is stir fried and therefore not cooked long enough to kill bacteria. Order hamburgers without lettuce and tomato when eating out.

Activity Level

Feeling fatigued after your bone marrow transplant is normal. You may not regain your full strength and ability to perform tasks for 8 to 12 months after transplant. Prioritize tasks. Save your energy for what is really important to you. Rest between activities and ask family and friends for help.

It is very important to continue your exercise program at home and try to increase it daily. The physical therapy department can help you with suggestions on your exercise program. Contact sports should be avoided. Also avoid any sports that require sudden or stressful movements of your arms above shoulder level while you have a Hickman catheter.

You may resume sexual relations with your loved one after your white cell and platelet counts are adequate. Please talk with your doctor or nurse regarding your counts and any restrictions on sexual activity.

Do not be alarmed if fatigue affects your interest in sex life at first. Fatigue may affect anyone this way. Many women will go through menopause after transplant. They may experience menopausal symptoms such as "hot flashes," vaginal dryness, and discomfort with intercourse. If this should occur, inform your nurse or doctor. Water-soluble lubricants may help vaginal dryness. Prolonged foreplay may increase sexual interest and increase vaginal lubrication. Hormone replacements may be given to treat these problems. Hormones can be continued until a woman reaches the normal age of menopause.

Psychosocial

Now that you are returning to the outside world, you may have new concerns. If you worked or were active outside the home, you may be bored staying at home. Your inability to fulfill all of your past roles may be frustrating to you and your family. Remember, recovery is a slow process. It is important that you and your family understand this.

If you are on prednisone for GVHD, you may have mood swings that may cause stress within your family. The drug can make you feel euphoric, and as the dose is decreased, you may feel depressed. It can also cause you to sleep poorly. If this happens, let your doctor know.

Once you are home, you may be more concerned about hair loss, weight loss or gain, and having to wear a mask. Your hair will grow back, and your appetite will improve. If you have taken prednisone, you may be heavier than normal and have a puffy face while on prednisone. When prednisone is stopped, the puffiness will go away. Prednisone does increase your appetite. Try to eat a well-balanced diet when on the drug.

You may be embarrassed to wear a mask in public. Keep in mind it's helping to prevent infection.

Many patients worry about being hospitalized, but reporting symptoms early may help to minimize hospital stays.

Check with your doctor before taking over-the-counter medications. Do not take aspirin, Empirin®, Alka-Seltzer® or any other aspirin-containing compound that might affect your platelets.

These are the discharge instructions currently in use at the Medical Center at the University of Calfornia; other centers may use somewhat different instructions. Consult your physician director about his/her particular preferences for discharge care information.

BONE MARROW TRANSPLANTATION NURSING CARE PLAN

Nursing diagnoses	Expected outcome	Nursing interventions
KNOWLEDGE DEFICIT of transplant process, treatment, prognosis, home management related to unfamiliarity with implications of transplant requirements for health maintenance.	Patient/family/ significant other(s), verbalize understanding of teaching related to transplant process.	1. Assess patient/ family throughout hospitalization to determine areas and extent of knowledge deficit. 2. Initiate patient/ family teaching utilizing a teach-ing/planning documentation record within first 24 hr. 3. Initiate patient information handbook on transplantation when he/she arrives on unit. 4. Initiate orientation to unit and isola-tion procedures.

*   *   *   *

High risk for injury related to **CHEMICAL INSULT TO BODY SYSTEMS** from administration of chemotherapy.	Absence of and/or stabilization of infection as a result of chemo-therapy toxicities Patient/family verbalizes understanding of possible toxicities and plan of care.	1. Refer to guidelines and toxicities for specific agents that patient is receiv-ing per chemotherapy manuals and/or protocols. 2. Premedicate patients prior to all chemo-therapy infusions with appropriate antiemetics per protocol. 3. Monitor for appro-priate agent toxicity. 4. Monitor patient and family level of understanding of protocol being utilized.

*   *   *   *

(continued)

BONE MARROW TRANSPLANTATION NURSING CARE PLAN (continued)

Nursing diagnoses	Expected outcome	Nursing interventions
High risk for injury related to **NEUTROPENIA** and **POTENTIAL FOR INFECTION**; absolute neutrophil count (ANC) less than 1,000 cells/cm^3	Absence and/or stabilization of infection. Patient/family verbalizes understanding of deficit and plan of care.	1. Monitor daily WBC and ANC, interpret values to patient/family. 2. Institute/maintain (compromised host or neutropenic precaution) isolation per hospital policy and document related teaching. 3. Monitor vital signs and temperature every 4 hrs or more frequently per patient status and nursing judgment. 4. Perform daily physical assessment of all body systems with high potential for infection.
	* * * *	
High risk for injury related to **THROMBOCYTOPENIA**; platelet (PLT) count less than 50,000 cells/cm^3	Absence and/or stabilization of bleeding as a result of thrombocytopenia. Patient/family verbalize understanding of deficit and plan of care.	1. Monitor daily PLT count and interpret values to patient/family. 2. Institute bleeding precautions per procedure and document related teaching. 3. Perform daily physical assessment and document signs/symptoms of bleeding. 4. Hema-test all body secretions (i.e., stool, urine, emesis).

(continued)

BONE MARROW TRANSPLANTATION NURSING CARE PLAN (continued)

Nursing diagnoses	Expected outcome	Nursing interventions
		5. For PLT count less than 10,000 cells/cm^3: limit activity, raise head of bed of bed 30°, monitor neuro signs and vital signs every 4 hr for signs/symptoms of acute bleeding and consult with MD regarding need for PLT transfusions.
		6. Perform neurological evaluation every 4 hrs if patient's platelets are below 10,000 cells/cm^3.
	* * * *	
High risk for **ALTERATION IN ORAL MUCOUS MEMBRANES** related to Stomatitis Gingivitis Infection Radiation therapy Dehydration	The integrity of the oral cavity will be maintained as well as possible. The patient will be able to participate in oral care.	1. Assess and document status of oral cavity every 4 hrs.
		2. Teach patient/family to perform oral care per unit policy qid.
		3. If patient develops lesions or discomfort, increase frequency of oral care to every 2–3 hrs.
		4. If severe pain develops, institute narcotics prn initially; if constant pain, give a continuous infusion to control pain.
		5. Set up suction (Yankauer) to clear oral secretions when patient unable to swallow comfortably.

(continued)

BONE MARROW TRANSPLANTATION NURSING CARE PLAN (continued)

Nursing diagnoses	Expected outcome	Nursing interventions
High risk for **ALTERATION IN NUTRITION,** less than body requirements, related to: Nausea Vomiting Anorexia Stomatitis Chemical injury GVHD	Patient's nutritional intake sufficient for age and size, weight stable and showing gradual increase after engraftment. Patient states or exhibits - decreased sensation of nausea and vomiting after engraftment or when mucous membranes are healed.	1. Assess and document dietary habits and history. 2 Identify the related etiology of patient's alteration in intake or discomfort and initiate preventive interventions. a. Encourage patient to eat/drink as tolerated and recognize patient's preference not to eat/drink. b. Eliminate unpleasant odors and unnecessary activity at meal times. c. Evaluate efficacy of antiemetic regimens; if appropriate, adjust agent's schedule or dose or make recommendations to physicians. 3. Reevaluate patients with prolonged nausea, vomiting, anorexia for other potential causes. 4. Initiate alternative interventions: antianxiety agents for prevention of nausea; administer appropriate pain medication to allow patient to try to eat and drink.

(continued)

BONE MARROW TRANSPLANTATION NURSING CARE PLAN (continued)

Nursing diagnoses	Expected outcome	Nursing interventions
		5. Assess for signs and symptoms of fluid and electrolyte imbalance.
		6. Assess and document patient's emesis for time, amount, duration and report any changes.
		7. Perform and record weights every day.
		8. Monitor need for implementation of hyperalimentation.
		9. Initiate calorie count/ diet consultation.
	* * * *	
High risk for **ALTERATION IN BOWEL ELIMINATION** (diarrhea) related to: Medications Infectious process. GVHD. Total body irradiation	Fluid and electrolyte balance will be maintained. Perianal area will remain intact. Patient demonstrates normal bowel pattern.	1. Assess and record time of stool, amount, consistency, presence of occult blood and any precipitating factors.
		2. Teach patient/family to perform perirectal care per unit protocol.
		3. Assess and document perianal area for redness, breakdown, lesions.
		4. Maintain accurate documentation of I&O, weights and abdominal girths if appropriate.
		5. If skin breakdown/lesions occur, institute dietary strategies to control or improve diarrhea.

(continued)

BONE MARROW TRANSPLANTATION NURSING CARE PLAN (continued)

Nursing diagnoses	Expected outcome	Nursing interventions
		6. Assess for signs/ symptoms of fluid and electrolyte imbalance.
		7. If skin breakdown/ lesions occur, institute the following orders: Sitz bath qid. Anusol® cream or other agent after each stool. Tucks® to perianal area after each stool.
	* * * *	
High risk for **ALTERATIONS IN INTEGUMENTARY SYSTEM** (skin rash, blisters) related to: GVHD Chemotherapy Radiation therapy	Skin will remain intact. Patient demonstrates normal skin pattern without rashes.	1. Evaluate skin integrity each shift. 2. Monitor changes in skin color—if rash or dry skin, start Eucerin Creme® or Aquaphor®. 3. If rash on hands or feet—start Silvadene® cream tid or qid if patient is not allergic to sulfa. 4. If skin is blistered, apply Burow's soaks at least bid as follows: 1 capful Burrow's solution to 2 qt tepid water; allow to soak for 15 mins; Follow with Silvadene cream; wrap with Kerlix®.

(continued)

BONE MARROW TRANSPLANTATION NURSING CARE PLAN (continued)

Nursing diagnoses	Expected outcome	Nursing interventions
		5. If chest, thighs, axillae, or groin are erythematous, apply Silvadene cream tid or qid.
		6. If pubic area or scrotum is erythematous, use nystatin cream to area qid. Do not place Silvadene on pubic area or scrotum—intense discomfort may ensue if applied to these areas. If patients remain uncomfortable, use baking soda and tepid or cool water soaks to pubic area or scrotum. Apply tid and prn for relief. Scrotal support for men may also provide relief.
		7. If head or face become dry or scaly, apply Aquaphor to areas tid to prevent dryness and remove scales; Aquaphor may also be applied to eyelids.
		8. Document all measures found to provide relief.
		9. Provide pain medication as needed to allow mobility.

(continued)

BONE MARROW TRANSPLANTATION NURSING CARE PLAN (continued)

Nursing diagnoses	Expected outcome	Nursing interventions
High risk for **ALTERATION IN PULMONARY PROCESS** (pneumonitis) related to Chemotherapy Radiation therapy Infectious process Idiopathic process	Normal pulmonary status will be maintained. Patient demonstrates normal breathing pattern.	1. Check respiratory rate and pattern of breathing every 4 hr. 2. Monitor breath sounds every 4 hr. 3. Monitor any new shortness of breath, nasal flaring, use of accessory muscles. 4. Apply pulse oximeter if short of breath or has increased respiratory rate. 5. Monitor level of anxiety during periods of shortness of breath. 6. Medicate as necessary to relieve symptoms.
	* * * *	
High risk for **ALTERATION IN CARDIAC OUTPUT** (pericardial effusion, cardiomyopathy) related to: heart sounds. Chemotherapy and/or Radiation	Cardiac hemodynamic status will be maintained within normal limits. Patient has normal heart sounds.	1. Monitor pulse and blood pressure every 4 hr. 2. Monitor for abnormal heart sounds, S3, rub, etc. 3. Monitor for pulsus paradoxus every 4 hr. 4. Initiate ECG after consult with MD if abnormal heart sounds noted. 5. Check for jugular venous distention. 6. Assess for edema. 7. Monitor daily weight.

(continued)

BONE MARROW TRANSPLANTATION NURSING CARE PLAN (continued)

Nursing diagnoses	Expected outcome	Nursing interventions
High risk for **ALTERATION IN RENAL PROCESS** (renal insufficiency, anuria, oliguria) related to: Chemotherapy GVHD Nephrotoxicity Antibiotics Antifungal agents Cy A	Renal function will be maintained. Patient has normal urinary output.	1. Monitor intake and output every shift. 2. Check all urine specimens for blood. 3. Measure specific gravity once every 24 hr. 4. Monitor laboratory results daily; check BUN and creatinine prior to administration of nephrotoxic agents. 5. Check for peripheral edema. 6. Check weight, abdominal girth daily.
* * * *		
High risk for **INEFFECTIVE COPING** related to: Changes in body image. Powerlessness Fear/anxiety Uncertain future	Patient/family verbalize feeling of an adequate sense of control in their lives and of a manageable level of anxiety, thus allowing them to function at satisfactory levels. Patient/family are able to perform activities of daily living (ADL) at or near admission level. Patient/family can identify support systems and how to utilize them most effectively.	1. Review with the patient/family their individual as well as group coping skills, noting any functional deficits that may require intervention; document in the nursing history. 2. Utilize a nursing history for ongoing assessment and development of nursing interventions. 3. Examine possible contributing factors (powerlessness, change in body image, anxiety, fear, depression); validate your assessment with patient and family.

(continued)

BONE MARROW TRANSPLANTATION NURSING CARE PLAN (continued)

Nursing diagnoses	Expected outcome	Nursing interventions
		4. Utilize appropriate nursing interventions as patient/family move through the various phases of crisis.
		5. Explore with patient/family the actual/potential support systems available in the hospital and at home. Help patient/family to identify patterns of anxiety (sources of stress) and most effective use of support systems.
		6. Consult with psychiatry, psychiatric liaison, clinical nurse specialist or social worker if needed.
		7. Allow time for patient to be alone or with family privately.
		8. Utilize hospital chaplain or patient's minister, priest or rabbi to assist with support.
		9. Utilize support system of friends and co-workers to help deal with crisis.

From "Care Plan for the Bone Marrow Transplant Patient," reprinted with the permission of the Department of Nursing at the Medical Center of the University of California, San Francisco, 1990.

CONCLUSION

The day of discharge is a happy day for patients and their families. Patients have survived an incredibly difficult hospitalization and are looking forward to resuming their normal life-styles.

However, the day of discharge is just the first step in the recovery phase. For some, the impact of treatment and follow-up care after hospitalization is difficult. There may be infectious complications that require hospitalization, multiple blood and platelet transfusions, extreme fatigue, and long-term side effects from the prednisone and cyclosporine that patients must take to prevent or control GVHD.

It is imperative that comprehensive discharge teaching be completed and the above issues discussed with patients and their families. The physical and psychological impact of this treatment can at times be overwhelming, and patients need a lot of encouragement and support from the interdisciplinary team after discharge.

The potential for cure is real. As researchers continue to look further into the prevention and treatment of complications, many more patients will be survivors, and their disease will be only a distant memory.

REFERENCES

Bennett, J., & Brachman, P. (1985). *Hospital infections* (p. 235). Boston: Little, Brown.

Bensinger, W. I., Buckner, C. D., Clift, R. A., Williams, B., Banaji, M., & Thomas, E. (1987). Comparison of techniques for dealing with major ABO-incompatible marrow transplants. *Transplantation Proceedings, 19* (6), 4605–4608.

Blume, K. Petz, L., (1983). *Clinical bone marrow transplantation* (p. 2). New York: Churchill Livingstone.

Bozdech, M. J. (1986). *Discharge instructions for bone marrow transplant patients.* San Francisco: University of California Medical Center.

Brown, H. N., & Kelly, M. J. (1976). Stages of bone marrow transplantation: A psychiatric perspective. *Psychosomatic Medicine, 38*(6), 439–446.

Burnett, A. K., & McDonald, G. A. (1987). Bone marrow transplantation. *Clinical transplantation: current practice and future prospects*, (pp. 171–197). Norwell, MA: MTP Press.

Carney, B. (1987). Bone marrow transplantation nurses' and physicians' perceptions of informed consent. *Cancer Nursing, 10*(5), 252–259.

Champlin, R. E., & Gale, R. P. (1984). The early complications of bone marrow transplantation. *Seminars in Hematology, 21*(2), 101–108.

Corcoran-Buchsel, P. (1986). Long-term complications of allogeneic bone marrow transplant: nursing complications. *Oncology Nursing Forum, 13*(6), 61–70.

Corcoran-Buchsel, P., & Ford, R. (1988). Introduction. *Seminars in Oncology Nursing, 4*(1), 1–2.

De Gregorio, M., Lee, W., Linker, C., Jacobs, R., & Ries, C. (1982). Fungal infections in patients with acute leukemia. *American Journal of Medicine, 73*(10), 543–548.

Eilers, J., Berger, A., & Petersen, M. (1988). Development, testing and application of the oral assessment guide. *Oncology Nursing Forum, 15*(3), 325–330.

Folsom, T., & Popkin, M. (1987). Current and future perspectives on psychiatric involvement in bone marrow transplantation. *Psychiatric Medicine, 4*(3), 319–329.

Ford, R., & Ballard, B. (1988). Acute complications after bone marrow transplantation. *Seminars in Oncology Nursing, 4*(1), 15–24.

Ford, R., McClain, K., & Cunningham, B. (1983). Veno-occlusive disease following marrow transplantation. *Nursing Clinics of North America, 18*(3), 563–569.

Freedman, S. (1988). An overview of bone marrow transplantation. *Seminars in Oncology, 4*(1), 9–14.

Gale, R. P. (1986). Potential utilization of a national HLA-typed donor pool for bone marrow transplantation. *Transplantation, 42*(1), 54–58.

Gale, R. P., Bortin, M., Van Bekkum, D., Biggs, J., Dicke, K., Gluckman, E., Good, R., Hoffman, R., Humphrey, E., Kersey, J., Marmont, A., Masoaka, T., Rimm, A., Van Rood, J., & Zwann, R. (1987). Risk factors for acute graft versus host disease. *British Journal of Hematology, 67*, 397–406.

Hickman, R., & Buckner, C. (1979). A modified right atrial catheter for access to the venous system in marrow transplant recipients. *Surgical Gynecology and Obstetrics, 148*, 871–875.

Hows, J., Yin, J., Marsh, J., Swirsky, D., Jones, L., Apperley, J., James, D., Smithers, S., Batchelor, J., Goldman, J., & Smith, E. (1986). Histocompatible unrelated volunteer donors compared with HLA non-identical family donors in marrow transplantation for aplastic anemia and leukemia. *Blood, 68*, 1322–1328.

Klemm, P. (1985). Cyclosporine A: Use in preventing graft versus host disease. *Oncology Nursing Forum, 12*(5), 25–32.

Linker, C. A. (1988, August). *Preliminary results in the Glaxo antibiotic study.* Paper presented at the University of California, San Francisco.

Martocchio, B. (1985). Family coping: Helping families help themselves. *Seminars in Oncology Nursing, 11*(4), 292–297.

McCullough, J., Rogers, G., Dahl, R., Therkelsen, D., Kamstra, L., Crisham, P., Kline, W., Bowman, R., Scott, E., Halagan, N., Williams, J., & Sander, S. G. (1986). Development and operation of a program to obtain volunteer bone marrow donors unrelated to the patient. *Transfusion,* July–August, 315–323.

McDonald, G. B., Shulman, H. M., Sullivan, K., & Spencer, G. (1986). Intestinal and hepatic complications of bone marrow transplant. Part 1. *Gastroenterology, 90*, 460–467.

McGlave, P. (1985) *Hospital Practice,* November 15, 292–297.

McGuire, T., & Almgren, J. (1987). Complications associated with bone marrow transplantation. *Highlights on Antineoplastic Drugs,* May/June, 16–20.

Murchinson, I., Nicholos, T. S., & Hanson, R. (1982). *The meaning and mythology of consent: Legal accountability in the nursing process* (2nd ed.). St. Louis: C. V. Mosby.

Parker, N., & Cohen, T. (1983). Acute graft versus host disease in allogeneic transplantation. *Nursing Clinics of North America, 18*(3), 569–577.

Petersen, F., Buckner, C., Clift, R., Nelson, N., Counts, G., Meyers, J., & Thomas, E. (1987). Infectious complications in patients undergoing marrow transplantation: A prospective randomized study of the additional effect of decontamination and laminar air flow isolation among patients receiving prophylactic systemic antibiotics. *Scandinavian Journal of Infectious Diseases, 19*(5), 559–567.

Pizzo, P., Commers, J., Cotton, D., Gress, J., Harthorn, J., Hiemenz, J., Longo, D.,

Marshall, D., & Robichaud, K. (1986). Approaching the controversies in antibacterial management of cancer patients. *American Journal of Medicine, 76*, 436–448.

Pizzo, P., & Schimpff, S. (1983). Strategies for the prevention of infection in the myelosuppressed or immunosuppressed cancer patient. *Cancer Treatment Reports, 67*(3), 223–234.

Rio, B., Andreu, G., Nicod, D., Arrago, J., Dutrillaux, R., Samama, M., & Zittoun, R. (1986). Thrombocytopenia in veno-occlusive disease after bone marrow transplantation or chemotherapy. *Blood, 67*(6), 1773–1776.

Rollins, B. J. (1986). Hepatic veno-occlusive disease. *American Journal of Medicine, 81*, 297–306.

Ruggiero, M. (1988). The donor in bone marrow transplantation. *Seminars in Oncology, 4*(1), 9–14.

Ruutu, T., Volin, L., & Elonen, E. (1988). Low incidence of severe acute and chronic graft versus host disease as a result of prolonged cyclosporine prophylaxis and early aggressive treatment with corticosteroids. *Transplantation Proceedings, 20*(3), 491–493.

Sambol, N. (1986). *Infection in the granulocytopenic host.* Paper presented at University of California, San Francisco.

Schryber, S., Lacasse, C., & Barton-Burke, M. (1987). Autologous bone marrow transplantation. *Oncology Nursing Forum, 14*(4), 74–79.

Storb, R., Prentice, R., Buckner, C., Clift, R., Appelbaum, F., Deeg, H., Doney, K., Hansen, J., Mason, M., Sanders, J., Singer, J., Sullivan, K., Witherspoon, R., & Thomas, E. (1983). Graft-versus-host disease and survival in patients with aplastic anemia treated by marrow grafts from HLA-identical siblings. Beneficial effect of a protective environment. *New England Journal of Medicine, 308*, 302–309.

Tutschka, P. J. (1987). Complications of bone marrow transplantation. *American Journal of Medical Science, 294*(2), 86–90.

University of California, San Francisco. (1986). *Bone marrow transplant information.* San Francisco: Author.

Wingard, J., Sostrin, M., Vriesendorp, J., Mellits, E., Santos, B., Fuller, D., Braine, H., Yeager, A., Burns, W., & Saral, R. (1988). Interstitial pneumonitis following autologous bone marrow transplantation. *Transplantation, 46*(1), 61–65.

Wolcott, D., Fawzy, F., & Wellisch, D. (1986). Psychiatric aspects of bone marrow transplantation: A review and current issues. *Psychiatric Medicine, 4*(3), 299–317.

Wolcott, D., Wellisch, D., Fawzy, F., & Landsverk, J. (1986). Adaptation of adult bone marrow transplant recipient long term survivors. *Transplantation, 41*(4), 478–483.

Wolcott, D., Wellisch, D., Fawzy, F., & Landsverk, J. (1987). Psychological adjustment of adult bone marrow transplant donors whose recipient survives. *Transplantation, 41*(4), 484–488.

PART III

Special Issues in Transplantation

CHAPTER 9

PEDIATRIC TRANSPLANT RECIPIENTS: SPECIAL NURSING CONSIDERATIONS AND CHALLENGES

Rosanne Perez-Woods
Eleanor A. Hedenkamp
Karen Ulfig
Danielle Newman
Vicki L. Fioravante

Care of children with transplants differs from that of adults in a number of ways: (a) Children's biophysical characteristics and responses depend on their developmental stage; (b) children's inability to understand fully the implications of transplants and engage in informed decision making compounds ethical and legal issues; (c) children's responses to separation, pain, bodily injury, and loss of control are developmentally specific; and (d) children's need for their parents' ongoing support is required as they experience the new and sometimes threatening hospital environment. Thus, nursing management must focus on both the children and the parents.

Ethical issues associated with transplants in the pediatric population raise significant concerns. Kanoti (1986) believes that transplantation is no longer an experimental therapy. However, problems associated with informed consent are profound. Experience with children's illness does not prepare families for the realities of what to expect following a transplant.

Transplant involves exchanging one difficult ethical problem for another. The terminal nature of end-stage disease is in itself coercive (Kanoti, 1986), as to refuse the possibility of transplant is an acceptance of certain death. To choose transplantation is to choose life; it is also to risk a long, painful intensive care unit (ICU) stay and possibility of death. Each family confronts the possibility of their child's death before and after transplant; few recognize how difficult the child's dying might be.

In addition to understanding the ethical issues and children's unique biophysiological responses, nurses must recognize the stressors associated with each developmental stage, accept the behavioral reactions, and provide support and assistance needed for successful coping. Children have developmentally specific responses to the stress of separation, loss of control, and bodily injury and pain associated with transplantation.

This chapter outlines indications for kidney, heart, liver, and bone marrow transplants in children and also provides recommendations for preoperative evaluation and nursing management of pediatric transplant patients. Differences in surgical techniques between adults and children are highlighted, and postoperative complications more prevalent in the pediatric kidney, heart, liver, and bone marrow transplant population are emphasized. Recommendations for postoperative nursing care include information about discharge planning, initial follow-up and long-term rehabilitation. Strategies to minimize separation and loss of control, decrease fear of bodily injury and pain, and maximize development and growth are integrated throughout the discussion. Table 9.1 provides a list of the nursing diagnoses for pediatric transplant patients.

INDICATIONS FOR TRANSPLANTATION IN CHILDREN

Kidney

As in adults, end-stage renal disease (ESRD) is the primary indication for kidney transplants in children. The incidence of ESRD, ages 1 to 15, is approximately 1.5 children per million. Congenital and hereditary diseases cause ESRD more frequently in children than in adults (Ettenger & Fine, 1986).

While dialysis remains an option for adults, kidney transplantation offers children with ESRD the best opportunity for life and normal growth and development. Potter et al. (1966) published the first documented results of pediatric kidney transplant.

Heart

The two main indications for heart transplantation in children are dilated cardiomyopathy and congenital heart disease (CHD) not amenable to other

TABLE 9.1 Nursing Diagnoses for Children Requiring Tranplants

Preoperative
  Knowledge deficit related to transplant process
  Anxiety
  Alteration in coping
  Alteration in family functioning
  Alteration in comfort
  Alteration in fluids and electrolytes
  Alteration in skin integrity (if total body irradiation is used prior to BMT)
  Alteration in diversional activity (isolation)
Early postoperative
  Impaired gas exchange
  Impaired tissue perfusion
  Alteration in cardiac output
  Alteration in clotting process
  Fluid volume disturbance
  Pain
  Alteration in consciousness
  Potential for infection
  Potential for bleeding
  Alteration in comfort
  Impaired tissue integrity
  Ineffective airway clearance
  Alteration in nutrition
Discharge
  Knowledge deficit
  Alteration in coping
  Alteration in self-concept and body image
  Alteration in reproductive competence
  Potential alteration in cognitive competence
  Potential for infection
  Potential alteration in nutrition
  Potential alteration in growth and development
  Potential alteration in family functioning
  Potential alteration in social competence

medical or surgical therapy. Children with CHD such as pulmonary atresia with the absence of the right and left pulmonary arteries, as well as those with pulmonary vascular obstructive disease, may also be considered for heart–lung transplantation. Children are considered for transplantation if their condition is such that death is expected within the next 6 to 12 months and there is no other appropriate medical or surgical therapy available. Infants born with hypoplastic left heart syndrome are an exception. Palliative surgery is offered for this condition; however, transplantation may offer less morbidity and a better outcome for some of these children. Between 1984 and 1988, 206 children younger than 9 years received heart transplantations; the current 1-year survival rate for pediatric heart transplantation is 85% (Heck, Shumway, & Kaye, 1989).

Liver

Biliary atresia is the leading indication for liver transplant in pediatric patients. The majority of these children have undergone one or more failed portoenterostomies (kasai procedures), and transplantation is their best hope for long-term survival. Other indications for transplantation in children include inborn errors of metabolism, cirrhosis, and fulminant hepatic failure (see Table 9.2 for complete listing).

Bone Marrow

Bone marrow transplantation (BMT) has progressed from an experimental therapy of last resort to the therapy of choice for certain diseases; it is a controversial therapy of curative potential for others. Immunological, hematological, malignant, metabolic, and congenital disorders are included in this group. Survival rates for BMT vary depending on the type of underlying disease.

Immunological Disorders

BMT has been used to treat infants with severe combined immunodeficiency disease (SCID). Allogeneic BMT with immunocompetent donor lymphoid

TABLE 9.2 Indications for Pediatric Liver Transplantation

Metabolic (inborn errors)
   Alpha-1-antitrypsin deficiency
   Alagille's syndrome
   Glycogen storage disease (types I and IV)
   Wilson's disease
   Tyrosinemia
   Hemochromatosis

Cirrhosis
   Biliary atresia
   Chronic active hepatitis
   Congenital hepatic fibrosis

Fulminant Disease
   Non-A, non-B hepatitis
   Drug-induced
   Viral

cells restores the immune function to infants born with defective T- and B-cell function. Bone marrow transplantation is the treatment of choice for children with SCID who have a sibling matched for human lymphocyte antibody (HLA) for bone marrow donation. Wiskott-Aldrich syndrome and other immunodeficient states, such as Chédiak-Higashi disease and DiGeorge syndrome (Goldsobel, Haas, & Steihm, 1987), have been reported to be successfully treated with allogeneic BMT.

Hematological Disorders

BMT has also been used to treat several pediatric hematological diseases. However, before BMT is selected over conventional therapy, careful consideration must be given to the risks and benefits of BMT versus the chronic effects of the original hematological disease and the quality of life following standard treatment.

Aplastic anemia, an idiopathic or acquired disorder characterized by bone marrow failure and resultant pancytopenia, may be primary or secondary to environmental factors such as viruses, drugs, or chemicals. Early BMT, using marrow from histocompatible donors, is the treatment of choice (Camitta, Storb, & Thomas, 1982). Children who have received multiple transfusions are at greater risk (50%) for rejecting the marrow and demonstrate decreased long-term survival rates (Bortin, Gale & Rimm, 1981; Sanders et al., 1986). Many children with aplastic anemia do not have an identical sibling who can donate marrow. Since BMT offers the greatest chance of surviving aplastic anemia, the use of alternate donors, such as partially matched relatives or matched nonrelatives, is currently being investigated in clinical trials (Thomas, 1988).

Fanconi's anemia is an autosomal, recessive, inherited disorder involving bone marrow failure, blood cell chromosome abnormalities, and congenital malformations. Early experiences using BMT as treatment for Fanconi's anemia yielded high morbidity and mortality rates due to conditioning-related toxicities and inherently defective repair mechanisms associated with this condition. However, recent research using modified conditioning regimens suggests improved survival rates (Deeg et al., 1983; Gluckman, Berger & Dutreix, 1984).

Thalassemia major is a genetic disorder resulting in severe hypochromic anemia. In the early 1980s, the first successful transplant for thalassemia was performed (Thomas et al., 1982). A recent investigation by Lucarelli et al. (1987) reported a 70% success rate. Since children can become iron overloaded and sensitized from chronic transfusion requirements, a more favorable outcome is achieved for these children if BMT can be performed early.

BMT was performed as a treatment for acute nonlymphoblastic leukemia (ANLL) in an 8-year-old girl who also had sickle cell anemia (Johnson et al., 1984). BMT provided for marrow reconstitution with elimination of the leukemia as well as the sickle cell anemia. BMT can potentially eradicate the hemoglobinopathy of sickle cell anemia and can potentially eradicate the disease. However, the use of BMT to treat sickle cell disease remains controversial because conventional supportive therapy can provide a fairly good prognosis and quality of life.

Although the role of BMT in the treatment of aplastic anemia is clear, its role in the treatment of inherited hematological disorders, such as sickle cell disease, thalassemia, and Fanconi's anemia, requires further definition and research. One exciting and highly experimental approach to treating genetic diseases such as inherited hemoglobinopathies is gene insertion therapy with autologous BMT. Gene insertion therapy provides the child's missing gene by inserting the gene into the autologous bone marrow cells, which are then transplanted into the patient.

Congenital and Metabolic Disorders

In addition to inherited immunodeficiencies and hemoglobinopathies, allogeneic BMT has been used with variable success to treat other congenital diseases, such as Diamond-Blackfan syndrome. These diseases result in spectrum bone marrow failure and resultant hematological or immunological instability (August et al., 1976). Other genetically acquired disorders that can involve metabolic abnormalities have been successfully treated with BMT, including Gaucher's disease, metachromatic leukodystrophy, mucopolysaccharidosis, and infantile osteopetrosis (August et al., 1976; Coccia, 1980; O'Reilly, Brochstein, Dinsmore, & Kirkpatrick, 1984).

Malignancies

Most experience with BMT, as part of cancer therapy, has been in treating hematological malignancies such as leukemia. Leukemias are cancers arising from malignant bone marrow stem cells, specifically immature white blood cells. The malignant overgrowth of leukemic cells results in the bone marrow's failure to produce functional blood cells. Thus, the ability to remove and replace the dysfunctional bone marrow and simultaneously eradicate cancerous cells is desirable.

Leukemia accounts for one third of cancers occurring in children (Poplack & Reaman, 1988). Leukemia affects children differently from adults. The majority of children with leukemia have acute leukemia characterized by a sudden onset of symptoms such as anemia, fatigue, joint pain, weight loss, bleeding, fever, infection, hepatosplenomegaly, and abnormal white counts. A diagnosis of leukemia is made when greater than 5% leukemia blast cells are seen on a bone marrow aspirate smear. Acute leukemia is further differentiated as lymphoblastic or nonlymphoblastic based on the type of malignant cell type.

Children with acute lymphoblastic leukemia (ALL) who achieve a sustained remission have approximately a 60% chance of surviving their disease when treated with conventional chemotherapy (Poplack & Reaman, 1988). For children who experience a relapse, BMT with a histoidentical donor is the recommended treatment once a second remission is attained. Allogeneic BMT performed during the second remission for these children can provide a 30% to 45% chance of disease-free survival (Butturini, Rivera, Bortin & Gale, 1987; Herzig et al., 1987; Johnson et al., 1981). Children with ALL and poor prognostic factors, such as leukemia spread to the central nervous system or mediastinum and certain chromosomal aberrations, have a 27% to 45% possibility of long-term survival with conventional chemotherapy (Butturini et al., 1987; Herzig et al., 1987; Johnson et al., 1987).

Treatment of ANLL with conventional therapy is improving, but survival rates remain much less optimistic than for ALL. When appropriate donors are available, allogeneic BMT is the preferred form of therapy.

Chronic myelogenous leukemia (CML), marked by accelerated phases and chronic phases, rarely occurs in children. Reported survival with BMT performed during the chronic phase is 60% to 70%, whereas survival with BMT performed during the accelerated phase is poor (Feig, 1986).

Autologous BMT is being investigated as treatment for pediatric cancers when a histoidentical donor is not available and conventional treatment has been ineffective in eliminating malignant disease. For some children, autologous BMT can offer a 25% to 30% chance of survival for otherwise incurable acute nonlymphoblastic leukemia (Cheson, Lacerna, Leyland-Jones, Sarosy, & Wittes, 1989). Autologous BMT as a therapeutic approach for resistant solid tumors is also being investigated. Neuroblastoma, the most common solid tumor occurring in children, is an aggressive malignant process arising from sympathetic nervous tissue. Using conventional therapy, the overall prognosis for children older than one year diagnosed with neuroblastoma is 10% to 20% (August et al., 1976; Philip et al., 1987).

PREOPERATIVE EVALUATION

When transplantation is presented as a treatment option, both children and their families face a decision with lifelong implications, uncertainties, and ambiguities. Children are offered the potential for achieving a cure of an otherwise fatal disease. Conversely, the transplant process can cause serious complications and long-term sequelae; and even after surviving the procedure, the risk of relapse and complications persists.

Transplantation must be realistically and honestly discussed with parents so that transplant is chosen because it is the best option. It is important to offer an overview of the long-term picture, the transplant procedure, and expectations for the postoperative period. Past experiences and coping styles of children and parents should be assessed and considered in the discussion. Coloring books, puppet play, photographs, and first-person stories from other recipients can help the teaching process. The decision-making process should involve discussion of diagnosis, age, donor availability, overall health status, treatment alternatives, risks and benefits, the transplant process, quality of life, time frames, commitment to long-term care, family dynamics, and social and financial responsibilities (Wiley & House, 1988). Psychosocial issues and reproductive options, such as sperm-banking for adolescent males, should be discussed with older children (Kaempfer, Hoffman, & Wiley, 1983).

Careful discussion and exchange of information is part of an ethical and legal obligation to obtain parental consent and age-appropriate child assent to perform transplantation. If children are to receive allogeneic transplants, the donors are usually siblings. Siblings are often ambivalent about donating; they want to help their brother or sister but resent the disruption of their lives and imposed fear and pain. Both children's feelings must be assessed regularly throughout the BMT process, especially if complications develop. The rights of both children must be protected when informed consent is obtained. Can siblings really say "no" when they are asked? Opportunities should be made available for siblings to express feelings and be supported in any decisions they make.

Pretransplant Evaluation

The pretransplant evaluation has two functions: It allows the transplant team to evaluate the potential transplant candidate, and it allows the team to educate the child and family about transplantation. Adult and pediatric evaluation processes are similar. They include a history, chart review, physical examination, interview, and laboratory evaluation. The following components are of special significance for the pediatric population.

Etiology

The type of problem determines the necessary assessment procedures. For hereditary problems, a careful family evaluation is necessary, especially if a living-related transplant is being considered. A living related donor's organ or marrow function must be determined to avoid donors who may be affected with a similar disease. A number of diseases occur in transplanted organs or marrow.

Prior Therapy

In BMT patients, prior therapy is reviewed because residual or anticipated toxicities may accumulate and intensify the toxic effects of the conditioning regimen.

Age

There is no lower age limit for transplantation in children. In children who have ESRD, transplant is delayed, as long as the child is doing well, until the child weighs more than 5 kg (Lum, Wassner, & Martin, 1985). Children weighing under 5 kg have problems with vascular thrombosis because of the small size of their vessels. Children who are old enough to have some understanding of the transplant process must be included in the preoperative educational process and offered the opportunity to assent. Children over 7 years are considered old enough to have their opinions taken seriously, although this varies with individuals (Kanoti, 1986).

Physical Findings

Children's physical condition affects understanding and reactions. Critically ill children may be depressed and exhausted, both physically and emotionally. Discussions should be brief to avoid fatigue. They should be offered when children are feeling rested and receptive; competing stimuli should be minimized. Children who have been previously healthy and are suddenly catastrophically ill may display more shock and grief than chronically ill children, who may have considered transplantation as a potential option. In children with cardiac problems, decreased cardiac output can impair understanding, thus requiring simple basic explanations. Play can supplement discussions in assessing children's levels of understanding and reactions. Meeting other children and families can be helpful in the decision-making process.

Maintaining adequate nutrition and maximizing growth potential is extremely difficult in children with ESRD (Lum et al., 1985). In very small children, severe growth and neurological retardation may be present. In addition, children with ESRD must have satisfactory urological function prior to transplantation. Pretransplant preparatory surgery may be needed if other urological abnormalities are found. Preexisting severe hypertension or chronic hypertension may require bilateral nephrectomy.

Physical findings associated with increased morbidity and mortality following cardiac transplantation include multiple organ involvement, cachexia, and elevated pulmonary vascular resistance (PVR), which might predispose to early right ventricular failure. One option for some children with elevated PVR who need a heart transplant is to receive a heart in which right ventricular hypertrophy has developed in response to the increased workload caused by pulmonary disease. Hearts of patients with cystic fibrosis who undergo heart–lung transplantation may be considered in this situation. All children must be free from infection at the time of transplant to prevent increased infection-related morbidity and mortality due to posttransplant immunosuppression.

PREOPERATIVE NURSING CARE

Once children are accepted as candidates for transplants, the waiting period begins. This time is difficult for children and their families for various reasons (Gold, Kirkpatrick, Fricker, & Zitelli, 1986). Great uncertainty exists without possibility of making long-term plans; the wait is for an unknown time, and children may die before donors are found. Parents may experience guilt related to waiting for another child's death or a sibling's agreement to donate marrow. Competing with others for donor organs or marrow and perceiving failure to protect their own children's health and safety is difficult for parents.

Some families publicize their situation, either for financial reasons or to emphasize the need for donors. Although some families feel relief in sharing the problem and having something to do, most feel that their privacy is invaded during a difficult and personal time. In addition, some families feel pressured to agree to future media demands because of the previous media access and support.

Preparation of children for transplantation is a complex problem because in many cases the transplant will occur at an unknown time with little preparation time when donors are found. Young children cope best when they are not given too much information too soon; after a short period of time, worrying and fretting replace productive coping. Older children are usually involved in ongoing discussions, but they may find the uncertainty and wait extremely difficult. Children should be allowed to pace themselves; information should be offered when it is requested but not forced on them if they are unwilling to listen. Masks and gloves, books about hospitalization and surgery, and coloring books can be helpful. Relief from the topic is also important; there is no need to discuss it daily.

Siblings also should be involved in preparation and discussion. Their needs are easily overlooked because of the sick child's demands. Conflicting feelings of fear and worry for the sick sibling and jealousy at the extra attention they receive are common.

Clinical nurse specialists play an important role during the waiting period. In consultation with the social worker and recreation therapist or child life worker, nurses offer help and support to parents in coping with a child's condition, medication regimen, and daily management, as well as providing continuity of care and information as events develop.

Admission to Hospital

There is usually joy and relief when donors are found. Children are admitted to the hospital, and the preparation for surgery is begun. Careful age and developmentally appropriate explanations of the special rooms and rules avoid misinterpretation and enhance cooperation. Parents are encouraged to bring cherished play items from home, such as dolls and video games, to create a less threatening environment. In addition to performing laboratory tests, pediatricians, surgeons, oncologists, and anesthesiologists complete history and physical examinations. Immunosuppression is also begun, and additional preparation is integrated into these activities.

Routine activities and tasks that children and parents, or caregivers, are expected to perform can be tiresome and unpleasant. However, these tasks add structure and consistency to the children's days and serve as signs that they are being cared for. These tasks encourage them to take interest in caring for themselves. Encouragement and compassionate assistance with difficult tasks enhances trust and adjustment. Creativity and rewards for completing tasks foster mastery and self-esteem. Play and quiet time are also important and are planned for in children's daily activities.

Children who are to receive BMT require a pretransplant conditioning regimen. Pretransplant conditioning regimens are similar to adult regimens and last for 4 to 8 days. The type of regimen depends on the underlying disease and prior treatment. Infants with severe combined immunodeficiency syndrome may not require a preoperative regimen because they lack the cellular immune responses necessary for rejection (Yeager, 1988). The side effects and nursing interventions to reduce discomfort are similar to those that adult patients experience. Children usually experience general malaise during the conditioning regimen and require a restful environment and parents to console them.

Parents often experience guilt related to children's discomfort and anticipate future problems. Skillful nursing management reassures the parents, allows them to express their feelings, and teaches them how to care for their children.

Care for sibling donors also requires skillful nursing management. Sibling donors often provide kidneys for transplantation or bone marrow. Care for the sibling kidney and bone marrow donors is similar to that for adult donors. Often the day of the donor's harvest is the same as the recipient's transplant. Parental anxiety over placing a healthy child at risk for the possible but uncertain benefit of another comes to fruition as they anticipate one child's return from the operating room and the other child's potentially life-saving transplant (Ruggiero, 1988).

INTRAOPERATIVE NURSING CARE

Children are taken to the operating room following appropriate sedation. During this time parents should accompany them as long as possible and not leave them alone with unfamiliar care providers. Optimally, clinical nurse specialists accompany children to the operating room waiting area. Children who appeared to have been sedated have later reported fear and anxiety associated with experiences that occurred while in the surgical waiting area. Thus, nurses should reduce children's exposure to patients experiencing other surgical procedures and conversations between health care providers related to patient care. Nurses must ensure that someone the children know and trust are with them until anesthesia is achieved.

SURGICAL PROCEDURE

The techniques for most transplants are the same for most children as for adults. Variations exist for the following:

1. Pediatric cardiac transplant patients with corrected levo-transposition of the great vessels (Reitz, Jamieson, Gaudiani, Oyer, & Stinson, 1982) and infants with hypoplastic left heart syndrome (Bailey, Concepcion, Shattuck, & Huang, 1986).

2. Pediatric kidney transplant patients whose iliac fossae (see site A in Figure 9.1) are not large enough to accommodate the kidneys from adult donors, requiring graft implantation using the recipient aorta and vena cava (site B) (Salvatierra, 1986). Figure 9.1 illustrates the two surgical modifications for pediatric kidney transplant procedures.

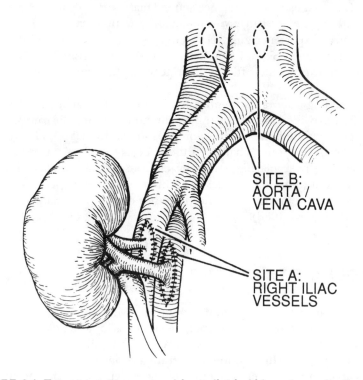

FIGURE 9.1 Two anastomoses used in pediatric kidney transplant procedure. *Site A:* **Iliac vessels, used when donated kidney fits into iliac fossa.** *Site B:* **Aorta/vena cava, used when an adult or large child's kidney is donated. Drawing by Bayard Colyear, medical illustrator.**

3. Pediatric cadaver kidneys grafted into adults and children as single units. This operation is similar except that patches of the donor aorta and vena cava are used for anastomosis (Salvatierra, 1986).

During surgery, preparations are made in the ICU to receive the children. In addition to the equipment needed for adults, pediatric equipment includes microcontainers for laboratory work, the correct size blood pressure cuff, catheters, and intubation equipment.

Keeping parents informed of operating room progress decreases their concern and stress. Clinical nurse specialists, social workers, or operating room staffs should plan brief, regular visits to families to keep them informed. If problems develop, families need information and support; uncertainty may be the most difficult aspect of waiting during surgery.

During surgery, families should also meet the nurses who will care for the children postoperatively. Primary nursing is invaluable for all transplant recipients but especially for children. This is an opportune time for nurses to review with families how children will look immediately after surgery, anticipated ICU visiting hours and routines, and special procedures following transplant. The first visit with the children is feared but also eagerly anticipated. Opportunity for parental visiting should be provided as soon as possible, even if only for a few minutes.

POSTOPERATIVE COMPLICATIONS

Many complications pediatric transplant patients experience are similar to those anticipated in adults following transplant. However, there are some specific differences.

Kidney

As with adults, postoperative complications include rejection, infection, hypertension, and the complications of immunotherapy. The long-term impact of steroids on growth requires monitoring and dosage adjustment to minimize the growth-retardant side effect of immunosuppression.

Heart

Following heart transplantation, many children have a dramatic recovery, reflecting the normal cardiac output of healthy hearts. Other children, particularly those with cachexia and multiorgan disease, have slower recoveries. Complications associated with heart transplants are similar to those expected in adult patients.

Liver

The risk of postoperative hemorrhage is increased in pediatric recipients. Because of the small size of the child's blood vessels, a protocol using dextran 40 is used to prevent capillary slugging and potential thrombus formation in the portal vein and hepatic artery. Aspirin and dipyridamole are instituted once children are started on oral feedings and continued for up to 3 months posttransplant. This therapy may predispose children to bleeding.

In addition, control of hypertension is especially important in pediatric patients whose clotting studies are somewhat prolonged for prevention of hepatic artery thrombosis. Hepatic artery thrombosis is the most common and most serious complication of liver transplantation in children and may occur as late as 3 months following transplant.

Bone Marrow

As with adults, postoperative complications may occur because of (a) prolonged lack of functional bone marrow (hemorrhage and infection); (b) side effects and organ toxicities from chemotherapy or total body irradiation (gastrointestinal mucositis, veno-occlusive disease, and renal, pulmonary, or cardiac complications); and (c) graft-versus-host disease (GVHD) secondary to allogeneic bone marrow transplantation. Complications may occur early within the first weeks after transplant or months later. Children may manifest long-term sequelae.

Primary cardiac failure is rare in children following BMT. However, children may experience cardiovascular disturbances such as altered blood pressure, altered cardiac output, and arrhythmias because of fluid and electrolyte shifts due to sepsis, bleeding, and hepatic or renal failure. Cardiac failure may occur acutely as a result of these disturbances or as a result of progressive multisystem failure.

Engraftment criteria are similar to those used for adults. Although engraftment is the hallmark of a successful transplant, some engrafted children still succumb to posttransplant complications and long-term health alterations. Table 9.3 describes these complications.

Children who survive BMT are at risk for neurological and endocrine dysfunction affecting growth, learning, and sexuality. BMT preparatory regimens used to treat pediatric malignancies often include total body irradiation, cranial radiation, and intrathecal chemotherapy and can damage the brain and central nervous system.

Although young tissues are more resilient after trauma, development may be impaired and late complications become more apparent as children grow and develop (Wiley & House, 1988).

TABLE 9.3 Significant Organ System Complications of BMT Conditioning in Children (Total Body Irradiation, High-Dose Chemotherapy)

System/complication	Onset (after BMT)	Nursing implications
Pulmonary Infection Interstitial pneumonia Cytomegalovirus *Pneumocystis carinii*	3–15 months	Assess signs and symptoms of fever, sepsis, cough, hypotension, routine vital signs Chest auscultation of breath sounds and aeration Monitor arterial blood gas and pulmonary function test (PFT) as needed Respiratory hygiene: cough and deep breath, hydration, suction
Lung Obstructive Restrictive	Variable	Assess cough, dyspnea, activity intolerance, routine vital signs Respiratory hygiene. Arterial blood gas (ABG), PFT
Neurologic Leukoencephalopathy	1–5 months	Assess neurologic status for signs and symptoms of lethargy, somnolence, dementia, seizures, coma, personality changes
Learning disabilities (associated with abnormal motor, perceptual, behavioral, and language performance)	Variable	Patient/parent counseling Assess progress with developmental tasks Inform school; special education classes may be necessary Follow closely to provide early intervention
Cataracts	1–5½ years	Patient/parent risk information Frequent eye examinations Ophthalmology referral
Endocrine Subnormal growth development, delayed puberty, infertility, sterility (associated with decreased adrenocortical and thyroid function and growth hormone production)	Variable	Careful monitoring of growth and development with charts Annual growth pattern review Assess reproductive and gonad status Patient/parent counseling and anticipatory teaching about infertility, sexuality, birth control, sperm banking, and growth hormone supplementation.

From: "Bone marrow transplantation in children" by F. Wiley & K. House(1988), *Seminars in Oncology Nursing, 4(1),* p.34. Copyright Grune & Stratton, Orlando, Florida. Reprinted by permission.

POSTOPERATIVE NURSING CARE

Postoperative nursing care of children depends on the type of transplant and the age and development of childen. Nursing care required by children during this period is similar to the care adult transplant recipients need. The next section describes differences related to biophysical differences in children and their developmental needs.

An important nursing diagnosis after heart transplantation is alteration in cardiac output. Pharmacological agents maintain hemodynamic stability and cardiac output (isoproterenol for its chronotropic effect; prostaglandin E_1 as a pulmonary vasodilator; dopamine, dobutamine, and epinephrine as positive inotropes; and nitroglycerin and nitroprusside to decrease afterload). Volume replacement with blood or blood products maintains the central venous pressure and left atrial or pulmonary artery pressures within normal limits. Left-sided monitoring of the heart may be indicated in infants because of their normally higher pulmonary artery pressures and immature pulmonary vasculature. Monitoring may also be needed in older children with pulmonary hypertension or pulmonary vascular changes.

Bleeding can frighten children; they should be calmed with reassurance that the bleeding will be controlled. Children also require frequent blood work following BMT and should have the minimum possible amount of blood drawn to limit additional blood losses. Children require nutritional support with intravenous total parenteral nutrition to meet the increased metabolic needs for healing and growth. In addition, children commonly require narcotic infusions such as fentanyl or morphine to relieve stomatitis.

Children have a larger ratio of body surface area to volume, higher fluid requirements per unit of body weight, and a larger proportion of extracellular fluid than do adults. These differences cause pediatric BMT patients experiencing blood vessel damage and fluid loss to be at increased risk of circulatory compromise (Hazinski, 1984). In addition, children are at increased risk for metabolic disturbances, coagulation abnormalities, and toxic drug or metabolite levels that can affect neurological function and compound blood and fluid losses.

Children are also at increased risk for impairment of respiratory function following transplant. Oxygenation and ventilation are managed in the traditional manner. Children usually remain intubated. Oxygen concentration, tidal volume and rate, and positive end pressure are decreased as children awaken from surgery and become stronger. Most children are extubated within 24 hours following the transplant.

Ineffective airway clearance of nasal and oral secretions, as well as bleeding, causes airway obstruction in all children requiring a transplant more frequently than in adults because of the small size of children's airways. Parents and children should be taught nasal and oral suction techniques to maintain patent airways while childen are bleeding or producing large thick secretions. Supplemental oxygen or intubation becomes necessary when children's airways are compromised.

Measurement of hourly output is an important nursing intervention to determine kidney perfusion and intravascular fluid status following all types of transplant. For infants and young children, a minimum acceptable urine output is usually 1 cc/kg/hr.

Hemorrhage and/or diffuse bleeding may occur as a result of coagulopathies and/or inadequate surgical hemostasis. Coagulopathies are common after cardiopulmonary bypass and induced hypothermia for heart transplant. Children with previous cyanotic heart disease or liver dysfunction may be especially at risk. Bleeding may be noted during endotracheal suctioning and in gastric drainage and urine as well as in chest tubes. Standard laboratory measurement of coagulation factors permits treatment with appropriate coagulation factors. Continued surgical bleeding with chest tube drainage of 10 cc/kg/hr for a child of less than 10 kg may require a return to surgery for exploration and hemostasis. If this happens, families need reassurance that this is a less critical procedure than the initial transplant.

As children awaken from anesthesia, neurological assessment confirms that they can move all extremities and respond to stimuli in an age-appropriate manner. The potential for pain after surgery is an important nursing diagnosis. Nurses continually assess pain and anxiety and the need for analgesia and sedation. Children's pain can affect their moods, activity levels, and compliance with other medical therapy. Pain assessment is more difficult in children than in adults; behavioral cues, information from parents, and observation of the effects of various interventions are all important. Increased heart rate, blood pressure, splinting respirations, and a tense, anxious facial expression are all potential cues that the children are experiencing pain. Children may deny pain or discomfort because they are unclear about what it means or because of guilt or fear of needles. Use of intravenous and oral analgesia and frequent reassurance and positive reinforcement that children are "doing a good job" and getting better are helpful. Intramuscular injections for pain should be avoided in children. Analgesia given before planned activity or therapy improves compliance and effectiveness. The children's ages and personalities and levels of preparation affect the need for sedation. Anxiety and tension precipitates or worsens pain; soothing and comforting measures such as stroking, cuddling, singing, or reading stories and using musical tapes decrease the need for sedation or analgesia. Toddlers and older children benefit from relaxation exercises; for very young children parental presence promotes a sense of feeling safe. Parental participation in care is important for all children; many parents appreciate specific suggestions on how they can best support and help their children.

Potential for infection and rejection are important nursing diagnoses following transplantation. Sterile technique is imperative while caring for wounds, invasive catheters, and lines. Most children are initially roomed alone with modified protective isolation. Parents should be allowed to visit without masks as soon as possible; young children need to see faces. Good handwashing is imperative when entering the room and after handling soiled items such as diapers.

Nursing assessment for infection is performed by obtaining daily cultures and white blood cell measurements and by observing wounds and insertion sites for signs of infection. Temperature is measured every 4 hours and as necessary. A mild fever can be significant since steroids may mask or reduce the pyretic response to infection.

The noninvasive diagnosis of rejection continues to be a source of great interest and research. In cardiac transplant patients, the endomyocardial biopsy as first described by Caves, Stinson, Billingham, and Shumway (1973) continues to be the diagnostic method of choice. Bahargava et al. (1987) found that children have no specific clinical signs of acute rejection. Signs of congestive heart failure (tachypnea, tachycardia, arrhythmias, irritability, edema, and poor feeding) strongly suggest the need for a biopsy following heart transplant.

Immunosuppression routines vary; cyclosporine A (Cy A), azathioprine, and steroids are often used. Cy A levels can vary greatly in children, and children frequently require a higher dose per kilogram than do adults to achieve the same blood levels. Additional antirejection drugs include anti-thymocytic globulin and OKT3, which may be given prophylactically or used to treat rejection episodes.

DISCHARGE AND REHABILITATION

Preparation for Discharge

Discharge preparation begins at the time of surgery, if not during the discussions prior to transplantation. Postoperative rehabilitation is promoted by instilling a sense of independence and self-sufficiency in children and their families during the postoperative period. The initial hospitalization will be the first of many; how it is perceived by children and their families can greatly affect future behavior and cooperation.

As children awaken and stabilize, the environment can be enhanced and personalized. Calendars, pictures, cards, and posters can brighten the walls. Furniture scaled for children such as potty chairs, high-chairs, low tables and chairs, and toys and equipment from home can make children feel more comfortable.

Occupational and/or physical therapy should be ordered as soon as possible to promote play, exercise, recreation, rehabilitation, and preparation for further medical intervention. Relaxation tapes and similar resources can be particularly helpful during biopsies, venipuncture, and similar stressful and uncomfortable painful procedures. Whenever possible, painful procedures should take place away from the place where children sleep. Once children associate pain with sleep, the potential for long-term sleep disturbances increases. Older children cope with stress better if they know exactly what is happening and have some control during the procedure. Using coloring books and videotapes specifically developed to explain procedures assists children in understanding what will happen and their role in the procedure.

Patient Education

Parents are usually elated in the early postoperative period, especially when their children demonstrate rapid signs of recovery. However, they are also uncomfortable, apprehensive, and not sure what role they will play in the future. Staff–parent conflicts are common during this period of rapid change and readjustment. Many parents develop tremendous knowledge and skill in caring for their chronically ill child; this knowledge and skill must be honored and respected and used in developing the nursing care plan. Parents of children who have suffered sudden unexpected illness and deterioration may still be attempting to come to some acceptance and understanding of what has occurred. Parents need to be encouraged to reestablish their parenting role as soon as possible.

Nursing care is organized around the knowledge deficit related to transplantation. Nurses should encourage parents to provide complete care as soon as possible. Tasks that parents can perform include cleaning toys and equipment, measuring and controlling intake and output, and performing diapering, bathing, feeding, and comforting activities.

Immediately after surgery, parents can begin to learn the actions, doses, and side effects of medications. The medication schedule should be adjusted to fit as easily as possible with the family schedule. Various techniques for giving medications to young children should be discussed. Older children should be responsible for learning about and taking their own medications with supervision as needed.

Home blood pressure monitoring, frequently difficult in young children, may be needed to assess for hypertension, a common side effect of immunosuppressive medications. This is a new and possibly frightening activity for some parents. The technique should be taught so that there is adequate time for practice before discharge. A blood pressure cuff of the correct size, a manometer, and a stethoscope should be provided. Digital blood pressure cuffs may be used for children if the appropriate cuff size is available.

Additional information critical for discharge planning includes long-term diet information, recipes, and an exercise plan. Suggestions for adapting favorite recipes and substitutions for others are usually needed and appreciated. In children receiving steroids, weight control is a potential problem, in part because of the increased appetite associated with steroid therapy. Postoperative activity restrictions and guidelines for increasing physical activity and stamina are helpful; older children enjoy exercise rehabilitation programs.

Many medical centers' staffs believe that it is necessary for parents to learn cardiopulmonary resuscitation (CPR). They are instructed to take the CPR course offered by the hospital or the local American Heart Association.

Prior to discharge, parents of young children should have the opportunity to provide 24-hour total care, with nursing guidance and support, to prepare them for discharge and their total care responsibilities. This also provides an opportunity to discuss questions and problems that have not been anticipated.

The family should be given an appointment for follow-up and a list of telephone numbers to call if any questions or concerns develop. A call should also be made to the nurse at the primary pediatrician's office to discuss the discharge plan and offer detailed instructions on any aspect of the child's home care unfamiliar to the office or clinic nurse. The list of telephone numbers given to the family should also be made available to the nurse so that appropriate information can be given to the family should a problem arise. Often a small celebration party is the last event prior to discharge.

Rehabilitation

Families who live a long distance from the transplant center may stay in the immediate area 2 to 6 months following discharge. Most families appreciate social service assistance in locating appropriate housing. Children are seen for follow-up twice weekly at first, then weekly, and eventually less frequently. Follow-up visits can be very tiring for childen. Bringing strollers, snacks, and some tapes and books or games can help. Parents may experience frustration because of the economic and emotional turmoil of the disruption in the family caused by the separation. Family counseling may be of great assistance, especially if siblings are at home.

Follow-up biopsies are usually performed on an outpatient basis. It is important to continue the strategies learned in the hospital to facilitate coping and cooperation during this procedure. Significant stress is associated with the biopsy procedure because of its discomfort and unpleasantness and the implications of the results.

Acute rejection is common after transplantation. Until the first rejection episode, most families hope that their child will not reject. Chronic rejection occurs in children as it does in adults, and older children and teens have required retransplantation.

General pediatric care can be returned to the primary pediatrician, but close communication must be maintained with the transplant team. One important variation from normal pediatric care occurs in relation to the immunization schedule. Infants and small children are routinely immunized against several communicable diseases. However, due to chronic illness, pediatric candidates for transplantation often fall behind in their immunization schedule and, in the case of infants, there simply is not enough time. Once children have undergone transplantation, the type of immunizations they receive must be closely monitored. Children must not receive any vaccine derived from a live virus. Therefore, they may not receive oral, (attenuated) polio vaccine (OPV, or Sabin's vaccine) or measles–mumps–rubella vaccine (MMR). They may receive the Salk polio injection and the diphtheria–pertussis–tetanus (DPT) vaccine (Sebesin & Williams, 1987). If other children in the family are due for immunizations, this should be discussed with the transplant team, as the child may shed virus following immunization.

Return to school is an important step in rehabilitation. Home teachers may be used immediately after the transplant, but children should return to regular school as soon as possible. Planning for return to school should include discussions with administrators, school nurses, and teachers. When medical permission is granted, information provided to school nurses, and teachers should be reinforced. Plans need to be made for medication or other treatment that must take place during school hours. Teachers may be apprehensive; they need to know what to expect and whom to call with questions and concerns. Written instructions reduce teachers' anxiety and encourage cooperation with the children's treatment and medication regimens.

Many children, especially adolescents, have an altered body image and concern over peer acceptance depending on the degree of biophysiological response to therapy. At the time of discharge, hair loss, weight loss, and skin changes from GVHD or radiation and physical changes from complications are apparent. Classmates have questions and may tease children because of ignorance, fear, or lack of understanding. Some children who have transplants may want to provide a question-and-answer session for their class a week or so following their return to school. This session has the potential of providing the information the children's classmates need and strengthening the children's self-image and relationships with peers.

Neurological complications—results of total body irradiation used to treat pediatric malignancies in conjunction with BMT—include leukoencephalopathy, myasthenia gravis, decreased general intelligence, and academic and cognitive dysfunction (Van der Wal, Nims, & Davies, 1988). Prolonged school absences and learning disabilities may lead to frustrations, peer rejection, and school performance problems. Pediatric BMT patients should be evaluated for academic and learning difficulties so that their families, teachers, and health teams can maximize the children's education and school integration.

Children who have received total body irradiation are also likely to experience endocrine dysfunction affecting the thyroid, pituitary, gonads, and growth hormone. Endocrine dysfunction results in delayed or impaired growth and development of secondary sex characteristics. Infertility and sexual difficulties become additional concerns as children enter adolescence and young adulthood. Many of these children find counseling of value.

Most families tend to be overconscientious in maintaining a clean environment and protecting the child from infections and contact with others. Following BMT, children should wear masks for about the first 100 days posttransplant. This practice alters body image and self-concept. Sensible precautions such as avoiding obviously ill individuals and large crowds, as well as good handwashing, are important.

In infants and small children, especially those attending preschool, diarrhea is common. Unresolved diarrhea rapidly results in poor absorption of immunosuppressive medications (i.e., Cy A) and can trigger episodes of rejection. Parents should have their children examined by their local pediatricians if they develop more than four or five watery stools in a 24-hour period. Stool cultures should be obtained, and if the diarrhea continues, it may be necessary to place the children on intravenous Cy A until the diarrhea is resolved.

Varicella zoster (chickenpox) is a particularly dangerous and potentially lethal illness in immunosuppressed children if not treated promptly. Because it is prevalent in school-age children and there is currently no vaccine against it, parents and teachers should promptly report any outbreak of this virus. If transplant patients are exposed to varicella zoster, they must receive varicella zoster immune globulin (VZIG) within 72 hours of exposure. The drug will not prevent the child from getting the virus, but it will lessen its severity.

If children are unknowingly exposed to varicella zoster and skin lesions appear, they should be hospitalized immediately and begin therapy with intravenous acyclovir. The drug is continued until all skin lesions are completely crusted. In addition, a reduction of the immunosuppressive therapy may be necessary.

Following total parenteral nutrition and the low microbial diet post-BMT children must be reintroduced to normal nutrition . This process often occurs at home. Vigilant monitoring of growth and development is a continued concern, since obesity secondary to steroid therapy and adequate nutrition for growth needs are problems.

Over time, there should be some relaxation of vigilance of isolation and infection control, and the child's activity and opportunity for independence should be increased. Often this begins with the child's return to school, which may be a difficult time for parents. Although the transplant's purpose is to allow children to live as normally as possible, decisions to allow them opportunities for independence (i.e., to attend camp following a transplant), provide significant stress for families.

Appearance and self-image changes secondary to chronic illness, transplantation, and drugs can have a profound impact on some children. This can be difficult to predict and can vary with age. A $2\frac{1}{2}$-year-old girl was asked to draw pictures of herself before and after a heart transplant. She found this to be a bizarre request since there would be no difference in the portraits—she was the same person. A 7-year-old boy was very upset by his cushingoid reflection in the mirror and was reluctant to return home and to school until his appearance became more normal. Obesity has become a serious problem for teens. Consultation regarding weight control and programs with beauticians and color consultants are both fun and rewarding for some recipients. Social workers, counselors, psychologists, or psychiatrists may be helpful in dealing with other problems. Some families have found family therapy helpful in coping with the changes and difficulties inherent in chronic illness and transplantation.

The medication regimen often affects physical growth. Height may be affected because of steroid therapy. Human growth hormone has not been effective, but changing steroids to an every-other-day schedule has been successful in some children.

The teen years are difficult because of normal developmental stressors. They are even more difficult for children with transplants. The importance of physical appearance and the normal striving for independence are complicated by posttransplant routines. Cooperation may become a serious issue because of the feelings of rebelliousness and invulnerability. Peer pressure may encourage experimentation with drugs, smoking, and alcohol. Career choices and long-term commitments such as marriage and childbearing must include consideration of having had a transplant. Contraceptive choices are limited because of the medications required and the risk of infection.

Finally, unexpected benefits of maturity, self-confidence, and empathy can be seen in children and their families. Parents report strengths and abilities that they never knew they had. Association with families of other children with catastrophic illnesses helps them to put their problems into perspective. Although they continue to worry about small things, they envy families who have only the small things to worry about. The coping strategies and personal strengths that children develop in the hospital carry over into their everyday activities, and they develop a unique appreciation of life. The mother of a 5-year-old girl, 3 years post–heart transplant, feared she might have been too optimistic about the experience with other parents, so she asked her daughter if another 2-year-old should get a new heart. "Of course she should" was the answer. "Even if it means she will have to take medicine every day for the rest of her life and go to the hospital for blood tests and biopsies?" the mother continued. "Of course she should" was the answer; "otherwise she'll be dead."

CONCLUSION

Transplantation provides hope for children with end-stage organ disease. Because of the relative newness of pediatric transplant procedures, few data are available on which to predict long-term outcomes. Significant questions exist related to sibling responsibility, longevity, childbearing, and career choices. Children and families experience the stresses of living with ambiguity and uncertainty. Despite efforts to achieve a normal daily routine, reminders (daily medication and frequent follow-up) occur frequently to suggest that the child is "different."

The reactions of families differ depending on whether children have been previously healthy or have experienced chronic illness. When children who have been previously healthy become critically ill, their families experience shock and grief because of the new diagnosis that may interfere with the families' abilities to cope and to integrate the complex information needed to make difficult decisions. Families whose children have been chronically ill may perceive illness as a normal state (Anderson, 1981). These families need recognition of their coping, knowledge, and abilities as well as support and information. For all families, the costs, emotional turmoil, time, and energy are enormous. For nurses, although the challenges associated with providing care for these children and families are significant, opportunities abound to make meaningful contributions to an improved quality of life.

ACKNOWLEDGEMENT

Special thanks to Fran Wiley, Dr. Feig, Dr. Valentino, and the pediatric BMT nursing staff at UCLA; the University of Michigan 7^W Mott Hospital BMT staff; Shirley Brown, Mindy McKinnon, Melissa Manlin, and the entire Ulfig family.

REFERENCES

Anderson, J.M. (1981). The social construction of illness experience: Families with a chronically ill child. *Journal of Advanced Nursing, 6,* 427–434.

August, C., King, E., Githens, J., McIntosh, K., Humbert, J., Greensheer, A., & Johnson, F. (1976). Establishment of erythropoiesis following bone marrow transplantation in a patient with congenital hypoplastic anemia (Diamond-Blackfan syndrome). *Blood, 48,* 491–498.

Bahargava, H., Donner, R. M., Sanchez, G., Dunn, J. M., Zaeri, N., Brickley, S., & Cavarochi, N. (1987). Endomyocardial biopsy after heart transplantation in children. *Journal of Heart Transplantation, 6*(15), 298–302.

Bailey, L., Concepcion, W., Shattuck, H.,& Huang, L. (1986). Method of heart transplantation for treatment of hypoplastic left heart syndrome. *Journal of Thoracic and Cardiovascular Surgery, 32,* 1–5.

Bortin, M., Gale R., & Rimm, A. (1981). Allogeneic bone marrow transplantation for 144 patients with severe aplastic anemia. *Journal of the American Medical Association, 245,* 1132–1139.

Butturini, A., Rivera, G. K., Bortin, M. M, & Gale, R. P. (1987). Which treatment for childhood acute lymphoblastic leukemia in second remission? *Lancet, 1,* 429–432.

Camitta, B., Storb, R., & Thomas, E. (1982). Aplastic anemia: Pathogenesis, diagnosis, treatment, and prognosis. *New England Journal of Medicine, 306,* 645–652, 712–718.

Caves, P. K., Stinson, E. B., Billingham, M. E., & Shumway, N. E. (1973). Diagnosis of human cardiac allograft rejection by serial cardiac biopsy. *Journal of Thoracic and Cardiovascular Surgery, 66,* 461.

Cheson, B, Lacerna, L., Leyland-Jones, B., Sarosy, G., & Wittes, R. E. (1989). Autologous bone marrow transplantation. *Annals of Internal Medicine, 110,* 51–65.

Coccia, P. (1980). Successful bone marrow transplantation for infantile malignant osteopetrosis. *New England Journal of Medicine, 302,* 7011–7018.

Deeg, H., Thomas, E., Applebaum, F., Buckner, C., Clift, R., Doney, K., Johnson, L., Sanders, J., Sullivan, K., & Witterspoon, R. (1983). Fanconi's anemia treated by allogeneic bone marrow transplantation. *Blood, 61,* 954–959.

Ettenger, R. B., & Fine, R. N. (1986). Pediatric renal transplantation. In M. Garovoy & R. Guttman (Eds.), *Renal transplantation* (pp. 399–435). New York: Churchill Livingstone.

Feig, S. (1986). Bone marrow transplantation in children with cancer and hematologic disorders. In V. Kelley (Ed.), *Practice of pediatrics.* Philadelphia: Harper and Row.

Gluckman, E., Berger, R., & Dutreix, J. (1984). Bone marrow transplantation for Fanconi's anemia. *Seminars in Hematology, 21,* 20–26.

Gold, L. M., Kirkpatrick, B. S., Fricker, F. J., & Zitelli, B. J. (1986). Psychosocial issues in pediatric organ transplantation: The parents' perspective. *Pediatrics, 77,* 738–744.

Goldsobel, A., Haas, A., & Steihm, E. (1987). Bone marrow transplantation in DiGeorge syndrome. *The Journal of Pediatrics, 111,* 40–44.

Hazinski, M. (1984). Children are different. In M. Hazinski (Ed.), *Nursing care of the critically ill child* (pp. 1–11). St. Louis: C. V. Mosby.

Heck C. F., Shumway, S. J. & Kaye, M. P. (1989). The registry of the International society for Heart transplantation: Sixth official report—1989. *Journal of Heart Transplantation 8,* 271–276.

Herzig, R. H., Bortin, M. M., Barrett, A. J., Blume, K. G., Gluckman, E., Horowitz, M. M., Jacobsen, S. J., Marmont, A., Masaoka, T., Prentice, H. G., Ramsey, N., Rimm, A., Ringden, O., Speck, B., Zwann, P., & Gale, R. (1987). Bone marrow transplantation in high risk acute lymphoblastic leukaemia in first and second remission. *Lancet, 305,* 786–788.

Johnson, F., Look, A., Gockerman, J., Ruggiero, H., Dalla-Pozza, L., & Billings, F. (1984). Bone marrow transplantation in a patient with sickle cell disease. *New England Journal of Medicine, 311,* 780–783.

Johnson, F., Thomas, E., Clark, B., Chard, R., Hartmann, J., & Storb, R. (1981). A comparison of marrow transplantation with chemotherapy for children with acute lymphoblastic leukemia in second or subsequent remission. *New England Journal of Medicine, 305,* 846–851.

Kaempfer, S., Hoffman, D., & Wiley, F. (1983). Spermbanking a reproductive option in cancer therapy. *Cancer Nursing, 6,* 31–38.

Kanoti, G. A. (1986). Ethical considerations in solid organ pediatric transplantation. *Transplant Proceedings, 18*(Suppl 2), 43–46.

Lucarelli, G., Galimberti, M., Polchi, P., Giardini, C., Politi, P., & Baronciani, D. (1987). Marrow transplantation in patients with advanced thalassemia. *New England Journal of Medicine, 316,* 1050–1055.

Lum, C., Wassner, S., & Martin, D. (1985). Current thinking in transplantation in infants and children. *Pediatric Clinics of North America 32,* 1203–1232.

O'Reilly, R., Brochstein, J., Dinsmore, R., & Kirkpatrick, D. (1984). Marrow transplantation for congenital disorders. *Seminars in Hematology, 21,* 188–220.

Philip, T., Armitage, J., Spitzer, G., Chauvin, F., Jagannath, S., Cahn, J., Colombat, D., Goldstone, A., Gorin, N., & Flesh, M. (1987). High dose chemoradiotherapy with bone marrow transplantation as consolidation treatment in neuroblastoma: An unselected group of Stage IV patients over 1 year of age. *Journal of Clinical Oncology, 5*(2), 266–271.

Poplack, D. G., & Reaman, G. (1988). Acute lymphoblastic leukemia in childhood. *Pediatric Clinics of North America, 35,* 930–932.

Potter, D., Feduska, N., Melzer, J., Garovoy, M., Hopper, S., Duca, R., & Salvatierra, O. (1986). Twenty years of renal transplantation in children. *Pediatrics 77,* 465–470.

Reitz, B. A., Jamieson, S. W., Gaudiani, V. A., Oyer, P. E., & Stinson, E. B. (1982). Method of cardiac transplantation in corrected transposition. *Journal of Thoracic and Cardiovascular Surgery, 23,* 293.

Ruggiero, S. (1988). The donor in bone marrow transplantation. *Seminars in Oncology Nursing, 4,* 9–14.

Salvatierra, O. (1986). Renal transplantation. In Walsh, Gitts, Perlmutter, & Stamey (Eds.), *Campbells' urology* (pp. 2534–2557). Philadelphia: W. B. Saunders.

Sanders, J., Whitehead, J., Storb, R., Buckner, C., Clift, R., Mickelson, E., Applebaum, F., Bensinger, W., Stewart, P., & Doney, K. (1986). Bone marrow transplantation for children with aplastic anemia. *Pediatrics, 77*(2), 179–186.

Sebesin S. M., & Williams, J. W. (1987). Status of liver transplantation. *Hospital Practice, 22,* 75–86.

Thomas, E. (1988). The future of bone marrow transplantation. *Seminars in Oncology Nursing, 4,* 74–78.

Thomas, E., Sanders, J., Borgna-Pignatti, C., DeStefano, P., Clift, R., Buckner, C., Papayannopoulou, T., Sullivan, K., & Storb, R. (1982). Marrow transplantation for thalassemia. *Lancet, 227.*

Van der Wal, R., Nims, J., & Davies, B. (1988). Bone marrow transplantation in children: Nursing management of late effects. *Cancer Nursing, 11,* 132–143.

Wiley, F., & House, K. (1988). Bone marrow transplant in children. *Seminars in Oncology Nursing, 4,* 31–40.

Yeager, A. (1988). Bone marrow transplantation in children. *Pediatric Annals, 17,* 698–714.

CHAPTER **10**

NEONATAL/INFANT HEART TRANSPLANTATION

Joyce Johnston

Cardiac transplantation in neonates and older infants is evolving into a realistic therapeutic option for treating severe uncorrectable congenital heart disease (CHD), including hypoplastic left heart syndrome (HLHS). HLHS is a uniformly fatal disease characterized by underdevelopment of the systemic pumping chamber. It represents 3% to 5% of all CHD and is the leading cause of death from CHD in the first week of life (Ferencz et al., 1985).

The relative immaturity of the newborn immune system, recent improvements in immunosuppressive regimes with the advent of cyclosporine, and early operative success have encouraged ongoing trials of cardiac transplantation in the very young (Bailey et al., 1986, 1988; Johnston, 1990; Starnes et al., 1987).

Cardiac transplantation in infants has been attempted sporadically in the past. In 1967, Kantrowitz et al. introduced cardiac transplantation in infants when his group transplanted the heart from an anencephalic infant into a 3-week-old baby with tricuspid atresia (Kantrowitz, Haller, Joos, Cerruti, & Carstensen, 1968). In 1968, Cooley and others transplanted the heart and lungs of an anencephalic infant to another baby with complete atrioventricular canal (Cooley et al., 1969). Both transplanted infants died within hours of the procedures.

In 1984, worldwide attention focused on the possibility of neonatal cardiac transplantation when a baboon's heart was transplanted into a newborn named Baby Fae at Loma Linda University Medical Center (LLUMC) (Bailey, Nehlsen-Cannarella, Concepcion, & Jolley, 1985). Although this effort was highly criticized, an important derivative of this xenotransplantation project was a markedly increased awareness of the potential benefits of organ transplantation during neonatal life and the need for newborn human donors. Neither the demand for nor the supply of newborn human organs existed prior to this time.

In a summary from the International Society for Heart Transplantation (ISHT) Registry compiled by Dr. Pennington, he reported that fewer than five children per year (0–18 years) received a heart transplant before 1980. In 1984, 37 children (0–18 years) underwent transplantation procedures in 15 reporting centers (Pennington, Sarafrin, & Swartz, 1985). Ten of the 37 children were 10 years old or younger. In 1989, the ISHT Registry report revealed that approximately 65 children (ages 0–1 year) and 25 children (ages 1–2 years) underwent heart transplantation between 1984 and 1988 (Kaye, 1989). A recent communication from the United Network for Organ Sharing (UNOS) revealed that on a given day in March 1989 there were 16 children (ages 0–5 years) awaiting heart transplantation.

DONOR PROCUREMENT

The clinical nurse in the neonatal or pediatric ICU setting has a pivotal role in recognizing and supporting potential infant or pediatric donors. The nurse must be aware that modern technology has made it possible for newborn infants to benefit from organ replacement as well as realize what constitutes brain death. At many levels, nurses have opportunities to share in the miracle of transplantation.

Primary causes of death for potential infant organ donors include acute neurological trauma, drug overdose, cerebral anoxia (including birth asphyxia) and sudden infant death syndrome (SIDS).

The criteria currently used at LLUMC to determine brain death in infants include coma, pupils that are fixed and dilated, absent oculocephalic reflex (doll's eyes), absent gag or corneal reflexes, and absence of sustained, spontaneous respiration when the $PaCO_2$ is greater than 60 mmHg.[1] These criteria must be met in the presence of normothermia without the effects of narcotics or elevated barbiturate levels (Ashwal & Schneider, 1987a, 1987b). Electrocerebral quiescence may confirm brain death but is not necessary for declaration. The absence of cerebral blood flow as demonstrated by radionuclide isotope studies can provide near-absolute information in suspected brain death (Drake, Ashwal, & Schneider, 1986). In most states, brain

[1]Preoxygenate with 100% oxygen for 10 minutes. Establish a pCO_2 of at least 40 mmHg prior to disconnection from ventilator. Disconnect ventilator and administer passive O_2 at 100% for at least 10 minutes unless there is danger of cardiovascular collapse, at which point the apnea test is aborted. Draw ABG 10 minutes later to verify that pCO_2 was greater than 60 mmHg.

death declaration requires documentation from two separate physicians; one preferably should be a neurologist.

Potential cardiac donors need to be free from infection (although they may have received antibiotic therapy), have an essentially normal electrocardiogram, and have an echocardiogram that shows a structurally normal heart with reasonable cardiac function (shortening fraction $\geq$ 28% is acceptable). Creatine phosphokinase isoenzymes should be assessed. The MB fraction should be below 10%. Donors need to be ABO-compatible and appropriately size-matched with the potential recipient. They should not be receiving excessive doses of inotropic support (i.e., dopamine 10–15 µg/kg/min). Chest trauma need not be an absolute contraindication to heart donation (Hetzer, Warnecke, & Schuler, 1986). Organs that have undergone prolonged resuscitation efforts, even in the face of asystole, should not be disqualified if the donor later becomes stabilized with evidence of reasonable cardiac function.

Care of the Potential Organ Donor

Nurses' involvement in the care of a donor begins with recognizing the potential for organ donation and initiating and facilitating this process. Because of their previously established rapport, nurses are often uniquely suited to introducing the option of donation and offering family support throughout the crisis. The first step, after recognition of the potential for organ donation, is to notify the appropriate regional procurement agency. In concert with the procurement agency, the bedside nurse participates in a team effort to manage the donor. The expected outcome will be to optimize the quality and quantity of recoverable organs from each potential donor. Recognition and physiologic support of a potential organ donor have become critical components of emergency and critical care nursing. If donor organs become damaged from improper management, donation of those organs is ultimately lost (Futterman, 1988).

The procurement agency requires specific information from caregivers who initiate the donation process. This information includes history of the present admission, age, sex, blood type, weight, current vital signs and medications, current blood gas analysis, recent laboratory studies, infectious disease status, and evidence of neurologic evaluation that established brain death.

Intensive care of the donor is mandatory to help ensure that potentially transplantable organs remain viable and functional. Once a patient has been declared legally brain-dead and is deemed suitable as an organ donor, therapy must be altered to preserve and support donor organ function rather than aimed at salvaging irrevocably damaged central nervous system tissue (Emery et al., 1986; Goldsmith & Montefusco, 1985).

Adequate organ perfusion and oxygenation, dependent in part on hemodynamic stability and maintenance of acid–base and fluid–electrolyte balance, are the major physiologic objectives in organ donor care (Futterman, 1988). Specific nursing actions include aseptic endotracheal suctioning, careful monitoring of fluid status, and administration of crystalloids, colloids, and/or blood products as needed.

Supportive care of the donor may include insertion of a central venous line for volume replacement, cannulation of an artery to monitor blood pressure and sample blood gases, ventilatory support, and insertion of a urinary catheter to monitor output. Each transplantation center has its own set of criteria for evaluating and supporting potential donor organs and will provide counsel to the referral center regarding optimal management principles. Table 10.1 outlines care of the potential donor at LLUMC.

Distant Organ Procurement

A request to transport a newborn donor to the transplant center may be made in an effort to reduce ischemic injury to the recovered heart. If this is not feasible, distant procurement can be accomplished. The obvious advantages of on-site procurement are decreased ischemic insult to the donor

TABLE 10.1 Care of the Potential Donor

Donor must fit inclusion criteria.
Care while awaiting parental consent and/or transport
  Maintain normal pH
  Maintain normal arterial blood gases
  Take measures to prevent atelectasis and/or pneumonia
  Maintain normothermia
  Maintain adequate blood pressure using up to 10 μg/kg/min of dopamine and/or
    fluid replacement
  Avoid blood transfusion; if transfusion is required, use washed red blood cells
  Give antibiotics if indicated

Required documents
  Parents' consent for organ donation
  Parents' consent for transport of body to LLUMC (when appropriate)
  Brain death certificate by two pediatricians or progress notes documenting brain
    death signed by two pediatricians
  Copy of death certificate
  Documentation of coroner's consent (also coroner's consent for transport to
    LLUMC)
  Consent for cremation if indicated
  Copy of donor chart
  Copy of CXR, echocardiogram (M-mode), and ECG

heart and better control of timing for the recovery process. Parents of small infants, however, may be reluctant to permit the transfer of their brain-dead child. Also, the coroner may not allow transfer. Distant organ procurement usually involves multiorgan recovery and requires a coordinated effort among a number of highly trained professionals in order to obtain donor organs of optimal quality (Wood & Shaw, 1988).

INDICATIONS FOR HEART TRANSPLANTATION

Indications for cardiac transplantation in neonates are gradually expanding as long-term survival with good quality of life improves. Indications other than HLHS for cardiac transplantation may include severe Ebstein's anomaly and pulmonary atresia with intact ventricular septum. Every effort is made to obtain an echocardiographic diagnosis of uncorrectable heart disease in utero so that the fetus may benefit by an increased time interval to locate a suitable donor organ while awaiting delivery if the option of transplantation is chosen (Johnston et al., 1990; Vincent et al., 1987). Table 10.2 indicates the current congenital or acquired defects that will be considered for treatment with cardiac transplantation at LLUMC. Tables 10.3 and 10.4 outline the current recipient inclusion and exclusion criteria at LLUMC.

TABLE 10.2 Cardiac Malformations in Early Infancy Acceptable for Consideration for Orthotopic Transplantation

Hypoplastic left heart syndrome (hypoplastic aortic tract complex)
Symptomatic severe Ebstein's anomaly with normal pulmonary arteries
Multiple obstructive rhabdomyomas
Pulmonary atresia/intact ventricular septum (large sinusoids[a])
Hypoplastic left heart equivalent
   D-TGA with hypoplastic RV and aortic tract
   Single ventricle with hypoplastic aortic tract
   L-TGA with single ventricle and heart block
Severe congenital or acquired cardiomyopathy
A-V canal with hypoplastic LV and mitral component (frequently associated with
   coarctation)
Single ventricle with subaortic obstruction (bulbo-ventricular foramen)
Severe intrauterine A-V valve insufficiency and ventricular dysfunction
Straddling A-V and tensor apparatus
Complex truncus arteriosus

[a]Diminutive right heart malformation must have normal-size right and left pulmonary arteries. Neonates unresponsive to PGE-1 may have systemic-pulmonary shunts while awaiting a donor.

TABLE 10.3 Recipient Inclusion Criteria

Gestational age greater than 36 weeks[a] and birth weight greater than 2,200 gm[a]
Cardiac evaluation:
  Diagnosis of HLHS or other lethal CHD for which there is no standardized
  treatment or the diagnosis of end stage cardiomyopathy made by attending
  pediatrician or pediatric cardiologist
  Echocardiographic confirmation of diagnosis
Stable metabolic and hemodynamic status while receiving PGE-1 and other supportive
  measures (cardiac inotropic drugs, mechanical ventilation, parenteral nutrition, etc.)
Psychosocial evaluation
  Candidate should reside within 45 min traveling time from LLUMC for a
  minimum of 6 to 12 months after transplantation
  Supportive family structure
  Candidate's family should be capable of long-term intensive care of the child and
  be able to support the exceptional needs of the child
No clinical suspicion of major sepsis
Normal neurological evaluation; may include head ultrasound/CT scan/EEG
Normal evaluation
  If BUN>30 and creatinine>1.5, pediatric nephrology consultation to exclude gross
  renal abnormalities
  Abdominal ultrasound study showing no significant renal malformations
Phenotypically normal

[a]Relative criteria.

TABLE 10.4 Recipient Exclusion Criteria

Marked prematurity[a] and low birth weight
Unclear cardiac diagnosis
Persistent acidosis of pH below 7.10 for > 2 hr
Sepsis
Abnormal neurological evaluation suggesting poor long-term prognosis
  History of blood sugar below 20 mg% for more than 30 min
  Gross central nervous system anomaly
Abnormal renal function
  Gross urinary tract anomaly
  Persistent and/or markedly elevated BUN and creatinine
Significant dysmorphy or genetic problem
Positive drug screen
Other considerations[b]
  Strong history of parental (custodial) alcohol and/or substance abuse
  Documented parental (custodial) child abuse or neglect
  Family situation unable to support long-term medical needs of recipient
  Parent (custodian) with cognitive/psychiatric impairment severe enough to limit
    comprehension of medical regimen

[a]Relative consideration.
[b]It is impossible to separate these considerations from what is in the dependent patient's best
interests medically. It is understood that federal guidelines exclude psychosocial considerations.

EVALUATION FOR ACCEPTANCE INTO THE TRANSPLANT PROGRAM

Evaluation for possible transplantation involves a multidisciplinary approach to determine if there are any other major systemic diseases or permanent underlying organ dysfunction that would exclude the transplant option. Neurologic compromise or significant dysmorphism would be contraindications for transplantation. A thorough assessment of infectious disease status is accomplished. Potential transplant recipients are screened for prior exposure to cytomegalovirus (CMV), human immunodeficiency virus (HIV), toxoplasma, Epstein-Barr virus (EBV), herpes simplex virus (HSV), and rubella. In addition, the infants receive CMV-negative blood products that have been washed and irradiated prior to administration. After a decision has been made to proceed with transplantation, the child is registered with regional organ procurement agencies and UNOS according to medical status, weight, and blood type.

The waiting period for a donor organ is uncertain. Prolonged waiting often results in significant emotional stress within the family. In addition to the uncertain wait for a donor, parents must learn to cope with their disappointment at the birth of a physically imperfect infant. Nurses and social workers involved with the family during this time are dealing with altered emotional responses. Interventions may include explaining the transplant process, listening to family concerns, and reassuring the parents that they can be comforted by knowing they have done everything possible to help their baby.

PREOPERATIVE NURSING CARE

Preoperative nursing diagnoses in the care of a newborn awaiting transplant focus on recognizing the potential for impaired cardiac function. A specific nursing intervention may include assessment of changes in the clinical manifestations of HLHS. The manifestations include peripheral duskiness, diminished peripheral pulses, and low blood pressure. The infants usually require continuous intravenous infusion of prostaglandin E_1 (PGE_1) for maintenance of a patent ductus arteriosus, which provides for systemic and coronary circulation. A careful balance of the ratio of systemic and pulmonary circulations is maintained with manipulation of ventilatory and pharmacologic support. Desired patient outcomes include spontaneous or controlled ventilation with a low FIO_2, while maintaining a $PaCO_2$ above 30 mmHg. Hypocarbia and hyperoxia are avoided since they decrease pulmonary vascular resistance and hence reduce systemic circulation. In the newborn, a PaO_2 of 40 mmHg provides an arterial saturation of approximately 80%, which is near the plateau of the fetal oxyhemoglobin dissociation curve and provides adequate oxygen transport to the tissues. The nurse monitors the side effects of PGE$_1$, which include cutaneous vasodilation, rhythm or conduction disturbances, hypotension, seizure-like activity, temperature elevation, and apnea.

In addition, another important nursing diagnosis relates to the parents' knowledge deficit about transplantation. The family meets with a multidisciplinary team that will outline their options, the transplant process, and the commitment involved. Parents are given radio pagers so that they can be notified when a suitable donor is located. Parents visit the ICU and become familiar with isolation procedures. They have opportunities to speak with other families who have experienced transplantation. Nurses provide preoperative teaching and give parents written materials that reinforce what they have heard. If distances between a potential recipient and the transplant center are great, there may be telephone communication. Because there is a severe shortage of infant donors, a potential transplant recipient is usually cared for in the referral facility until a suitable donor is identified. At that time, donor and recipient may be transported to the transplant center simultaneously, or distant procurement of the donor organ may be accomplished while the recipient is transferred to the transplant center.

SURGICAL PROCEDURE

The operative method for cardiac transplantation in neonates and young infants is the same as for adults, with the option of utilizing profound hypothermic circulatory arrest (Bailey, Concepcion, Shattuck, & Huang, 1986). The patient's chest is opened through a midsternal incision, and the pericardium is opened in the midline. Extracorporeal perfusion is accomplished by inserting a venous cannula into the right atrium. An arterial cannula is placed through the distal main pulmonary artery into the patent ductus arteriosus. Perfusion is begun, and the patient is cooled to a core (rectal) temperature of 20°C.

The hypoplastic heart is excised, with the posterior atrial walls and septum left in place. The cardiectomy requires transection of the main pulmonary artery and aorta. The donor heart is implanted beginning with the atrial septum and continuing around the right and left atria. The portion of donor aorta distal to the arch vessels is joined to the opened recipient aorta. The pulmonary arterial anastomosis follows. The cardiac transplantation procedure itself is usually uneventful. Ischemic time, myocardial preservation techniques, and overall condition of the donor heart prior to transplantation will ultimately influence the integrity of the donor heart (Futterman, 1988). In the Loma Linda experience, cold ischemic time has been in excess of 8 hours with good recovery of cardiac function in the recipient. Traditionally, in adults, a 4-hour ischemic time has been the accepted upper limit of normal. Perhaps the smaller mass of the infant heart allows for better myocardial preservation.

The recipient has two vascular access lines in place. One is a double-lumen central venous line, and the other is a low central arterial line. These lines are positioned at least 6 to 8 hours prior to transplantation, usually in the left groin. An intravenous cyclosporine infusion (0.25 mg/hr) is commenced by way of the venous line. Posttransplantation, the heart must adapt to the absence of autonomic innervation. Consequently, it is often necessary to augment function with intravenous catecholamines such as isoproterenol and/or dopamine until hemodynamic parameters stabilize (Funk, 1986; Shinn, 1985).

POSTOPERATIVE NURSING CARE

Following transplantation, the neonatal or young infant recipient is cared for in the intensive care unit (ICU). The usual hospital stay is 2 to 3 weeks. Protective isolation including mask, gown, and 3-minute handwashing is enforced. Routine postcardiac surgical management is employed and may include mechanical ventilation and cardiac inotropic drugs (Bailey et al., 1990). On rare occasions, peritoneal dialysis has been employed early in the postoperative period when there was compromised distal aortic perfusion prior to operation (Bailey et al., 1990).

An important nursing diagnosis for these infants is potential for decreased cardiac output. Nursing interventions include assessment for tachycardia, tachypnea, and/or signs and symptoms of cardiac tamponade. Other interventions include maintenance of an acceptable heart rate in the denervated heart, usually by manipulation of inotropic drugs or use of a pacemaker. Prevention of fluid overload is primarily ensured by accurate intake and output measurements, daily weights and evaluation of chest x-rays to assess the pulmonary vasculature.

Another nursing diagnosis, respiratory impairment secondary to airway secretions, is also important during the early postoperative period. Meticulous pulmonary toilet is essential for the prevention of pneumonia and atelectasis. Nursing interventions include careful asepsis with tracheal suctioning and vigorous chest physiotherapy. There is an effort to extubate the infants as soon as possible postoperatively to avoid infectious sequelae.

Potential renal dysfunction may also occur postoperatively. Strict attention to intake and output measurements, control of inotropic drugs, and monitoring of electrolyte and cyclosporine A (Cy A) levels are important nursing actions. Cy A is known to have potential nephrotoxic side effects, although such effects seem somewhat less severe in newborns (Bailey et al., 1990).

Acute Rejection

Infants undergoing cardiac transplantation in the neonatal period are unique hosts in regard to their immune systems. They are receiving immunosuppression while their immune apparatuses are still evolving. This immaturity of the newborn's immune system may afford an optimal window of time in which the rejection response may be less acute (Johnston et al., 1990). However, the potential for injury due to acute rejection is still an important nursing diagnosis. It is normal that the body's immune system recognizes the graft tissue as foreign. Most infants have an average of two to three episodes of rejection, the majority occurring within the first 6 months posttransplant.

Monitoring Rejection

Criteria for assessing acute cardiac rejection have been divided into clinical, echocardiographic, electrocardiographic, radiographic, and laboratory parameters (Johnston & Mathis, 1988). Careful clinical evaluation and correlation of these parameters are required. Clinically, an unexplained persistent increase in resting heart rate, presence of a third heart sound, arrhythmias, tachypnea, and/or diaphoresis may alert the caregiver to the potential for graft rejection.

Hepatomegaly may also be evident. Babies with this condition usually become irritable, with poor feeding and/or lethargy. The M-mode echocardiogram usually shows rapidly increasing left ventricular posterior wall and septal wall thickness. There may be a decreasing left ventricular fiber shortening fraction. Pericardial effusion may be present. A simple 12-lead ECG is obtained twice weekly in hospital and with each clinic visit. Voltage, representing measurement of the QRS complex in the limb leads and chest leads, is plotted on a graph. The ECG will often show a significant reduction (approximately 20%) in voltage at times of rejection. Changes in the ECG that have been identified with rejection episodes include conduction system abnormalities, such as development of a new bundle branch block, and/or arrhythmias, including second-degree heart block.

Chest x-rays and laboratory tests also provide useful information. On chest x-rays, rejection is diagnosed based on advancing global cardiomegaly with or without pulmonary edema and/or pleural effusion (Toomey et al., 1988). Laboratory measurements may show an increase in spontaneous blastogenesis, but one must differentiate between rejection and infection. When lymphocytes are stimulated by an antigen, they synthesize new proteins and become "blasts," thus the term spontaneous blastogenesis (Johnston & Mathis, 1988). Immune stimulation, as a result of infection or rejection, will increase the spontaneous blastogenesis level. Also, any significant elevation of CK isoenzyme–MB fraction is evaluated.

An infant recipient who is suspected of having acute rejection is placed on a rejection protocol based on the degree of hemodynamic compromise. Histologic confirmation of rejection is generally not sought due to potentially hazardous complications of the biopsy procedure in the newborn age group. Reversal of the symptoms within 24 hours following the institution of treatment substantiates the diagnosis of rejection.

Control of the Immune Response

Cy A is the primary immunosuppressive medication employed. Parents learn that the drug has potential nephrotoxic side effects and that it may cause elevated blood pressure. Blood pressure is monitored regularly in the hospital and with each clinic visit in the outpatient setting. Routine blood testing is performed to monitor kidney function. To date, there has been no evidence of severe long-term renal dysfunction in infants who have undergone cardiac transplantation at LLUMC. If Cy A levels become elevated, the baby may develop a bulging fontanel, become irritable, and develop systemic hypertension. Parents learn that the cyclosporine dose is prescribed based on information obtained from blood levels. The Cy A dose is initially maintained between 300 and 400 ng/ml of whole blood (monoclonal antibody measuring parent compound only).

Azathioprine is another drug used that suppresses the immune system. Parents are taught that azathioprine can make the child more susceptible to infection. The white blood cell count is monitored to determine a safe level of administration. At LLUMC, azathioprine is initially started at 2–3 mg/kg/day, and at 6 months posttransplant, the dose is reduced to 1 mg/kg/day. At one year, azathioprine is discontinued if the infant is less than 30 days of age at time of transplant.

Like Cy A, steroids help prevent rejection by suppressing immune system activity. Steroids are given intravenously for several days at times of presumed rejection. Infants will have increased appetites and will want to drink more fluids while receiving steroids. Because steroid therapy may cause fluid retention, the baby's blood pressure and weight may increase, and the baby may become extremely irritable. The fontanel may also begin to bulge. There may be increased pulmonary vasculature on chest x-rays. The baby usually requires diuretic therapy at this time. If rejection occurs in the outpatient setting, clinic visits may become more frequent.

Infection

Potential for infection is another ongoing nursing diagnosis. Nursing responsibilities include monitoring for and prevention of infection. Protective isolation is maintained at all times, and infected health care workers are not allowed to care for the infants. Strict aseptic technique is employed when caring for and handling invasive lines. All infants undergoing transplantation at LLUMC receive immunosupportive therapy in the form of intravenous gamma globulin during the perioperative period. Broad-spectrum antibiotics are routinely administered during the first postoperative week as a prophylactic measure. There are regular assessments with TORCH (a screen for toxoplasmosis, rubella, CMV, and HSV) and EBV titers, as well as routine surveillance of the white blood cell count for early detection of infection.

Optimal nutritional status is also critical in protection from infection and is closely monitored by the nurse.

ROLE OF THE NURSE IN DISCHARGE PLANNING AND CLINIC FOLLOW-UP

Although families have learned about transplantation preoperatively, they will still have a knowledge deficit related to home care of the infant recipient. Therefore, discharge planning begins early. Parents learn about the consequences of the transplant process: denervation, risk of acute rejection, and increased risk of infection with immunosuppression. During the hospital stay, parents learn to use a stethoscope to determine the infant's heart rate, rhythm, and respiratory rate. They are also required to have CPR instruction prior to the infant's discharge from the hospital. Parents are taught to recognize signs and symptoms of rejection, and the nursing staff helps them become familiar with the medication regimen so that by the time of projected discharge, they feel comfortable administering medications and understand drug side effects.

Nurses should be aware of patient care considerations after hospital discharge and during long-term follow-up. These considerations include the family's commitment to ongoing outpatient clinic visits and the effects that this commitment will have on family dynamics. The parents must also deal with the knowledge that answers to such concerns as longevity and development of ischemic heart disease in the children are unknown at this time.

After discharge, the infant is followed in the outpatient cardiac transplant clinic, initially twice weekly. Parents have 24-hour access to transplant coordinators, who answer questions and facilitate the baby's outpatient follow-up care. The baby receives all well baby care in the transplant clinic.

Psychosocially, there is a great commitment required on the part of the family and the caregivers for the continued well-being of these infants after transplantation. Families have been required to relocate near the transplant center for 6 months to accommodate postoperative surveillance. This poses both financial and social hardships. Many insurance agencies view transplantation in the infant as "investigational" and will not cover their clients.

CONCLUSION

Cardiac transplantation in the newborn/infant age group involves a committed team effort as well as active family participation. The results of early, short-term follow-up (4 years) are encouraging. At the time of this chapter's preparation, 67 infants at LLUMC (<6 months of age) have undergone cardiac allotransplantation; 50 of these infants are surviving at 1 to 55 months posttransplant (75%). These infants are experiencing improved quality of life without apparent negative side effects from immunosuppression. Because of the relative immaturity of the immune system in this age group, long-term graft survival may be enhanced. Transplantation offers these infants the promise of normal cardiovascular function. However, despite major technologic advances in the transplantation field, a serious imbalance remains between the number of potential transplant candidates and the number of available replacement organs. Increased public awareness and professional education may help to ameliorate this paucity of organs. Health care professionals and families should consider organ donations before terminating artificial support for a brain-dead infant (Bailey et al., 1988).

REFERENCES

Ashwal, S., & Schneider, S. (1987a). Brain death in children: Part 1. *Pediatric Neurology, 3*, 5–10.

Ashwal, S., & Schneider, S. (1987b). Brain death in children: Part 2. *Pediatric Neurology, 3*, 69–77.

Bailey, L., Assaad, A., Trimm, F., Nehlsen-Cannarella, S., Kanakriyeh, M., Haas, G., & Jacobson, J. (1988). Orthotopic transplantation during early infancy as therapy for incurable congenital heart disease. *Annals of Surgery, 208*, 279–286.

Bailey, L., Concepcion, W., Shattuck, H., & Huang, L. (1986). Method of heart transplantation for treatment of hypoplastic left heart syndrome. *Journal of Thoracic and Cardiovascular Surgery, 92*, 1–5.

Bailey, L., Johnston, J., & Cardiac Transplant Team (1990). Infant cardiac allotransplantation. In *Infant Heart Transplantation Protocol*. (Available from Cardiac Transplant Department, Loma Linda University Medical Center, Schuman Pavilion, Room 1636, P. O. Box 2000, Loma Linda, CA 92354).

Bailey, L., Nehlsen-Cannarella, S., Concepcion, W., & Jolley, W. (1985). Baboon-to-human cardiac xenotransplantation in a neonate. *Journal of American Medical Association, 254*, 3321–3329.

Bailey, L., Nehlsen-Cannarella, S., Doroshow, R., Jacobson, J., Allard, M., Hyde, M., Bui, R.,& Petry, E. (1986). Cardiac allotransplantation newborns as therapy for hypoplastic left heart syndrome. *New England Journal of Medicine, 315*, 949–951.

Cooley, D., Bloodwell, R., Hallman, G., Nora, J., Harrison, G., & Leachman, R. (1969). Organ transplantation for advanced cardiopulmonary disease. *Annals of Thoracic Surgery, 8*, 30–46.

Drake, B., Ashwal, S., & Schneider, S. (1986). Determination of cerebral death in the pediatric intensive care unit. *Pediatrics, 78*, 107–112.

Emery, R., Randall, C., Levinson, M., Riley, J., Copeland, J., McAleer, M., & Copeland, J. (1986). The cardiac donor: A six year experience. *Annals of Thoracic Surgery, 41*, 356–362.

Ferencz, C., Rubin, J., McCarter, R., Brenner, J., Neill, C., Perry, L., Hepner, S., & Downing, J. (1985). Congenital heart disease: Prevalence at live birth. *American Journal of Epidemiology, 121*, 31–36.

Funk, M. (1986). Heart transplantation: Postoperative care during the acute period. *Critical Care Nurse, 6,* 27–44.

Futterman, L. (1988). Cardiac transplantation: A comprehensive nursing perspective. Part 1. *Heart and Lung, 17,* 499–510.

Goldsmith, J., & Montefusco, C. (1985). Nursing care of the potential organ donor. *Critical Care Nurse, 5,* 22–29.

Hetzer, R., Warnecke, H., & Schuler, S. (1986). The donor heart: Procurement, selection, and preservation. *Transplantation Proceedings, 18,* 27–30.

Johnston, J. (1990). *Cardiac transplantation in early infancy.* Unpublished manuscript. (Available from Cardiac Transplant Department, Loma Linda University Medical Center, Loma Linda, CA 92354)

Johnston, J., & Mathis, C. (1988). Determination of rejection using non-invasive parameters after cardiac transplantation in very early infancy: The Loma Linda experience. *Progress in Cardiovascular Nursing, 3,* 13–18.

Johnston, J., Sakala, E., & Loma Linda University Heart Transplant Group. (1990). Neonatal cardiac allotransplantation facilitated by in utero diagnosis of hypoplastic left-sided heart syndrome: A case report. *The Western Journal of Medicine, 152*(1), 70–72.

Kantrowitz, A., Haller, S., Joos, H., Cerruti, M., & Carstensen, H. (1968). Transplantation of the heart in an infant and an adult. *American Journal of Cardiology, 22,* 782–790.

Kaye, M. (1989, April). The Registry of the International Society for Heart Transplantation: 6. Official Report—1989, Paper presented in Munich, Germany. April 1989.

Pennington, D., Sarafrin, J., & Swartz, M. (1985). Heart transplantation in children. *Heart Transplant, 4,* 441–445.

Shinn, J. (1985). New issues in cardiac transplantation. In M. K. Douglas & J. A. Shinn (Eds.), *Advances in cardiovascular nursing* (pp. 185–195). Rockville, MD: Aspen Systems Corp.

Starnes, V., Stinson, E., Oyer, P., Valantine, H., Baldwin, J., Hunt, S., & Shumway, N. (1987). Cardiac transplantation in children and adolescents. *Circulation, 76,* 43–47.

Toomey, F., Bailey, L., Bui, R., Kanakriyeh, M., Petry, E., Mathis, C., Johnston, J., Mace, J., Grill, B., & Klooster, M. (1988). Chest radiography in infant cardiac allotransplantation. *American Journal of Roentgenology, 150,* 369–372.

Vincent, R., Menticoglou, S., Chanas, D., Manning, F., Collins, G., & Smallhorn, J. (1987). Prenatal diagnosis of an unusual form of hypoplastic left heart syndrome. *Journal of Ultrasound Medicine, 6,* 261–264.

Wood, P., & Shaw, R. (1988). Multiple organ procurement. In J. G. Cerilli, *Organ Transplant and Replacement,* (pp. 322–336). Philadelphia: J. B. Lippincott.

CHAPTER 11

A BRIDGE TO TRANSPLANTATION: MECHANICAL SUPPORT DEVICES TO RESTORE FAILING CIRCULATION

Kathleen L. Grady
Doris M. Sandiford-Guttenbeil
Barbara A. Williams

The concept of assisting and replacing the heart is not new. As early as 1812, scientists contemplated ways to improve perfusion of body organs by developing a "substitute for the heart" (DeVries, 1983).

Scientists have since developed a variety of mechanical assist devices to support the failing heart while the patient's heart recovers or while the patient awaits cardiac transplantation (Starnes et al., 1988). Mechanical assist and replacement devices in use today are the intra-aortic balloon pump (IABP), ventricular assist device (VAD), and the total artificial heart (TAH).

Kantrowitz used the first IABP in dog models in 1953. He reported preliminary results with improved circulatory status in two patients in 1968 (Kantrowitz et al., 1968). The IABP is the most widely used conventional assist device today and provides adequate circulatory support for short periods of time for many patients with heart failure.

A VAD or TAH can completely support the circulation and maintain temporary systemic perfusion. The first VADs to assist the failing heart were developed during the early 1960s and applied clinically to a small series of patients during the mid-1960s (DeBakey, 1971). Additional devices were developed and tried clinically during the 1970s (Bernhard et al., 1979; Holub et al., 1979; Pierce et al., 1981). Success in patients with postcardiotomy or postinfarction cardiogenic shock was limited. Pierce used a VAD to support eight patients with right and/or left ventricular failure and achieved long-term survival (4–18 months) in half of the group (Pierce et al., 1981). Bernhard reported a survival rate of 25% in his group of eight surgical patients who required VAD support (Bernhard et al., 1979). With improvements in patient selection, biomaterials, and technology, morbidity and mortality rates have improved over the years.

Cooley and associates implanted the first VAD as a bridge to heart transplantation in 1978 (Norman et al., 1978). Unfortunately, the patient died a few days later of infection. In 1984, Portner and his colleagues successfully bridged a patient with an electrically powered VAD by supporting the left ventricle with a left ventricular assist device for the first time (Portner, 1985). With concurrent and successful development of heart transplantation, the use of temporary assist devices increased during the 1980s.

In 1957, Akutsu and Kolff (1958) implanted the first TAH into a dog. During the 1960s, researchers developed methods to power hearts, and they improved blood-surface interface problems by developing Biomer, a segmented polyurethane. Cooley implanted the first artificial heart in a human in 1969 (Akutsu, & Koiff, 1958). The patient received a human heart transplant 64 hours later but died of pneumonia 32 hours after transplantation. Many years of improvements in design, biomaterials, and technology followed.

In 1981, scientists began implanting artificial hearts again. During the 1980s, DeVries implanted four permanent Jarvik-7 total artificial hearts. Three of the four patients achieved relatively long-term survival (112-620 days), but they subsequently died of severe thromboembolic complications that led to multiorgan failure with or without sepsis (DeVries, 1988). Since the mid-1980s, the TAH has been successfully used as a bridge to heart transplantation (Joyce et al., 1986).

The newest approach to cardiac assistance is through the use of transformed skeletal muscle. With a procedure called cardiomyoplasty, the surgeon detaches the latissimus dorsi from the tendons that connect it to the back and arm, passes it into the chest cavity, and wraps the muscle around the damaged portion of the ventricle (Magovern et al., 1988). The skeletal muscle, with its nerve and blood supply intact, must then be trained for 4 to 6 weeks to contract and relax by an internal pacemaker (Magovern et al., 1988). Unfortunately, the time required to train the skeletal muscle is too long for most patients who need it.

The Combined Registry for the Clinical Use of Mechanical Ventricular

Assist Pumps and Total Artificial Hearts reports that as of December 31, 1989, 400 patients from 62 centers (32 in the U.S.) required circulatory support as a bridge to orthotopic cardiac transplantation (Pae, 1990). Of the 400 patients, 92 received univentricular support, 130 received biventricular support, and 178 were bridged with the TAH (Pae, 1990). Of the 400 patients, 272 (68%) underwent heart transplantation, and 163 (60%) of the 272 patients were discharged from the hospital.

Researchers are encouraged by improved survival rates. Interestingly, Pae & Pierce, (1989) found that shorter durations of mechanical support were associated with better outcomes. The most common complications seen after VAD or TAH implantation are bleeding, infections, thromboembolism, and multiorgan failure (Pennington et al., 1989)

The remainder of this chapter describes indications, types of devices in use today, preoperative preparation, implantation, complications, and postoperative nursing care for patients with a ventricular assist device or total artificial heart.

INDICATIONS FOR DEVICE IMPLANTATION

Before discussing the indications for VADs and TAHs, it is important to understand IABP limitations. The IABP, the most widely used conventional assist device, often provides adequate circulatory support for short periods. The IABP can be easily inserted in the operating room or percutaneously at the bedside. The IABP has three purposes: to increase oxygen supply to the myocardium, to decrease the workload of the left ventricle, and to increase cardiac output (CO) and perfusion of vital organs (Patacky, Garven, & Schwirian, 1985)

However, for some patients the IABP does not offer adequate circulatory support because it cannot generate cardiac output independent of left ventricular function (Weintraub & Thurer, 1983). Another limitation is the difficulty in tracking dysrhythmias to maintain adequate systemic perfusion. Severe peripheral vascular disease may prevent insertion of the catheter (May, 1987). Aortic valve insufficiency and aortic aneurysm are two contraindications for using the IABP. Many patients with deteriorating cardiac function may not receive sufficient hemodynamic assistance from the IABP with or without the use of inotropic drugs.

A VAD can completely support the heart and maintain systemic perfusion. The goal of ventricular support is to decrease workload and myocardial oxygen consumption and thereby allow time for metabolic recovery of the heart (Pae, Pierce, Pennock, Campbell, & Waldhausen, 1987). Perfusion is also improved to other organs, and if ventricular recovery does not occur, circulation can be maintained until a donor heart is found.

Current indications for VADs are

1. Postcardiotomy pump failure with the patient unable to come off cardiopulmonary bypass (CPB) after an IABP trial.
2. Acute cardiogenic shock in the medical patient with potentially reversible left ventricular failure and trial with IABP, such as acute myocarditis, myocardial infarction (MI).
3. Cardiac transplant candidate with a deteriorating clinical condition receiving maximum inotropic support, followed by an IABP trial while an active search for a donor heart continues (Starnes et al., 1988; Williams, Lough, & Shinn, 1987).

Patients with the indications listed above have failing hearts even after all conventional medical therapies have been tried to reverse their condition. They have ventricular failure accompanied by cardiogenic shock and exhibit the following:

- Cardiac output <2.0 L/min, cardiac index <1.8 L/min/m^2 with vasopressors.
- Systolic aortic pressure <90 mmHg.
- Age and weight limits variable.

Additionally, patients with left ventricular failure exhibit

- Left atrial pressure (LAP) >18–25 mmHg.
- Right atrial pressure (RAP) <15 mmHg.
- Inability to decrease systemic vascular resistance (SVR) below 1,200 dynes/sec/cm^{-5} with afterload reducing agents, (e.g, nitroprusside).
- Failure to improve condition with an IABP or having a contraindication to the use of an IABP.

Patients with right ventricular failure exhibit

- Left atrial pressure <15 mmHg despite volume loading to an RAP of 25 mmHG because not enough preload can be delivered to the left ventricle.
- Irreversible acidosis, hypoxia, and hypercarbia.
- Unresponsiveness to treatment with isoproterenol and prostaglandin E$_1$ (PGE$_1$) (Pae et al., 1987).

The TAH has been used both as a permanent replacement device and as a bridge to heart transplantation to support patients whose hearts are failing. However, complications such as thromboembolism and infection have limited the use of the TAH as a permanent heart replacement (Davis, Rosenberg, Snyder, & Pierce, 1989). Short-term use of the TAH reduces the risk of developing these complications.

As a temporary device, the TAH is currently used as a bridge to heart transplantation in patients with a variety of situations leading to irreversible heart failure. Patients who require TAH implantation may suffer from coronary artery disease (often presenting as postcardiotomy cardiogenic shock), valvular or congenital heart disease, dilated cardiomyopathy, doxorubicin (Adriamycin®) cardiotoxicity, or myocarditis that does not respond to conventional therapy. These patients must also meet criteria for heart transplantation (See Chapter 5, p. 131). The specific hemodynamic criteria outlined in the indications for use of the VAD are also applicable for the TAH. Selection of a device depends upon the potential reversibility of myocardial failure, access to devices or experimental protocols, surgical expertise, and risks associated with the available devices.

DESCRIPTION OF MECHANICAL ASSIST DEVICES

VADs

Circulatory support for the failing heart is provided as follows: Left ventricular support is provided by a left VAD (LVAD), and support for the failing right ventricle is provided by a right VAD (RVAD). When both ventricles fail, biventricular support is necessary, and a BiVAD is used. Blood flow is diverted from the heart via cannulae that are placed in the left atrium or the left ventricle (LV) and the right atrium. Blood is pumped back into the body through cannulae that are placed in the ascending or transverse aorta and pulmonary artery on the right side of the heart. Devices may be implanted internally or extracorporeally. (See Figures 11.1–11.3).

Advantages of VADs are retention of the natural heart (with the potential for weaning from the device), maintenance of left-to-right circulatory balance, retention of endocrine function, and retention of regulatory function.

VADs use roller, centrifugal, pneumatic, or electrically powered systems. Roller pumps (the earliest VAD designs) use peristaltic occlusion to remove blood from the atrium and pump it back into the aorta, similar to a CPB machine. Advantages cited by users of the roller pump include simplicity, availability, and low cost. Others express concern about thromboembolism and the need for anticoagulation, as well as blood trauma, flow limitations based on cannula size, and nonpulsatility (Pae et al., 1987). (See Figure 11.4)

Centrifugal (vortex) pumps incorporate two magnetic cones that couple and rotate to propel blood forward in a circular motion (Mulford, 1987). The nonocclusive design of centrifugal pumps is favored by surgeons because it reduces blood trauma. In addition, they are readily available, cost-effective, and simple to operate, and they seem to require less systemic anticoagulation, although necessary levels are not well defined. Unfortunately, thrombi have been found in the vortex pump system and systemic embolization has occurred (Pae et al., 1987). Centrifugal pumps are also nonpulsatile. (See Figure 11.5.)

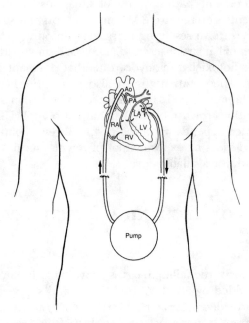

FIGURE 11.1 External left ventricular assist device. Drawing by Bayard Colyear, medical illustrator.

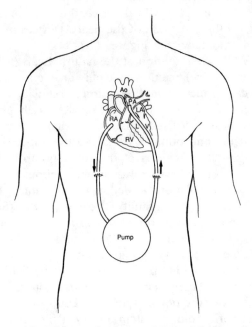

FIGURE 11.2 External right ventricular assist device. Drawing by Bayard Colyear, medical illustrator.

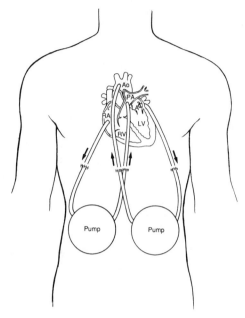

FIGURE 11.3 External right and left ventricular assist device. Drawing by Bayard Colyear, medical illustrator.

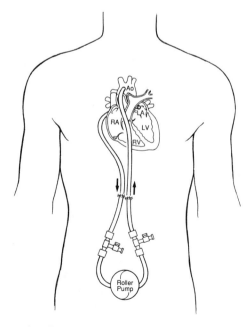

FIGURE 11.4 External roller-pump-powered system. Drawing by Bayard Colyear, medical illustrator.

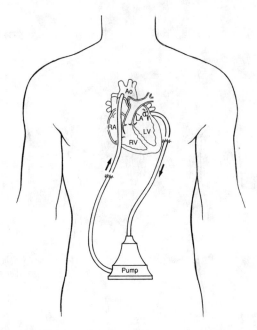

FIGURE 11.5 External centrifugal-pump-powered system. Drawing by Bayard Colyear, medical illustrator.

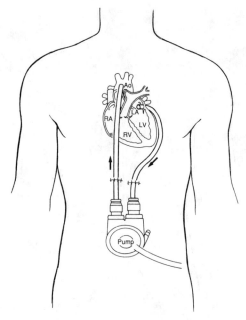

FIGURE 11.6 External pneumatic-pump-powered system. Drawing by Bayard Colyear, medical illustrator.

Pneumatic pumps are air-driven and provide pulsatile flow. Compressed air is provided by a console through tubing into a saclike device enclosed in a rigid housing. Air exhaust and the application of vacuum as needed result in collapse of the saclike device and entry of blood into the pump. Positive pressure from the console causes ejection of blood into the aorta or pulmonary artery. All of these devices require an investigational device exemption (IDE) from the Food and Drug Administration (FDA) for use. Factors such as complexity, cost, and limited availability have had an impact on their use. Advantages of pneumatic assist devices include reduced blood trauma and reduced potential for thromboembolism (Pae et al., 1987). (See Figure 11.6.)

Finally, an electromechanically driven pump is being clinically tested after the FDA granted an IDE exemption in 1984 (Portner et al., 1989). The electrically powered NOVACOR device is implanted in the left upper quadrant of the abdomen and connected to the heart by conduits that traverse the diaphragm. With the LVAD, blood is removed from the left ventricle and returned to the ascending aorta. It is connected to a console via a percutaneous lead that provides electrical power and automatic control (see Figure 11.7). This device provides total systemic circulatory support with a stroke volume of 70 ml and output of up to 10 L/min. It is autoregulatory, requiring minor adjustment over a wide hemodynamic range including during dysrhythmias. The NOVACOR pump is capable of filling and pumping during ventricular fibrillation (Williams et al.,1987).

TAH

There are also a variety of TAHs being investigated. All of the TAHs are pneumatically driven. Examples of hearts implanted in humans include the Jarvik heart, the Unger heart, the Penn State heart, the Berlin heart, and the Phoenix heart (Joyce et al.,1986). The most common TAH is the Jarvik-7 heart.

There are two sizes of the Jarvik-7 TAH. The Jarvik 7-100 has a stroke volume of 100 ml, and the Jarvik 7-70 has a stroke volume of 70 ml. The Jarvik-7 is composed of two ventricles that are attached to the natural atria via cuffs and to the great vessels via Dacron grafts. Each ventricle contains a multilayer polyurethane diaphragm with a rigid housing. Two mechanical tilting disk valves provide unidirectional blood flow. Drive lines are connected from the base of each ventricle to the heart driver. Air is intermittently pulsed from the heart driver through tubing to the ventricles (DeVries, 1988). (See Figures 11.8 and 11.9.)

Control of heart rate, pressurization, and percentage of time spent in systole is adjusted via controls on the driver (Mays, Williams, Barker, Hastings, & Devries, 1986). During diastole, air is vented out of the ventricle on the lower side of the diaphragm. As the diaphragm collapses, blood enters the ventricle from the atrium on the upper side of the diaphragm. During systole, air is pulsed into the underside of the ventricle and blood is ejected. Resistance from valves and the pulmonary or peripheral vasculature must be

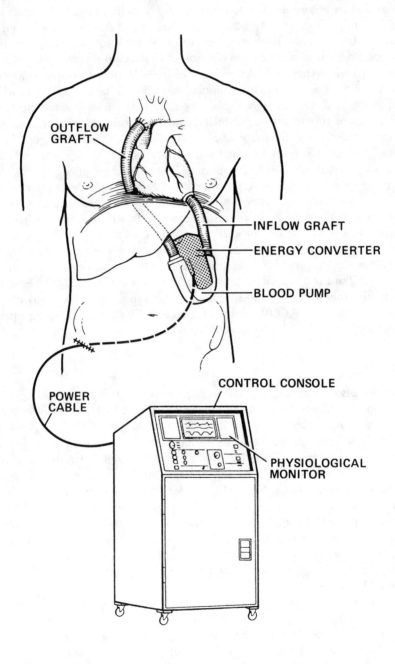

FIGURE 11.7 Internal electrical-pump-powered system (NOVACOR). (Printed with permission from NOVACOR Division of Baxter Healthcare Corporation, Oakland, California.) Drawing by Bayard Colyear, medical illustrator.

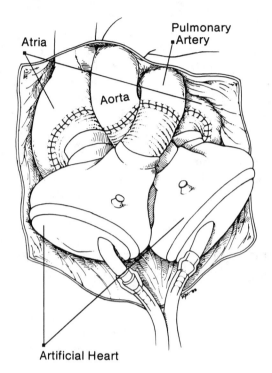

FIGURE 11.8 Attachment of the Jarvik-7.

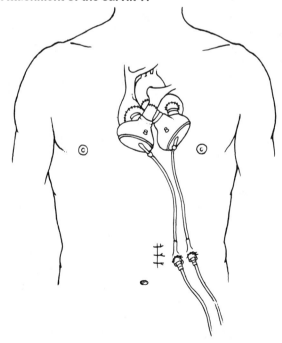

FIGURE 11.9 Location of the Jarvik-7.

overcome during systole. With increased venous return, stroke volume increases to the maximum allowable volume of the ventricle (DeVries, 1988).

Monitoring of the Jarvik-7 TAH is accomplished via a computer with a software program called COMDU: Cardiac Output Monitor and Diagnostic Unit. TAH heart rate, right and left fill volume, right and left cardiac output, and diastolic and systolic waveforms are displayed on a CRT screen and stored on a floppy disc at preset intervals (Mays et al., 1986). Driver and COMDU activated alarms are built into the system and triggered by changes in cardiac output and air pressurization of the ventricles. Use of the primary or reserve air tanks activates less critical alarms. In addition, changes in displayed waveforms and patient condition signify problems that require attention.

PREOPERATIVE NURSING PREPARATION FOR DEVICE IMPLANTATION

When the decision is made to implant a VAD or TAH in a patient, certain protocols are set into motion. The team of trained physicians, nurses, and bioengineers involved in inserting the device and caring for the patient is notified and assembled. Team mobilization includes:

- Staffing of the surgical suite for the procedure.
- Assembly of equipment for implantation.
- Staffing of the ICU with device-trained nurses for postoperative care.
- Assignment of a private room and setup with special equipment necessary for postoperative care.

The routine preoperative preparations of the VAD or TAH candidate include

- Informed consent.
- Completion of preoperative checklist (e.g., identification band on patient, consent signed, appropriate tests completed, vital signs, height and weight on chart).
- Completion of preoperative laboratory tests (complete blood count, chemistry profile, coagulation profile, type and cross-match of blood, etc.) and a chest x-ray.
- Administration of preoperative medications as indicated (e.g., sedative, prophylactic antibiotics as needed).
- Mobilization of patient (includes transport of IABP if indicated).
- Possible placement of patient on local and national waiting lists for heart transplantation (the physician may also wait until the patient is hemodynamically stable postoperatively).
- Completion of additional laboratory tests as indicated for pretransplant requirements.

Physicians implanting the device obtain informed consent. In many cases, the patient has become so ill that a family member must sign the consent.

INTRAOPERATIVE PROCEDURES

Examples of two mechanical support devices are the LVAS (Left Ventricular Assist System, NOVACOR) and TAH (Jarvik-7). Preparation for surgery involves the insertion of lines for monitoring hemodynamic status. Monitoring is performed via a central venous catheter and an arterial line. Additional peripheral lines are placed for fluid, blood, and medication administration. A Foley catheter is used to monitor urine output. Also, the patient is intubated and has a nasogastric tube placed. Once the patient has been anesthetized, a midline sternotomy is performed, and CPB is begun.

LVAS: NOVACOR

Major components of the LVAS are a balanced energy converter, a dual pusher-plate, a sac-type blood pump, and an electronic control and power-monitoring console. The implanted package includes the integrated energy converter/pump unit, two bioprosthetic valves, woven Dacron inflow and outflow conduits, and a percutaneous venting tube carrying the electrical leads (*NOVACOR*, 1987).

The device is placed in a pocket fashioned within the anterior abdominal wall in the left upper quadrant with an inflow conduit to the left ventricular apex and an outflow conduit to the ascending aorta (Starnes et al., 1988). The control console is located extracorporeally, connected to the implanted energy converter via an extension cable and the percutaneous leads. The LVAS operates in synchronous counterpulsation, synchronizing to and effectively decompressing the left ventricle.

TAH: Jarvik

Before implantation of the Jarvik-7 TAH, the pericardium is opened, and the ventricles and valves are removed at the atrioventricular groove (DeVries & Joyce, 1983). The atrial cuffs are sewn in place and Dacron grafts are measured and sewn to the pulmonary artery and aorta. Before the artificial ventricles are connected, the anastomoses are tested via injection of blood under pressure to identify leaks.

The portion of the cuffs and grafts that attach to the Jarvik ventricles are referred to as quick connects because they simply snap onto the artificial ventricles. The left ventricle is snapped on first, and its drive line is brought out below the costal margin. Then the right ventricle is connected, and its drive line is positioned and brought out next to the left drive line.

Subsequently, air is removed from the ventricles, all lines are connected, and the TAH begins to pump slowly. The left ventricle is started first, followed by the right ventricle, in order to prevent pulmonary edema. Once adequate right and left cardiac output is obtained and hemostasis is achieved, CPB is discontinued, chest tubes are placed, and the incision is closed.

POSTOPERATIVE MONITORING AND COMPLICATIONS

Postoperative Patient Monitoring

During the early recovery stage, post-VAD or -TAH implantation, nurses responsible for patient care perform a thorough patient assessment, check and evaluate the operation of device systems, and adjust for deficits according to physician orders. The nurses monitor routine vital signs and observe the patient for signs of hemorrhage; fluid, electrolyte or acid–base imbalances; and changes in respiratory, renal, neurological, or liver function. If the patient has a TAH, a Swan-Ganz catheter and ECG monitoring are not used.

Complications

Complications following device implantation partially depend on the patient's preimplantation status. If the patient had renal and/or hepatic failure secondary to heart failure, return to normal renal and hepatic function is often dramatic and fairly rapid. Respiratory, neurologic, and nutritional insufficiencies caused by "low-perfusion state" are slower to improve (Starnes et al., 1988).

The same management used for preoperative blood pressure control, fluid and electrolyte balance, and nutrition must continue after device implantation. For example, nurses continue to administer antihypertensives or vasopressors as indicated. Sodium nitroprusside and other vasoactive drugs are titrated to maintain normal blood pressure and decrease stress on suture lines. Nurses monitor fluid balance, and diuretics are administered as needed to decrease heart failure in VAD patients and to remove excess fluid in VAD and TAH patients. Some patients may need ultrafiltration when diuresis alone cannot remove fluid. In addition, hemodialysis may be indicated if renal dysfunction does not respond to improved renal perfusion.

Nurses need to assess patients' nutritional status and should encourage patients to take fluids and food by mouth. Nutritional supplementation such as enteral feedings or total parenteral nutrition (TPN) is administered as necessary.

Complications After VAD Implantation

Within the VAD group of patients, complications also vary with different designs, implantation techniques, patient care protocols, and power systems. Rose described complications causing death in a group of 79 patients with insertion of a roller-pump-driven left (n = 72) and right (n = 7) heart assist device after a variety of cardiac surgical procedures (Rose, Connolly, Cunningham, & Spencer, 1989). Causes of death included severe coagulopathy, refractory arrhythmias, biventricular failure, pulmonary embolism, irreversible neurological injury, multi-organ failure, and sepsis (Rose et al., 1989). Thirty-two patients were weaned from the device, and 21 (29%) were long-term survivors.

Bolman used a centrifugal pump in nine patients prior to transplantation (Bolman et al., 1989). Complications resulting in death while on the device included biventricular failure and brain death. Seven patients underwent transplantation and were long-term survivors. Other surgeons reported bleeding requiring reoperation, hemolysis, and thrombi in the pump system (Pae et al., 1987).

Complication data from cardiac surgical patients who required pneumatically powered VADs have also been reported. Thirty patients at one midwestern institution who could not be weaned from CPB received a pneumatic VAD (Pennington et al., 1989). Bleeding, biventricular failure, and multiple organ failure were the cause of death in patients (n = 14) who died. Biventricular failure, bleeding, respiratory failure, renal failure, and infection were also reported in several patients in this series of 30.

Portner and his colleagues (1989) have recently reported on use of the electromechanically driven LVAS. As of April 1990, 65 patients who were hemodynamically unstable have received LVAS support. The most common complications were bleeding, infection, right ventricular failure, and renal failure.

Each assist device has unique potential problems. In common, ventricular failure, bleeding, thromboembolism, multiorgan failure, and sepsis seem to occur at varying rates in patients with assist devices. Patient selection, timing of device implantation, choice of anticoagulation protocols, and prevention and treatment of multiorgan failure and infection remain as high investigational priorities.

Complications After TAH Implantation

Complications associated with TAH implantation have also been reported in several series of patients (Cabrol et al., 1989; Griffith, 1989; Joyce et al, 1986, Pae & Pierce 1989). Joyce examined data regarding TAH implantation at 13 centers around the world. Eight different types of TAHs were implanted; data were reported on 26 patients. The most significant postoperative problem was bleeding. Renal failure with the need for hemodialysis was also a frequent complication. Cerebrovascular accidents (CVAs) and transient ischemic attacks (TIAs) were reported. The CVAs occurred in patients with permanent TAH implantation. Infection of the drive lines or pneumonia also occurred commonly. Griffith (1989) and his colleagues have experience with TAH implantation in 16 patients.

Fourteen of these patients underwent cardiac transplantation. One patient died of infection and another from bleeding before transplantation.

Patients bridged with the TAH who died after transplantation often succumbed to infections (e.g., mediastinal infection [Griffith, 1989]), rejection, and oncologic complications (e.g., Kaposi's sarcoma [Cabrol et al., 1989]). Cabrol tentatively found that survival after transplantation in bridge patients was comparable to patients without TAH implantation (Cabrol et al., 1989).

Pae and Pierce (1989), in the "Combined Registry for the Clinical Use of Mechanical Ventricular Assist Pumps and the Total Artificial Heart," reported the following complications for TAH and VAD patients ($n = 124$) precluding transplantation: bleeding, kidney failure, respiratory failure, infection, thrombus/ embolus, disseminated intravascular coagulation, hemolysis, neurologic events, and inadequate cardiac output.

As with VAD implantation, researchers emphasize the need for strict patient selection criteria, coagulation control, and careful management of hemodynamic, respiratory, and renal parameters.

NURSING CARE OF THE PATIENT WITH A VAD OR TAH

The device-trained ICU nurse assigned to monitor the device is responsible for its setup, calibration, timing, recording, and troubleshooting. At some institutions, bioengineers or perfusionists may have postoperative responsibilities for device management. Along with assisting in patient care, the nurse's duties include the following:

- Monitoring hemodynamic status.
- Recognizing and maintaining optimum device function.
- Adjusting for changes in the patient's status (dysrhythmias, pump failure, or a cardiac arrest [VAD only]).
- Recording data on device flow sheets. (See Figure 11.10. for sample of NOVACOR flow sheet and photo of NOVACOR device.)
- Tabulating device research data.
- Mobilizing patients for transport (battery mode for assist device/TAH).
- Preventing and recognizing infections.

Figure 11.11 illustrates the drive console, monitoring equipment, and invasive lines for a patient immediately after TAH implantation. Table 11.1 lists an RN orientation plan for care of patients with a VAD or TAH.

Nurses who care for VAD/TAH patients must incorporate nursing diagnoses related to cardiopulmonary function into their care. As the patient stabilizes after surgery, cardiac output can decrease secondary to complications such as mediastinal bleeding with tamponade and hypovolemia.

NOVACOR LVAS CLINICAL TRIAL

PARTICIPATING INSTITUTION ______________ ____________________

Case # ____________________ Patient ID # ______________

LVAS PARAMETERS
Start a New Form for Each Shift
Please Read the Instructions for Completing this form
To be Completed in Real Time by the LVAS Operator/Monitor
Use Form # 13 B for Comments (See Instructions)

Date ______________ Shift Period __________ to ________

TIME	Heart Rate	ECG Rythm	LVAS Control Settings						LVAS Function			Pressures										Cardiac	Comm.
			Fill Rate		ECG	Fill Delay	Disrh Adapt	Fixed Rate	Stroke Vol.	Pump Outflow	Res. Vol.	Left Ventricular			Arterial			CV	Pulmonary Artery			Output	on Form
			End of Fill	Eject Delay	QRS - Eject		E or D					Syst.	Dias.	End Dias.	Syst.	Dias.	Mean	Mean	Syst.	Dias.	Mean		13 B
hh:mm	bpm		%	ms	ms	ms		bpm	mL	L/min	mL											L/min	(X)

Signature ______________________ Signature ______________________

(Print Name, Title) ______________________ (Print Name, Title) ______________________

DCP(3/87) - FORM #13A

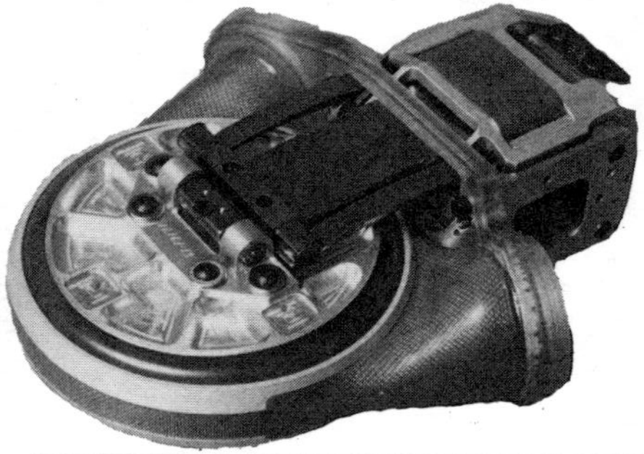

FIGURE 11.10 NOVACOR device and data sheet. (Printed with permission from NOVACOR Division of Baxter Healthcare Corporation, Oakland, California.)

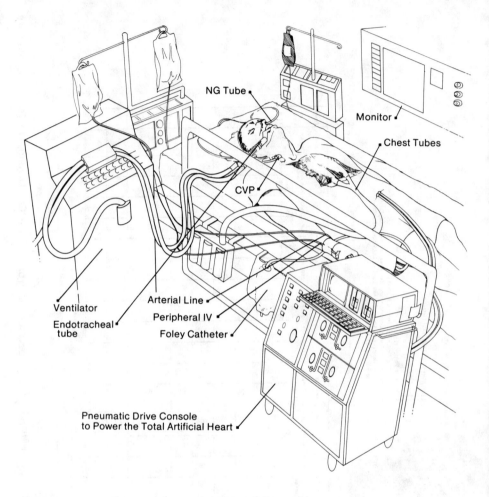

FIGURE 11.11 TAH implantation, major tubes and equipment.

Appropriate nursing interventions relate to monitoring chest tube drainage, volume replacement, and hematologic parameters (hemoglobin/hematocrit and coagulation profile). In addition, LVAS patients may experience right ventricular failure and require increased inotropic/vasodilator support or RVAD placement. Nurses must carefully assess early biventricular function in LVAS patients for signs of improvement, stabilization, or deterioration. Fine tuning of device parameters optimizes cardiac output and blood flow to vital organs. In addition, vasoactive drugs can be used to reduce hypertension and improve peripheral blood flow. With the achievement of hemodynamic stability, as exhibited by adequate cardiac output, blood pressure, and perfusion of

TABLE 11.1 Orientation Plan for Care of Patients with a VAD or TAH

Introduction and overview
  History
  Mortality statistics
Selection of candidates and preoperative preparation
  Diagnoses and criteria
  Preparation for implantation
Description of devices and surgical implantation
  VADs
  TAH
Postoperative monitoring of patients with a VAD or TAH
Complications after device implantation and related nursing care
Equipment and nursing responsibilities
  Review of nursing policies and procedures
  Hands-on training session

other body organs, the patient can begin to recover and rehabilitate while awaiting heart transplantation.

Respiratory dysfunction due to preoperative pulmonary edema, surgical intervention, and accumulation of airway secretions is also improved after device implantation. Nursing interventions involve assessing the adequacy of respiration and weaning from the ventilator as soon as possible. Many devices generate noise, making pulmonary auscultation difficult. Assessment of respiratory rate, pattern of breathing, dyspnea, and subjective findings such as shortness of breath (SOB) are vital to patient management. Monitoring arterial blood gases (ABGs) and oxygen saturation provide additional information. Clearing airway secretions also improves respiratory function and reduces the potential for infection.

Potential for infection is a critical nursing diagnosis for the patient. Invasive intravenous and device lines, lack of mobility, and cardiac cachexia put the patient at high risk for infection. The nurse assesses temperature and all body systems every 8 hours (more frequently as needed). Nurses also assess intravenous lines and wound sites for signs of infection during dressing changes every 24 hours. The practice of good handwashing and aseptic technique for dressing changes is imperative. Nurses care for patients in private rooms and screen all visitors. Most patients receive prophylactic antibiotics for a few days immediately after implantation. The presence of an infection may require changes in antibiotic therapy after culture and sensitivity results are obtained. If the infection involves device lines or the device itself, surgical removal and replacement may be necessary.

Patients are also at risk for CVAs: potential for alteration in cerebral tissue perfusion related to embolization. Nurses should expect patients to be mentally alert and able to follow commands with normal sensation and movement. Neurological assessment and maintainance of anticoagulation are paramount in caring for patients at risk for CVAs. Thorough neurological assessment should be performed frequently. Coagulation profiles should be drawn and therapy adjusted to maintain adequate anticoagulation. In addition, seizures have been observed in TAH patients with high cardiac outputs. Therefore, nurses correlate any changes in neurological status with device parameters and cardiac output.

As mentioned earlier, patients may experience renal and hepatic dysfunction secondary to heart failure. After surgery for device implantation, nurses carefully assess patients for improvement or deterioration in these organ systems. Ultrafiltration and/or hemodialysis may be indicated to temporarily support failing kidneys.

In addition, patients will still have alteration in nutritional status secondary to cardiac cachexia and the inability to meet nutritional needs immediately after surgery. As previously stated, recovery will be a slow process. Dietary consultation should be instituted immediately so that parenteral and later enteral support may be provided.

Impairment of skin integrity and alteration in mobility will continue to be important nursing diagnoses after device implantation. As patients stabilize hemodynamically, they can be turned in bed and assisted to a chair. VAD and TAH patients must be carefully observed during initial turning to identify torsion or compression of the atria or conduits and subsequent decreases in cardiac output. The TAH will become stabilized in the chest with the development of adhesions within several days of surgery, and patient mobilization can be more actively pursued. Patients with long-term TAH or LVAS implantation are capable of participating in active exercise programs (including bicycling on a stationary bicycle). Rehabilitation during the pretransplant phase promotes rapid recovery after cardiac transplantation.

Patients and families may experience anxiety and have difficulty coping with device implantation. The patient will also most likely experience difficulty sleeping. Assessing the level of anxiety and coping methods, allowing patients and families to verbalize their concerns, and allowing them to participate in care are important nursing interventions. Planned times for rest and sleep with minimal to no interruptions are essential.

Finally, patients and families will have a knowledge deficit about device implantation and cardiac transplantation. Assessing deficits and providing information are important nursing interventions. Nurses need to determine patient and family "readiness" to learn and provide information with sufficient, but not too much, detail so that they can prepare for and understand the therapy in which they are about to participate.

A nursing care plan for care of device patients is included at the end of this chapter.

PREPARATION FOR HEART TRANSPLANTATION

After patients have stabilized, and while waiting for a donor heart, nurses can provide extensive pretransplant teaching and initiate rehabilitation. When a donor becomes available, the transplant physician notifies the nurse caring for the patient, and the nurse institutes routine preoperative preparations including

- Informed consent.
- Preoperative checklist.
- Preoperative laboratory tests and chest x-ray.
- Preoperative medication.
- Mobilization of patient (battery mode for support device/TAH).
- Tabulation of device research data.

CONCLUSION

Using mechanical support devices for critically ill heart patients has opened challenging frontiers for nurses: to adapt and work with new technologies, to work with bioengineers and others outside the health care profession, and to train for the unknown by extrapolating from animals to humans.

With increased use of circulatory support devices, the specialty area of critical-care nursing is still evolving. Pioneers in the use of VADs and TAHs must share their knowledge with all heart transplant centers. Medical teams must continue to define patient selection criteria, improve technology, and improve patient management to improve patient survival (Termuhlen, Swartz, & Pennington, 1988).

A transplant center that wishes to set up and activate a device team must do the following:

- Contact a device manufacturer.
- Select appropriate device team members.
- Write a proposal for review by hospital administration, medical chiefs, and institutional review boards. In addition, the state government may require a Certificate of Need (CON).
- Write department protocols and nursing policies and procedures.
- Implement device training programs involving formal classes, hands-on training sessions, animal laboratory, dry runs, and reviews.
- Follow up with regular evaluation of the program.
- Share results via abstract presentation and publication.

NURSING CARE PLAN: MECHANICAL ASSIST DEVICE PATIENT

Nursing diagnosis	Expected outcome	Nursing interventions
ALTERATION IN CARDIAC OUTPUT (CO) related to problems with device pump timing or dysfunction (e.g., loss of trigger, dysrhythmias (VAD only) Mediastinal hemorrhage Changes in patient position Ventricular failure (VAD only)	Patient will exhibit hemodynamic stability as exhibited by Adequate CO and BP Adequate cerebral, renal, and peripheral perfusion Mentally alert Urine output >30 cc/hr Adequate peripheral pulses. Absence of pul- monary and/or peripheral edema Minimal chest tube drainage Normal hemoglobin and hematocrit	1. Monitor and record BP, heart rate and rhythm (VAD only), CVP, CO, stroke volume (SV), and other pump parameters. 2. Auscultate heart sounds (VAD only) and assess for presence of peripheral pulses, peripheral edema, and skin temperature and color. 3. Auscultate breath sounds twice per shift and prn and obtain arterial blood gases prn. 4 Record intake and output. 5. Assess level of consciousness, movement, and sensation. 6. Assess for postoperative bleeding. Observe and record chest tube drainage. Monitor hemoglobin/ hematocrit and coagulation profile. Assess for other potential sources of bleeding (e.g., nasogastric aspirate) Administer blood products as needed. 7. Maintain adequate preload (e.g., with crystalloids, colloids, and blood products prn) or administer diuretics if CVP elevated. 8. Administer medications to decrease afterload (e.g., Hydralazine®) prn and observe effects. 9. Administer medications to control dysrhythmias, prn and observe effects, change trigger mode prn (VAD only).

(continued)

NURSING CARE PLAN: MECHANICAL ASSIST DEVICE PATIENT (continued)

Nursing diagnosis	Expected outcome	Nursing interventions
		10. Readjust timing for changes in position or 20% change in heart rate (VAD only).
	* * * *	11. No CPR.
ALTERATION IN RESPIRATORY FUNCTION (impaired gas exchange) related to Pulmonary edema Surgery Ineffective clearance of airway secretions	Patient will exhibit adequate gas exchange: ABGs within normal limits Clear breath sounds Normal pattern of respiration Clearance of airway secretions	1. Auscultate breath sounds (*note:* device noises may make this assessment difficult). 2. Assess other respiratory parameters: respiratory rate, pattern of breathing, presence of SOB, PND. 3. Monitor ABGs and oxygen saturation prn. 4. Suction endotracheal tube Q2 hrs and prn. 5. Turn or tilt patient side to side (if tolerated hemodynamically). 6. Wean from ventilator and extubate as soon as possible. 7. After extubation: Administer oxygen prn. Encourage coughing and deep breathing. Administer pain medication as ordered.
	* * * *	
ALTERATION IN FLUID AND ELECTROLYTE BALANCE related to Trauma of surgery Postoperative bleeding Diuretic therapy	Balanced I&O No weight gain >2 lb/day Electrolyte values within normal limits	1. Observe vital signs, CVP, and machine parameters for signs of hypo- or hypervolemia. 2. Monitor and record electrolyte values. 3. Assess I&O carefully. 4. Weigh patient daily. 5. Administer diuretics prn and evaluate. 6. Administer IV fluids and evaluate. 7. Observe for peripheral edema.

(continued)

NURSING CARE PLAN: MECHANICAL ASSIST DEVICE PATIENT (continued)

Nursing diagnosis	Expected outcome	Nursing interventions
* * * *		
POTENTIAL FOR INFECTION related to Invasive lines and cables Lack of mobility Alteration in nutritional state	Patient will be free of infection as exhibited by Afebrile Clear lung fields No drainage from incisional sites All cultures negative	1. Limit room traffic and use good handwashing technique. 2. Monitor temperature, auscultate lungs, check sputum for color, amount and texture. 3. Check all incisions for redness, swelling, tenderness, pain, or exudate and change dressing using aseptic technique. 4. Administer antibiotics as ordered. 5. Obtain cultures of sputum, urine, blood, and wounds prn.
* * * *		
POTENTIAL FOR ALTERATION IN CERE-BRAL TISSUE PERFUSION related to embolization	Patient will be mentally alert and able to follow commands with normal sensation and movement.	1. Perform neurological assessment frequently. 2. Orient patient to person, place, time, as needed. 3. Observe for possible seizure activity. 4. Correlate other parameters (e.g., machine function, cardiac output) with changes in level of consciousness. 5. Obtain coagulation profile as ordered prn. 6. Administer anticoagulants as ordered.
* * * *		
POTENTIAL FOR KIDNEY AND LIVER DYS-FUNCTION related to Organ dysfunction prior to device implantation Trauma of surgery	Patient will exhibit Urine output >30cc/hr Serum BUN and crea-tinine within normal limits Urine for creatinine clearance within normal limits.	1. Monitor and record I&O. 2. Monitor and record serum lab values (BUN, creatinine, bilirubin, SGOT, SGPT, GGT, alkaline phosphatase). 3. Weigh patient daily.

(continued)

NURSING CARE PLAN: MECHANICAL ASSIST DEVICE PATIENT (continued)

Nursing diagnosis	Expected outcome	Nursing interventions
	Serum total bilirubin and liver enzymes within normal limits.	4. Restrict fluid intake prn. 5. Observe for changes in skin color.
	* * * *	
ALTERATION IN NUTRITION (less than body requirements) related to 　Cardiac cachexia 　Inability to take in 　food immediately 　after surgery	Patient will maintain positive nitrogen balance and sufficient caloric intake to meet nutritional needs.	1. Consult with dietitian to determine current nutritional status. 2. Perform a calorie count prn. 3. Administer oral, enteral, or parenteral feedings as ordered. 4. Allow patient personal preferences regarding food choices. 5. Encourage family to bring in favorite food items.
	* * * *	
POTENTIAL IMPAIRMENT OF SKIN INTEGRITY related to 　Impaired preoperative 　and postoperative 　mobility 　Cardiac cachexia	Patient will be free of skin breakdown and decubiti.	1. Assess and document condition of skin and mucous membranes every shift. 2. Turn or tilt patient (if hemodynamically stable) every 2–4 hours and prn. 3. Perform mouth care every 2–4 hrs and prn. 4. Use special mattresses, sheepskin, etc., prn. 5. Massage bony prominences prn. 6. Assist patients to chair and ambulate if possible. 7. Provide adequate hydration and nutrition.
	* * * *	
ALTERATION IN MOBILITY and decreased ability to perform activities of daily living related to 　Prolonged bed rest 　Device implantation	Patient will maintain adequate joint mobility and muscle tone. Patient will perform activities of daily living (ADLs).	1. Assess joint mobility and muscles strength and tone. 2. Consult with physical therapist and perform passive and active range-of-motion exercises as soon as possible. 3. Encourage participation in active exercise program. 4. Assist patient in the perfor-

(continued)

NURSING CARE PLAN: MECHANICAL ASSIST DEVICE
PATIENT (continued)

Nursing diagnosis	Expected outcome	Nursing interventions
		mance of ADLs with increasing independence.
		5. Institute occupational therapy consultation for diversional activities.
		6. Monitor nutritional status.
	* * * *	
POTENTIAL FOR SLEEP PATTERN DISTURBANCE related to Device machinery noises Frequent patient monitoringr Anxiety Medications	Patient will have adequate rest and normal sleep patterns.	1. Explain device/machinery noises to patient. 2. Group nursing activities and allow periods for rest and sleep. 3. Coordinate other daily activities, consults, and visits to allow for rest and sleep. 4. Orient patient to times for wakefulness and sleep. 5. Administer sedatives/ hypnotics prn. 6. Provide a calm, therapeutic atmosphere.
	* * * *	
ANXIETY AND ALTERATION IN COPING related to Lack of privacy and depersonalization Dependency Sensory overload Media publicity Waiting for transplantation Removal of one's native heart and implantation of a device (TAH only) Fear of unknown	Patient will communicate feelings and anxiety.	1. Assess patient's emotional status and coping. 2. Allow patient to verbalize fears and frustrations. 3. Encourage patient to make decisions regarding care. 4. Be supportive, helpful, encouraging to patient and family. 5. Encourage family to bring patient's personal belongings from home. 6. Allow patient and family privacy and assist with media coverage per hospital policy and patient/family wishes. 7. Utilize all resources available (e.g., social work, occupational therapy, and pastoral care).
	* * * *	

(continued)

NURSING CARE PLAN: MECHANICAL ASSIST DEVICE PATIENT (continued)

Nursing diagnosis	Expected outcome	Nursing interventions
KNOWLEDGE DEFICIT about device implantation and cardiac transplantation	Patient and family will demonstrate knowledge regarding device implantation and cardiac transplantation.	1. Assess patient and family regarding knowledge and deficits. 2. Educate patient and family about device implantation and heart transplantation. 3. Be sensitive to readiness to learn. 4. Provide overview, give details as indicated. 5. Use discussion and written materials. 6. Involve surgeons, social work, others prn in teaching process.

ACKNOWLEDGEMENTS

We are grateful to Peer M. Portner, PhD, Novacor Division, Baxter Healthcare Corporation; and Roque Pifarre, MD, Professor and Chairman, Department of Thoracic and Cardiovascular Surgery, Loyola University Medical Center for their assistance and encouragement.

REFERENCES

Akutsu, T., & Kolff, W. (1958). Permanent substitutes for valves and hearts. *Transactions: American Society of Artificial Internal Organs. 4*(6), 230–235.

Bernhard, W. F., Berger, R. L., Stetz, J. P., Carr, J. G., Colo, N., McCormick, J. R., & Fishbein, M. C. (1979). Temporary left ventricular bypass: factors affecting patient survival. *Cardiovascular Surgery, 60*, I-131–I-141.

Bolman, R. M., III, Cox, J. L., Marshall, W., Kouchoukos, N., Spray, T. L., Cance, C., Genton, R. E., & Saffitz, J. (1989). Circulatory support with a centrifugal pump as a bridge to cardiac transplantation. *Annals of Thoracic Surgery, 47*, 108–112.

Cabrol, C., Solis, E., Muneretto, C., Pavie, A., Gandjbakhch, I., Bors, V., Szefner, J., Leger, P., & Cabrol, A. (1989). Orthotopic transplantation after implantation of a Jarvik-7 total artificial heart. *Journal of Thoracic and Cardiovascular Surgery, 97*, 342–350.

Davis, P. K., Rosenberg, G., Snyder, A. J., & Pierce, W. S. (1989). Current status of permanent total artificial hearts. *Annals of Thoracic Surgery, 47*, 172–178.

DeBakey, M. E. (1971). Left ventricular bypass pump for cardiac assistance. *American Journal of Cardiology, 27*, 3–11.

DeVries, W. C. (1988). The permanent artificial heart—four case reports. *Journal of the American Medical Association, 259*, 849–858.

DeVries, W. C., & Joyce, L. D. (1983). The artificial heart. *Clinical Symposia, 35*, 4–32.

Griffith, B. P. (1989). Interim use of the Jarvik-7 artificial heart: Lessons learned at Presbyterian-University Hospital of Pittsburgh. *Annals of Thoracic Surgery, 47*, 158–166.

Holub, D. A., Hibbs, C. W., Sturn, J. T., Fuqua, J. M., Edmonds, C. H., McGee, M. G., Fuhrman, T. M., Trono, R., Igo, S. R., & Norman, J. C. (1979). Clinical trials of an abdominal left ventricular assist device (ALVAD): Progress report. *Transactions: American Society of Artificial Internal Organs, 25*, 197–204.

Joyce, L. D., Johnson, K. E., Pierce, W. S., DeVries, W. C., Semb, B. K. H., Copeland, J. G., Griffith, B. P., Cooley, D. A., Frazier, O. H., Cabrol, C., Keon, W. J., Unger, F., Bucherl, E. S., & Wolner, E. (1986). Summary of the world experience with clinical use of total artificial hearts as heart support devices. *Journal of Heart Transplantation, 5*, 229–235.

Kantrowitz, A., Tjonneland, S., Freed, P. S., Phillips, S. J., Butner, A. N., & Sherman, J. L. (1968). Initial clinical experience with intraaortic balloon pumping in cardiogenic shock. *Journal of the American Medical Association, 203*, 113–118.

Magovern, G. J., Heckler, F. R., Park, S. B., Christlieb, I. Y., Liebler, G. A., Burkholder, J. A., Maher, T. D., Benckart, D. H., Magovern, G. J., Jr., & Kao, R. L. (1988). Paced skeletal muscle for dynamic cardiomyoplasty. *Annals of Thoracic Surgery, 45*(6), 614–619.

May, D.R., & Adams, M.A. (1987). Ventricular assist devices—A bridge to cardiac transplantation. *AORN Journal, 46*(4), 633–646.

Mays, J. B., Williams, M. A., Barker, L. E., Hastings, L., & DeVries, W. C. (1986). Diagnostic monitoring and drive system management of patients with total artificial heart. *Heart and Lung, 15*,466–475.

Mulford, E. (1987). Nursing perspectives for the patient receiving postoperative ventricular assistance in the critical care unit. *Heart and Lung, 16*, 246–257.

Norman, J. C., Cooley, D. A., Kahan, B. D., Keats, A. S., Massin, E. K., Solis, R. T., Luper, W. E., Brook, M. I., Klima, T., Frazier, O. H., Hacker, J., Duncan, J. M., Dacso, C. C., Winston, D. S., & Reul, G. J. (1978). Total support of the circulation of a patient with post-cardiotomy stone-heart syndrome by a partial artificial heart (ALVAD) for 5 days followed by heart and kidney transplantation. *Lancet, 1*,(8074), 1125–1127.

NOVACOR left ventricular assist system: Operator's manual. (1987). Available from NOVACOR Medical Corporation 7799 Pardee Lane Oakland, CA. 94621.

Pae, W. E., & Pierce, W. G. (1989). Combined registry for the clinical use of mechanical ventricular assist pumps and the total artificial heart: third official report—1988. *Journal of Heart Transplantation, 8*(4), 277–280.

Pae, W. E., Pierce, W. S., Pennock, J. L., Campbell, D. B., & Waldhausen, J. A. (1987). Long-term results of ventricular assist pumping in postcardiotomy cardiogenic shock. *Journal of Cardiovascular Surgery, 93*, 434–441.

Patacky, M. G., Garvin, B. J., & Schwirian, P. M. (1985). Intra-aortic balloon pumping and stress in the coronary care unit. *Heart and Lung, 14*(2), 142–148.

Pennington, D. G., McBride, L. R., Swartz, M. T., Kanter, K. R., Kaiser, G. C., Barnes, H. B., Miller, L. W., Naunheim, K. S., Fiore, A. C., & Willman, V. L. (1989). Use of the Pierce-Donachy ventricular assist device in patients with cardiogenic shock after cardiac operations. *Annals of Thoracic Surgery, 47,* 130–135.

Pierce, W. S., Parr, G. V., Myers, J. L., Pae, W. E., Bull, A. P., & Waldhausen, J. A. (1981). Ventricular-assist pumping in patients with cardiogenic shock after cardiac operations. *New England Journal of Medicine, 305,* 1606–1610.

Portner, P. M., Oyer, P. E., McGregor, C. G. A., Baldwin, J. C., Ream, A. K. Wyner, J., Zusman, D. R., & Shumway, N. E. (1985). First human use of an electrically powered implantable ventricular assist system. *Artificial Organs, 9A,* 36.

Portner, P. M., Oyer, P. E., Pennington, D. G., Baumgartner, W. A., Griffith, B. P., Frist, W. R., Magilligan, D. J., Noon, G. P. Ramasamy, N., Miller, P. J., Jassawalla, J. S. (1989). Implantable electrical left ventricular assist system: Bridge to transplantation and the future. *Annals of Thoracic Surgery, 47,* 142-150.

Rose, L. M., Connolly, M., Cunningham, J. N., & Spencer, F. C. (1989). Technique and results with a roller pump left and right heart assist device. *Annals of Thoracic Surgery, 47* 124–129.

Starnes, V. A., Oyer, P. E., Portner, P. M., Ramasamy, N., Miller, P. J., Stinson, E. B., Baldwin, J. C., Ream, A. K., Wyner, J., Shumway, N. E. (1988). Isolated left ventricular assist as a bridge to cardiac transplantation. *Journal of Thoracic Cardiovascular Surgery, 96,* 62–71.

Termuhlen, D. F., Swartz, M. T., & Pennington, D. G. (1988). Predictors for weaning patients from ventricular assist devices. *ASAIO Transactions, 34,* 131–139.

Weintraub, R. M., & Thurer, R. L. (1983). The intra-aortic balloon pump—a ten year experience. *Journal of Heart Transplantation, 3,* 8–15.

Williams, B. A., Lough, M. E., Shinn, J. A. (1987). Left ventricular assist device as a bridge to heart transplantation: A case study. *Journal of Heart Transplantation, 6*(1), 23–28.

CHAPTER **12**

PSYCHOSOCIAL ISSUES OF TRANSPLANT RECIPIENTS

Nancy Deeds Meister
Kimberly Stephens

Studies have indicated that quality of life following transplantation is good (Lough, 1986). Despite these findings, significant psychosocial problems may remain or develop for some patients following a transplant procedure. Interpersonal conflicts, employment difficulties, and financial struggles are just a few of these possible patient and family concerns. This chapter will discuss potential psychosocial problems and provide the nurse with a plan of care for transplant patients and their families. Postoperative issues will be emphasized. For more information regarding preoperative issues—for example, candidate selection criteria and living related kidney donation—refer to the appropriate organ-specific chapter in this book.

PSYCHOSOCIAL ASSESSMENT

Psychosocial assessment enables the nurse to understand the patient's psychologic patterns and social experiences (Parkinson, 1980). Having identified a patient's intellectual, social, and emotional needs, the nurse can then proceed with an individualized plan of care that will address these needs.

Upon admission to the hospital, the transplant nurse conducts a thorough patient interview to obtain information regarding the recipient's physical and psychosocial history. Due to the time constraints of many transplant surgeries, such as kidney, heart, lung, and liver, this interview is often brief. In such instances, valuable information can often be obtained from the family, the transplant nurse coordinator, or the social worker who was involved in the recipient's preoperative evaluation. An excellent resource for kidney transplant recipients is that of the patient's dialysis nurse and/or social worker.

During the interview, the nurse learns about the patient's anxiety level, capacity to learn, and expectations of hospitalization. Other important areas to assess include (a) the patient's potential for compliance, (b) the extent of the patient's social support system, (c) the patient's developmental stage, (d) the patient's self-image, (e) the patient's and family's coping styles, and (f) the patient and family's financial situation.

In addition to the nursing assessment, a social worker or psychiatrist may conduct a more in-depth psychological evaluation. In the program at the University of Arizona, the Minnesota Multiphasic Personality Inventory (MMPI), the Wechsler Intelligence and Memory Scale, and the Health Locus of Control are used. The MMPI is a standard personality measure. The Wechsler Memory Scale assesses verbal and visual-spatial memory looking at both hemispheres to determine whether there might be problems learning the medical regimen. The Health Locus of Control indicates valuing of one's health and is used as an indicator of compliance.

These test results may be used when selecting candidates or identifying potential psychosocial concerns postoperatively. Knowledge of a patient's personality variables and coping styles can help the transplant team become more sensitive to the recipient. Also, awareness of learning deficits are critical to health care providers because a successful transplant relies heavily on the patient and/or family's ability to understand and comply with the medical regimens after discharge from the hospital.

Patient Compliance

A successful organ transplant depends on patient and family compliance. Unfortunately, studies have failed to provide a clear explanation of the mechanism by which compliance with a prescribed medical regimen is facilitated. Therefore, the transplant nurse must be able to detect potential compliance problems prior to discharge.

An indicator of compliance may be how the person has complied with past medical treatment.

- Does the patient take medications as prescribed?
- Has the patient adjusted medication according to physician orders in the past?
- What are the patient's beliefs about self-healing or alternative therapies?
- Are these beliefs compatible with the medical program?
- Was the patient fully committed to the preoperative medical regimen?

Mills, Barnes, Rodell, and Terry (1985) conducted a study to evaluate the impact of a patient education program to assess the patient's knowledge regarding his/her illness and to identify obstacles to compliant behavior after discharge. A regression analysis of predictors of overall compliance scores after discharge demonstrated that indicators of motivation were most highly correlated with compliance.

Research by Stone (1979) demonstrated that caring relationships by health care professionals effect higher compliance rates in their patients. Therapeutic nurse–patient relationships can be achieved when the primary nursing model is utilized. The primary nurse is responsible for planning for the patient's needs through nursing care plans, conferences, referrals, and collaboration.

Primary nursing includes involving both the patient and the family in care (Ciske, 1979). Patients perceive their primary nurse as someone who takes a special interest in their needs, a nurse advocate. This caring relationship often encourages compliance with prescribed treatment.

In pediatric transplantation, family compliance is critical since children cannot be fully responsible for medication administration (Gold, Kirkpatrick, Fricker, & Zitell, 1986). One or both parents must be fully committed to the program. Unstable family situations can leave children vulnerable to non-compliance and consequent transplant complications. Preadolescent or adolescent transplant candidates present a particular nursing challenge because it is difficult to predict if they will become noncompliant when they establish independence and separation from their parents.

Support System

A significant other is an individual in one's life to whom the most meaning or importance is given. It is a person who is loved, respected, and valued and who in turn loves, respects, and values the person to a degree greater than in other relationships (Tedrow, 1984). People undergoing transplantation experience an increased need for love and support from their significant others. It is the transplant nurse's responsibility to identify the patient's support system and facilitate its effectiveness during the hospitalization.

Once the presence of a support system is established, the degree of involvement or commitment to the patient can then be evaluated. Sometimes family members have good intentions, but their actions are ineffective. If the nurse evaluates a patient as not having enough social support, it is important to determine whether the patient wants support or is comfortable being self-sufficient. The nurse might help a patient identify someone who can provide support, thereby helping to create a support system. For example, a referral may be made to the transplant team social worker if further assistance is necessary.

Developmental Stage

Assessing the patient's developmental stage in order to understand issues that the patient and family might face is important (Herz, 1980). Children with chronic illness or a history of congenital problems will need counseling to change established family patterns. The parents will need help to learn when to let go and allow the child recipient some independence. Power and control within the family shift as the child moves out of the sick role and needs less parental protection (McCollum, 1981). A person in his/her 20s is attempting to establish autonomy and independence from the family, establishing a career and developing relationships that may lead to marriage and children. The need for transplantation forces that person back into dependence on his/her family. Conversely, a person at or near retirement may view the transplant as "bonus time" to travel or enjoy grandchildren. Unfortunately, a person who is at midlife is usually at the height of career and family responsibilities and will be pulled in many directions after transplant.

Self-Image

As mentioned in previous chapters, an organ transplant cannot function properly without the use of immunosuppressive drugs. These potent anti-rejection medications often cause side effects that change one's physical appearance. Weight gain, round puffy face, acne, and hirsutism are the most common changes.

The adolescent recipient may be particularly concerned about these changes. During adolescent development, there is increased awareness of the body, sexual maturation, an acceptance of sexuality, and integration of a new body image. The adolescent who has received a transplant must deal with the normal changes in his or her body as well as the superimposed abnormal changes resulting from the transplant (Starkman, 1980).

These physical alterations can result in psychosocial problems for the transplant recipient. Patients may fear that their significant other will no longer find them attractive. A poor sense of body integrity may cause the recipient to withdraw from friends and family. Some patients become so unhappy with their appearance that they stop taking their immunosuppression medications, resulting in transplant rejection and possible loss.

Coping

The patient's coping mechanisms are important to the nurse, social worker, and support staff. Patients may be asked to identify what has helped them through difficult times in the past. For example, "I take one day at a time" or "It could be worse" or "I see it as a challenge" or "my family" or "God." Patients typically use these same coping mechanisms before and after transplant surgery. Patients can also learn new ways of coping from staff or other patients.

Most centers offer inpatient and outpatient support groups. Regularly scheduled meetings are organized and facilitated by nurses, social workers, and sometimes by patients. The transplant experience creates a natural bond for patients. There is no one best format for the group. Groups range from being highly therapeutic to purely educational.

Some transplant centers combine patients who are waiting with those who have received a transplant. Significant others are usually included in this group process. A structured format allowing for voluntary participation but not demanding participation is optimal.

The University of Arizona's support group format allows each member opportunities to share his/her experiences with transplantation. It is an open group that alternates between having discussions that are not topic-specific to having educational themes. The goal of the group is mutual support and reinforcement of life-style changes. The group also meets socially for lunch and participates in organ donor awareness and other advocacy programs.

Finances/Employment

The financial impact of a transplant can be devastating for some patients and their families. Often candidates do not want to be a financial burden on their families. Many come to the evaluation process with a history of financial problems; they may be living on social security or disability. Pretransplant financial distress does not go away after surgery; it remains a long-term issue. It can also become a new issue posttransplant if the patient cannot return to work and commercial insurance expires.

The Consolidated Omnibus Reconciliation Act of 1986 (COBRA) requires employers to provide employees with continued health insurance benefits for 18 months after termination. Unfortunately, the ex-employee must pay 102% of the insurance premium. This can be difficult when experiencing an income gap or reduced income. Many transplant families consider continued health insurance coverage to be more important than making mortgage payments. Long-term transplant recipients often lose coverage and have only Medicare. Their disability often puts them over income for state Medicaid programs. Medicare will not cover medication costs except for the first year for Medicare-funded heart, kidney, and liver transplants. Immunosuppression costs, which can average as much as $6,000 per year, can create a serious problem for some patients.

With the current private health insurance system in the United States, some transplant patients will continue to have financial and social problems that patients in Great Britain, Canada, and Australia do not have. These countries have national insurance plans. A study from Australia showed that 53% of patients after heart transplant had returned to full or parttime employment (Harvison et al., 1988). However, in a U.S. study of 40 patients after heart transplant, Meister, McAleer, Meister, Riley, and Copeland (1986) reported that only 32% returned to work, while 25% elected retirement and 6% were "insurance disabled." The insurance disabled group is defined as those patients physically able to work and desiring to work but unable to do so because of financial limitations. The authors concluded that more people could return to work if they could retain their insurance while doing so. The variables related to work status were length of disability prior to transplant, age, control over working conditions, and type of health insurance. Transplant recipients have reported various employment problems, including employer resistance regarding return to work, redefinition of the job, being locked into the same job for fear of not getting insurance coverage, and job discrimination.

The Federal Rehabilitation Act of 1973 prohibits employers who receive federal funds from discriminating against handicapped employees. However, this applies to a small number of employers. Strategies by transplant recipients to get around these problems include going on a spouse's group insurance plan, creative funding, doing volunteer work, or helping a spouse start a business. Education of the community about the rehabilitation of transplant recipients is needed. Changes need to be made in the insurance system to include those who are uninsurable.

After identifying patient financial problems, the University of Arizona Transplant Program developed a fund to pay for living expenses during the 3-month posttransplant period. A patient started the fund, which patients and families continue to support. The fund is also used for transportation to enable patients to return to the center for their yearly checkup. In some instances, the fund is used for medications on a limited basis. Many transplant centers have funds similar to this one.

This type of funding is usually limited and cannot help people who have no way to pay for their transplants. The social worker advises families on possible fund-raising techniques but never participates in fund raising for an individual. As organ transplantation becomes more common, fund raising will become more difficult.

COMMUNITY RESOURCES

Social workers are valuable members of transplant teams because they combine clinical assessment and counseling skills with community resource linkage. Since many patients are referred from out of town to the transplant center, the family needs assistance with decisions regarding housing, school districts, child care, transportation, and a general community orientation. These interventions are similar to those provided by other medical social workers, but there is less emphasis on discharge planning and more emphasis on long-term patient and family follow-up.

Developing community resources for patients and families is another aspect of the role of the social worker. Because most transplant centers/hospitals do not have housing facilities, the social worker can become involved in making discount agreements with motels and apartment complexes. Most hospitals provide information on the housing facilities available and city maps to orient families. Social workers can send letters to families prior to moving near the transplant center and advise them about what they should bring and what is available. Such guidance helps them in knowing what to expect and lessens the stress of traveling to an unfamiliar area.

COUNSELING

The transplant nurse is responsible for identifying the patient's psychosocial needs and developing a plan of care aimed at resolving those needs. Education is provided throughout the recipient's hospitalization in preparation for their discharge. Appropriate nursing interventions include encouraging patients to talk about their feelings and providing emotional support. A sample nursing care plan is located at the end of this chapter.

The transplant social worker counsels patients who express a need or who require additional emotional support beyond that which the nursing staff is able to provide. A social worker's counseling role includes availability at times of crisis or complications when patients are readmitted to the hospital.

A patient who is experiencing significant depression, marital problems, or an alcohol or drug dependency problem that may interfere with compliance should be referred to the transplant team psychologist or psychiatrist.

CONCLUSION

Allender, Shisslak, Kasniak, and Copeland (1983) identified six stages of psychological adjustment from evaluation through hospital discharge after heart transplantation. These stages include

- The evaluation period, with anxiety about acceptance into the transplant program.
- The stressful waiting period, with fear of death.
- The immediate postsurgical period, in which there is some pain but also elation about receiving the donor organ.
- The first rejection episode or other complication, when the patient and family realize that having a transplant means having less control over life because of the medical regimen.
- The recovery phase, when patients adjust to life as transplant recipients and begin accepting health monitoring and life-style changes.
- Hospital discharge, which includes gradually breaking the tie with 24-hour nursing care and establishing a self-care routine at home.

The University of Arizona expanded the phases to seven. The last phase is the patient's return to the home of origin. Concerns during this final stage include separating from the transplant center, returning to work, and reestablishing relationships with friends and family at home. The transplant nurse and social worker, along with other transplant team members, help patients and families make these transitions.

NURSING CARE PLAN FOR PSYCHOSOCIAL ISSUES

Problems	Patient behaviors	Expected outcome	Nursing interventions
1. **NONCOMPLIANCE** related to Inadequate knowledge Lack of motivation Lack of/or ineffective support system Anxiety Side effects of medication	Failure to adhere to prescribed treatment by direct observation Patient statement Family statement Development of transplant rejection, infection, or other complications. Failure to attend scheduled clinic appointments Partially used medications	**Short-term** Transplant recipient will demonstrate understanding and ability to perform prescribed treatment **Long-term** Transplant recipient will demonstrate behaviors consistent with goals of of posttransplant regimen	1. Assess causative factors: Negative experiences with health care system Recent changes in life-style (work, finances, family) Side effects of medications. 2. Allow patient to verbalize feelings toward expected/prescribed regimens. 3. Consult physician for medication dose reduc-tion and/or time of administration, e.g., medications that cause drowsiness to be taken at bedtime. 4. Provide transplant care instruction of: Medication administration Signs and symptoms of rejection/infection

(continued)

NURSING CARE PLAN FOR PSYCHOSOCIAL ISSUES (continued)

Problems	Patient behaviors	Expected outcome	Nursing interventions
			Nutrition Exercise 5. Individualize teaching approach by acknowledging patient's age, level of understanding, visual/hearing deficits, and level of anxiety. 6. Positively reinforce all efforts to learn and perform self-care. 7. Provide referrals if necessary to social worker or psychiatrist, physical therapist, or dietitian.
		* * * * *	
ANXIETY related to Unfamiliar surroundings/ procedures Threat to transplant integrity (rejection episode) Interpersonal conflict	Subjective patient statement: "I feel nervous." "I feel scared." Objective behaviors: Withdrawal Crying	**Short-term** Transplant recipient will recognize anxiety and its cause. **Long-term** Transplant recipient will utilize effective coping	1. Assess level of anxiety. 2. Assist patient in identifying source of anxiety. 3. Provide emotional support: Stay with patient Reassure Speak slowly and calmly (continued)

NURSING CARE PLAN FOR PSYCHOSOCIAL ISSUES (continued)

Problems	Patient behaviors	Expected outcome	Nursing interventions
Financial concerns	Irritability Restlessness Increased blood pressure Increased respiratory rate Insomnia Decreased appetite Nonverbal behaviors Wringing hands Poor posture Avoidance of eye contact Pacing	to achieve psychosocial and physical comfort	4. Decrease environmental stimuli: Take person to quiet room. Consult doctor for possible pharmacologic treatment if necessary Limit contact with anxious friends or family 5. When anxiety is decreased, assist patient to learn effective coping: Relaxation techniques Deep breathing Soothing music Problem solving 6. Initiate referrals as indicated.

Carpenito, L.J. (1987). *Nursing diagnosis: Application to clinical practice, Second Edition,* (pp. 116–126, 408–416), Philadelphia: J.B. Lippincott. Kim, M.J., McFarland, G.K., & McLane, A.M. (1989). *Pocket guide to nursing diagnoses, Third Edition.* (pp. 86–89, 196–199). St. Louis: Mosby.

REFERENCES

Allender, J., Shisslak, L., Kasniak, A., & Copeland, J. (1983). Stages of psychological adjustment associated with heart transplantation. *Journal of Heart Transplantation,* 2(3), 228–231.
Carpenito, L.J. (1987). *Nursing diagnosis: Application to clinical practice,* 2nd Edition (pp. 116-126, 408-416.) Philadelphia: J.B. Lippincott.
Ciske, K. L. (1979). Accountability: The essence of primary nursing. *American Journal of Nursing, 79,* 891–894.
Gold, L. M., Kirkpatrick, B. S., Fricker, F. J., & Zitell, B. J. (1986). Psychosocial issues in pediatric organ transplantation: the parents' perspective. *Pediatrics, 77,* 738–744.
Harvison, A., Jones, B. M., McBride, M., Taylor, F., Wright, O., & Chang, V. P. (1988). Rehabilitation after heart transplantation: The Australian experience. *Journal of Heart Transplantation, 7*(5), 337–341.
Herz, F. (1980). The impact of death and serious illness on the family life cycle. In E. A. Carter & M. McGoldrick (Eds.), *The family life cycle: A framework for family therapy.* New York: Gardner Press.
Kim, M.J., McFarland, G.K., & McLane, A.M. (1989). *Pocket guide to nursing diagnoses,* 3rd Edition (pp. 86-89, 196-199.) St. Louis: Mosby.
Lough, M. E. (1986). Quality of life issues following heart transplantation. *Progress in Cardiovascular Nursing, 1,* 27–33.
McCollum, A. T. (1981). *The chronically ill child: A guide for parents and professionals.* New Haven; CT: Yale University Press.
Meister, N. D., McAleer, M. J., Meister, J. S., Rilery, J. E., & Copeland, J. G. (1986). Returning to work after heart transplantation. *Journal of Heart Transplantation,* 5(2), 154–160.
Mills, G., Barnes, R., Rodell, D. E., & Terry, L. (1985). An evaluation of an inpatient cardiac patient/family education program. *Heart and Lung, 14*(4), 400–406.
Parkinson, M. H. (1980). Psychosocial assessment. In J. Luckmann & K. C. Sorensen (Eds.), *Medical-surgical nursing: A psychophysiologic approach.* Philadelphia: W. B. Saunders.
Starkman, M. N. (1980). Psychological problems resulting from parent-to-adolescent renal transplantation. *General Hospital Psychiatry, 2,* 289–293.
Stone, G. (1979). Patient compliance and the role of expert. *Journal of Social Issues, 35,* 34–60.
Tedrow, M. P. (1984). Interdependence: Theory and development. In C. Roy (Ed.), *Introduction to nursing: An adaptation model* (2nd ed.). (pp. 306–322). Englewood Cliffs, NJ: Prentice-Hall.

CHAPTER **13**

REVIEW OF QUALITY OF LIFE AFTER TRANSPLANTATION

Kathleen L. Grady
Anne Jalowiec

IMPORTANCE OF QUALITY OF LIFE

As health care becomes more sophisticated, health care providers become increasingly capable of prolonging the lives of patients with serious chronic illnesses by using advanced technological procedures. However, patients are then often subjected to burdensome treatment regimens that cause major life-style upheavals, and so the question arises, "Does the increased survival time of these patients necessarily reflect a better quality of life?" Increasingly, therefore, quality of life (QOL) questions surface in choosing one treatment regimen over another, in evaluating the effectiveness of various treatment protocols, in clinical and ethical decisionmaking, and in health policy matters (Dean, 1985). Hence, longer survival time can no longer be the sole outcome indicator for making decisions about the effectiveness of treatment protocols or about the choice of treatment options (Wenger, Mattson, Fursberg, & Elinson, 1984).

It is thus obvious that the issue of QOL is becoming a central theme in treating chronic illness with sophisticated technological treatments such as transplantation of organs and tissues.

CONCEPT OF QUALITY OF LIFE

Even though the salience of QOL for chronic illness patients is recognized, QOL has remained an elusive concept to define and measure. McDowell and Newell (1987) feel that this occurs because "the concept is intuitively familiar" and therefore everyone knows what QOL is, so why bother defining it? However, examination of some conceptual definitions offered for QOL belies the idea that health care professionals intuitively know what QOL is and what it is not.

Examples of conceptual definitions found in the literature are as follows: Evans and his associates (Evans, Hart, & Manninen, 1984; Evans, Manninen, Garrison et al., 1985; Evans, Manninen, Maier, Garrison, & Hart, 1985) saw QOL as having two main dimensions: one objective (e.g., patient survival, employment status, ability to work, health status, functional impairment), and one subjective (e.g., patient well-being, life satisfaction, and psychological affect). Croog et al. (1986) based their assessment of QOL on five measures: sense of well-being, life satisfaction, physical emotional state, intellectual functioning, and performance of and satisfaction with social roles.

Wenger, Mattson, Fursberg, and Elinson (1984) define QOL in terms of three major components: functional capacity, perceptions, and symptoms. Subcomponents of functional capacity include the ability to carry out the activities of daily life; functioning in social, intellectual and emotional domains; and the ability to maintain economic status. Perceptions are defined as an individual's view of his/her situation and include perceptions of general health status, level of well-being, and satisfaction with life. Symptoms of the disease per se, those induced by treatment or concurrent illnesses, or those ameliorated by the intervention, constitute the third major component of QOL. The presence of symptoms is also likely to influence both functional capacity and perceptual views of QOL.

Sechrest and Pitz (1987) felt that QOL should be broadened to include significant others in the patient's life (spouses, children, intimate friends, co-workers). Ware (1984) proposed five elements to measure QOL: disease, personal functioning, psychological distress/well-being, general health perceptions, and social role functioning.

Thus, review of the literature on QOL shows only two main points of agreement that QOL is a multidimensional concept and that health and functional ability are primary determinants of how good a person's QOL is.

MEASUREMENT OF QOL

Since it is difficult to define QOL precisely, this in turn has caused problems in measuring it. Measurement issues have focused on two main considerations: (1) Should QOL be measured objectively or subjectively and (2) what are the important dimensions to include in assessing QOL and how does this differ for various patient populations?

Objective versus Subjective Measurement

Whether to measure QOL by objective or subjective means is an evolving and somewhat confusing issue. When QOL has been discussed in the literature, it has sometimes referred to using objective indicators versus subjective indicators. Commonly used objective indicators of QOL include income and socioeconomic status, which are more easily quantified, whereas subjective indicators usually refer to one's feelings about different aspects of one's life, which are more difficult to quantify (Levine & Croog, 1984).

At other times, the issue of objective versus subjective measurement has been addressed by obtaining an opinion about the patient's QOL from someone such as the health care provider versus getting the patient's own opinion. Overlap and confusion between these two measurement approaches may occur. For example, measuring functional ability as one aspect of QOL could be seen as either an objective or subjective approach depending on how it is measured (quantitatively vs. qualitatively) and also on who does the assessment (patient vs. physician).

The thinking in this field today recognizes the contributions of both objective and subjective indicators and provides a more comprehensive understanding of a person's QOL. Therefore, assessment of QOL should include both types of approaches.

Dimensions of Quality of Life

Similarly, there has been confusion and controversy about which are the important dimensions to measure in assessing QOL. Early studies looked only at physical functional ability in patients with chronic illness, or the ability to hold a job or return to work (i.e., more objective types of indicators). Then there was a growing emphasis on measuring the person's satisfaction with various aspects of his/her life; this became such a major focus in QOL research that life satisfaction was often equated with QOL. Overlap between these two concepts does exist, but some researchers feel that life satisfaction and QOL are not necessarily the same thing.

Therefore, dimensions of QOL that have been measured show that, in addition to life satisfaction, the following factors are also exceedingly important: physical and social activity, quality of relationships, number of social support resources, educational level, time and money for recreational activities, ability to get around outside the home easily, peace of mind, realization of career goals, energy to do the things the patient wants to do, health and happiness of family members, financial security and independence, ability to prepare sufficiently for old age, quality of the home and neighborhood environment, adequate sexual activity, good body image, absence of pain and other physical symptoms, and low stress with adequate coping (Ferrans & Powers,1985).

Since there is a limit to what can be measured in one QOL assessment, investigators have to determine what the important dimensions are given the population being examined and the resources available to evaluate QOL. Thus, QOL is indeed an important factor to examine in the chronic illness population. Although the concept still eludes precise definition, measurement must include both objective and subjective indicators, using a multidimensional approach to assessment.

Transplant patient populations have been the focus of QOL studies over the last several years. Kidney transplant patients were among the first populations to be studied, and there is also a growing body of knowledge about heart and liver transplant patients. Fewer studies have been conducted with the bone marrow transplant population. This chapter presents a representative review of the literature on QOL in kidney, heart, liver, and bone marrow transplant patients.

QOL AFTER KIDNEY TRANSPLANTATION

Studies on QOL after kidney transplantation have often compared kidney transplant patients to dialysis patients. Both objective and subjective indicators have been examined, and various dimensions of QOL have been emphasized by different research teams. An array of statistical techniques has been used to analyze the data and derive conclusions.

As part of the National Kidney Dialysis and Kidney Transplantation Study, Evans and his team (1984,1985) conducted the most comprehensive study on kidney transplant patients and compared the QOL of 144 renal transplant patients to 715 dialysis patients from 11 dialysis and transplant centers in the United States. Four major types of variables were examined: sociodemographic data, medical data, and both subjective and objective data on QOL. The results of this nationwide study were reported in several publications that focused on different comparisons of the data, both within the transplant group and between the transplant and dialysis groups.

Evans, Hart, and Manninen (1984) addressed whether subjective and objective indicators of QOL differed in patients with successful renal transplants based on whether they had cadaveric grafts ($n = 70$) versus living donor grafts ($n = 74$). Subjective indicators of QOL were based on the patient's perception of socioeconomic level, well-being (measured by the Index of Well-being), life satisfaction (Index of Overall Life Satisfaction), and psychological affect (Index of Psychological Affect). Objective indicators of QOL were physical functional status, based on the care provider assessment using the Karnofsky Index, and patient-reported ability to work.

The living-donor graft recipients showed a somewhat higher QOL than did the cadaveric-graft recipients on all indicators of QOL except psychological affect; however, none of the differences was significant. Therefore, the type of graft did not affect the QOL of renal transplant patients. However, the data reported were only for successful transplantations whereas 78% of failed renal transplants came from cadaveric grafts. The type of graft did affect the patient's QOL since patients with cadaveric grafts had lower survival rates, lower graft retention rates, and poorer rehabilitation profiles. Thus, it is only after the graft takes and the patient survives that it does not make any difference in the patient's QOL whether the graft came from a cadaver or from a living donor.

Evans, Manninen, Garrison et al. (1985) compared the QOL of renal transplant patients to all three kinds of dialysis patients noted above and found that transplant recipients consistently reported a significantly higher QOL than did any of the dialysis patients.

About 74% of the transplant recipients were able to work, compared to only 28% to 59% of the dialysis patients. In addition, 79% of the transplant recipients functioned at nearly normal levels, compared to only 48% to 59% of the dialysis group. Younger age, more education, and less co-morbidity were significantly related to better objective indicators of QOL. Transplant patients also had significantly higher scores on subjective indicators of QOL (well-being, life satisfaction, and psychological affect) than did any of the dialysis patients. Caucasians and younger and more educated patients scored significantly better on subjective indicators of QOL.

Simmons, Anderson, and Kamstra (1984) compared the QOL of 55 renal transplant patients (1 year posttransplant) to 321 dialysis patients from multiple centers in the Midwest. QOL covered physical, emotional, and social well-being. Physical well-being was measured by uremic symptoms, ability to perform daily activities, number of days hospitalized, and self-rated health perception. Indications of emotional well-being were self-esteem, depression, independence, control over destiny, and well-being. Social well-being was measured by vocational rehabilitation.

Simmons et al. (1984) found that the renal transplant patients scored significantly better on all indicators of physical, emotional, and social well-being. Compared to the dialysis patients, the renal transplant patients reported fewer uremic symptoms, less difficulty with daily activities, better health perception, less depression, better self-esteem, greater independence, more control over their destiny, and greater well-being. In addition, 78% of the male transplant patients were working, compared to only 32% to 54% of the male dialysis patients. Further, kidney transplant patients were significantly happier with their treatment than was either dialysis group.

Simmons, Abress, and Anderson (1988) later reported on the QOL of 113 kidney transplant patients from a prospective study in which patients were randomized to either experimental immunosuppressive therapy (cyclosporine with prednisone, $n = 64$) or conventional therapy (antilymphocyte globulin, prednisone, azathioprine; n = 49). Physical, emotional, and social well-being were again measured, in addition to satisfaction with health and social roles, worry about health, happiness with life, and family and sexual adjustment.

The Simmons et al. (1988) study showed that patients on cyclosporine scored significantly better on satisfaction with life, health, happiness, and emotional well-being, partly because they had fewer episodes of rejection and infection and fewer side effects. Simmons et al. discount the possibility that these results are due to a "steroid high." They point out that if the main causative factor was a steroid high, then the patients on conventional therapy (who received higher doses of steroids) should have scored better on well-being than did the cyclosporine patients, when in fact the opposite was found.

In one of the few studies done by nurses, Hathaway, Winsett, and Peters (1987) examined adjustment to illness in 97 renal transplant patients, using Derogatis's Psychosocial Adjustment to Illness Scale, which measures psychological adjustment to an illness in seven domains: health care, vocational, domestic, sexual, family relationships, social, and psychological.

Hathaway et al. (1987) found no significant differences in adjustment between males and females except in the psychological domain, where women reported more distress. Patients who identified a significant other in their lives were better adjusted in three of the seven domains: family and sexual relationships and vocational. The salience of a social support system for coping better with various illness-related stressors has often been documented in the literature. Patients who were working scored significantly better on vocational, domestic, and social adjustment; the relationship of employment to better adjustment has also been reported in other studies.

Hathaway et al. (1987) also compared the adjustment scores for renal transplant patients with previously established norms for dialysis patients and found, unexpectedly, that the transplant patients scored significantly better on only two of the seven domains: health care and domestic. Thus, although renal transplant patients often express greater satisfaction with their life posttransplant, this is not always reflected in better adjustment to the impact of the illness in all of the domains often affected by a serious chronic illness, nor is the expected rehabilitation potential of these patients necessarily achieved. Therefore, some of these findings would seem to indicate that patients trade off having to deal with some kinds of problems while on dialysis for having to deal with other kinds of problems posttransplant because of the complex medication and follow-up regimen.

Parfrey et al. (1987) compared the QOL of 97 renal transplant patients and 82 dialysis patients based on the following indicators: symptoms, activity level, well-being, general affect, life satisfaction, and subjective QOL. They developed a questionnaire composed of selected items from six other well known tools plus a new scale for symptoms.

Using age-matched patients, they found that the transplant recipients scored significantly better than the dialysis patients on activity level and on objective QOL but not on subjective QOL or life satisfaction. The investigators felt that transplant patients may have unrealistic expectations of transplant, which then influences their lower perceptions of QOL and causes them to be less satisfied with their lives posttransplant.

QOL AFTER HEART TRANSPLANTATION

QOL in the heart transplant patient population has been examined with increasing frequency over the last 5 years. There are, however, only limited QOL data available for heart–lung transplantation because the number of procedures performed is small, and length of survival as the primary outcome still requires extensive research. Investigators examining QOL in heart transplantation have used a variety of approaches to measurement, thus making meaningful comparisons among studies difficult. Populations examined in the literature have included heart transplant patients at a single institution, a comparison of heart transplant patients at two institutions, and comparisons between patients with heart transplantation and patients with coronary artery bypass grafting, kidney dialysis, and renal transplantation.

One of the earliest attempts to evaluate QOL in heart transplantation was a study by Christopherson, Griepp, and Stinson (1976), wherein rehabilitation of 56 patients who survived more than 6 months was examined. Through the use of medical records and data collected from patients and family members, they categorized patients according to the following rehabilitation statuses: competitive employment, retirement by choice, student status, homemaker, and disability. They found that 51 of 56 patients (91%) were successfully rehabilitated and thus able to lead physically and psychologically active lives equivalent to abilities attained before the onset of severe cardiovascular disease. Interestingly, only 26 of 51 patients (46%) returned to full-time employment.

In a preliminary report from an ongoing study, Hunt (1985) evaluated QOL through use of the Nottingham Health Profile (NHP) in patients before and after transplantation. The NHP measures perceived distress in six domains: pain, physical mobility, energy, emotional reactions, sleep and social isolation, and the impact of problems on daily activities, such as employment and personal relationships. Hunt found that perceived distress was very high before transplantation, especially in the domains of energy, physical mobility, and sleep and social isolation, all of which are reflections of poor health. After transplantation, significant improvement occurred in all six domains; and for 34 patients who completed the tool at 3, 6, 9, and 12 months posttransplant, the improvement was sustained over time.

At about the same time, Evans, Manninen, Maier, et al. (1985) reported on their QOL research on two major studies of heart transplant patients and kidney transplant and dialysis patients. Data were collected from 859 dialysis patients, of whom 144 had received renal transplants, and 59 patients who were heart transplant recipients. One of the tools used to assess objective indicators of QOL was the Karnofsky Index, which assesses functional impairment (the ability to perform activities of daily living); the physician completed this tool. The second tool used was the Sickness Impact Profile (SIP), a 136-item tool completed by the patient that assesses functional disability in 12 physical and psychosocial domains: body movement, mobility, ambulation, intellectual function, social interaction, emotional behavior, communication, sleep and rest, nutrition, usual daily work, household management, and leisure activities. Also, patients were asked about their ability to work. Subjective indicators of QOL were determined from the Index of Psychological Affect, the Index of Overall Life Satisfaction, and the Index of Well-Being.

Analysis of Evans's data revealed that for all objective indicators of QOL except functional impairment, heart transplant recipients scored lower than kidney transplant recipients. Thus, heart transplant recipients were in poorer health and less able to return to work than were kidney transplant recipients. Kidney dialysis patients ranked lower than both transplant recipient groups for objective indicators of QOL. Subjectively, heart transplant patients also ranked lower than kidney transplant patients on well-being, psychological affect, and life satisfaction.

Wallwork and Caine (1985) performed a preliminary prospective study to compare QOL between heart transplant recipients and coronary artery bypass graft (CABG) patients. Wallwork and Caine used the NHP and a QOL questionnaire with 30 questions assessing the following areas: symptoms, occupation, financial concerns, life-style, and expectations. Data analyzed in this study were collected from patients before surgery and at 3 months to 1 year after surgery. Before surgery, heart transplant patients were found to be significantly less healthy than CABG patients in four of the six domains (physical mobility, sleep, energy, and social isolation). After surgery, both groups identified significant improvement in their health profiles in all domains. Interestingly, heart transplant patients reported fewer problems with lack of energy and fatigue at 1 year after transplant than did CABG patients. Wallwork and Caine attributed this finding to the fact that transplant patients receive a "new" heart, whereas CABG patients have "repaired" hearts. By 1 year after surgery, 70% of the 30 CABG patients and 56% of the 24 transplant patients had returned to work.

In 1985, Lough, Lindsey, Shinn, and Stotts also examined QOL and life satisfaction as reported by heart transplant patients. A questionnaire was mailed to 100 adult heart transplant recipients who were between 6 months and 14 years posttransplant; 75 patients responded. The questionnaire covered QOL and life satisfaction, life change since heart transplantation, and symptom frequency and distress. From the 75 questionnaires that were returned, Lough et al. determined that patients were highly satisfied with their QOL after surgery. Positive feelings of life change including improvement in health, physical endurance, and self-accomplishment, were reported.

Lough et al. (1985) analyzed symptom frequency and symptom distress by dividing patients into two groups: those who received the immunosuppressant regimen of azathioprine and corticosteroids versus those who received cyclosporine and corticosteroids. The most frequent symptoms reported by patients in the azathioprine group were fragile skin and bruises (60%), while the most frequent symptom in the cyclosporine group was excessive hair growth (45%). The most upsetting symptoms in both groups were impotence and decreased interest in sex. Lough et al. pointed out, however, that the number of reported symptoms and the degree of distress due to these symptoms seemed to have little impact on the patients' subjective evaluation of their overall QOL or life satisfaction.

There is very little predictive research in the heart transplant literature; however, Brennan, Davis, Buchholz, Kuhn, and Gray (1987) published a pilot study that attempted to predict QOL based on pre- and postsurgical factors. A group of 11 patients who were at least 9 months posttransplant was examined using the QOL questionnaire developed by Lough and her colleagues (1985). Brennan et al. (1987) found that their results were similar to those of Lough and her group in that patients were more satisfied with their QOL after transplant than before. In addition, psychiatric diagnoses were recorded for each patient prior to transplant. Patients with a personality disorder had a lower QOL score than did patients without a personality disorder. This finding may be due to a problem with compliance with the medication regimen, which was identified in the three patients with personality disorders. Also, there was a trend toward positive change in QOL, especially job-related QOL, in patients who had shorter hospital lengths of stay and who required one or no hospital readmissions during the first year after transplant.

QOL AFTER LIVER TRANSPLANTATION

Studies of QOL in the liver transplant population are not as numerous as in other transplant groups. However, with liver transplant survival rates approaching 80% with the use of cyclosporine, outcomes related to QOL are more frequently being examined (Schade, 1987). The examination of QOL in the liver transplant population has usually included data gathered from children and adults after surgery. In one study, the liver transplant population was compared to patients with stable Crohn's disease to control for the effects of chronic illness (Tarter et al., 1984). Investigators from early studies limited their examination of QOL to objective dimensions, including survival and return to work. Later on, interviews and questionnaires were developed to identify patient perceptions of their QOL and life satisfaction.

Liver transplant recipients who survived from 1 to 14.5 years posttransplant (*n* = 44) were assessed for QOL by Starzl et al. in 1979. They defined
QOL as survivability and what patients had done with their lives posttransplant. Eighteen of the 44 patients (41%) died after 1 year, with an average
survival of only 2 years. As a group, these patients experienced many medical complications and poor rehabilitation, spending 56% of their time in the
hospital after the first year until death. The 26 patients who were still alive
at the time of the study had superior rehabilitation according to Starzl et al.
These 26 patients spent only 5% of their time in the hospital after the first
year posttransplant and returned to work or school. Starzl stated that long-
term prognosis could be determined in a patient by 1 year after transplantation and that social and vocational outcomes were dependent on graft function.

A more recent study by Williams, Vera, and Evans (1987) was conducted to
examine outcome, cost, length of hospital stay, and extent of rehabilitation in
liver transplant patients. Williams and his colleagues examined hospital
records of 55 consecutive patients who underwent transplantation from 1982
to 1985. One-year survival for these patients was 69%. The investigators
defined rehabilitation as full (return to full-time school, work, or home
responsibilities) or partial (improved physical activity and well-being without
a return to pre-illness activities). Of the 1-year survivors (*n* = 38), 79% experienced full rehabilitation. Further, Williams et al. stated that the costs
associated with liver transplantation were justified when compared with
patients who had end stage liver disease who did not receive transplants.

Tarter et al. (1984) used a series of standardized psychometric tests to
examine QOL after liver transplantation. They examined cognitive capacity,
emotional well-being, and social and behavioral functioning. Of paramount
concern in this study was the potential reversibility of hepatic encephalopathy, a frequent sequela of chronic liver disease. Ten liver transplant
patients (mean age = 28) were compared with ten patients with stable
Crohn's disease (mean age = 39) to control for the effects of chronic illness
on test results. Cognitive function was evaluated through a series of
standard tests that examined intelligence, attention, learning, memory, perceptual ability, psychomotor skills, and language. The MMPI and 16PF (Personality Factor) were used to evaluate personality and psychopathologic
characteristics. Finally, the SIP was used to evaluate physical and psychosocial functional disability.

The two groups did not differ significantly on tests of cognition, psychiatric
profile, or functional disability. However, when data from the liver transplant
patients were compared with normative population data, Tartar et al. (1984)
found that the liver transplant patients presented with moderate anxiety,
somatic distress, frustration, depression, worry, and withdrawal. Likewise,
functional disability, including lack of rest and sleep, decreased appetite and
eating, reduced work capacity and recreation, were found in the liver transpl-

ant patients. Tarter et al. concluded that the liver transplant patients have a basically positive prognosis regarding QOL.

In 1988, Colonna et al. reported on QOL in 28 adults and 32 children who were between 6 months and 3 years post–liver transplant. Objective and subjective indicators of QOL were studied. Researchers developed a questionnaire, to which 97% of the patients responded. Colonna et al. found that patients experienced improved QOL after liver transplantation. Whereas only 32% of adult patients were working before surgery, 75% were gainfully employed afterward. Likewise, activity tolerance improved significantly in both children and adults from before to after surgery. Although one third of the patients reported hirsutism, hypertension, and edema as their most common side effects after transplant, 75% were completely satisfied with the overall transplant experience. Sixty-seven percent of patients rated their posttransplant QOL as excellent; while pretransplant, 47% rated their QOL as intolerable.

More recently, Starzl et al. (1988) examined rehabilitation in a select group of liver transplant recipients. Patients with alcoholic cirrhosis (n = 56) underwent transplantation between 1969 and 1987, 41 of them during the cyclosporine era. For the 41 patients, 1-year survival was 69%, not statistically different from 625 cyclosporine-era patients who had received transplants for other causes of end-stage liver disease. More important, 61% of the alcoholics who received transplants survived more than 6 months, and of these, only 2 returned to drinking. Twenty-seven of the cyclosporine-era patients were rehabilitated and returned to jobs either as homemakers or outside the home.

QOL AFTER BONE MARROW TRANSPLANTATION

Literature on QOL in patients having bone marrow transplants (BMT) is sparse and is based mainly on anecdotal records and case studies, focusing mainly on symptomatology or on psychiatric aspects of bone marrow transplantation. Wolcott, Fawzy, and Wellisch (1987) point out that the following factors have made it difficult to perform systematic studies on BMT patients: the variety of bone marrow transplant regimens, the fairly small number of transplants done at any one center, the relatively high patient mortality following this procedure, and the fact that many BMT recipients live a far distance from the center.

Only one study was found that did a comprehensive assessment of the impact of BMT on the patient's life. Wolcott, Wellisch, Fawzy, and Landsveux (1986) examined the adaptation of 26 adult BMT recipients who had survived at least 1 year. Diagnosis was evenly split between aplastic anemia and leukemia. Variables studied were perceived health status, symptoms, moods, social role function, self-esteem, life satisfaction, and relationships with BMT donors and family members. Some of the results were compared with those of the donors.

A slight majority of the BMT recipients rated their health posttransplant as good. The most commonly reported symptoms were dry and sore mouth, diarrhea, and itchy skin. About one third of the patients reported a high number of infections, mainly colds. The Wolcott et al. (1986) study showed that three fourths of the BMT recipients were well satisfied with their activity level and their relationships posttransplant. Posttransplant social role function in the BMT recipients was, in fact, similar to that of a healthy general population used for comparison. It was also found that those BMT recipients who had higher self-esteem also had fewer problems with negative moods, felt that their health was better, and were better able to function in social roles.

The BMT recipients in the Wolcott et al. (1986) study felt that there was little change in their relationships with their donors compared to pretransplant; essentially the same view was held by the BMT donors. Interestingly, a higher quality of recipient–donor relationship correlated significantly with better self esteem and with better social role function in the recipient. The authors suggest that the recipient–donor relationship might be highly sensitive to changes in the recipient's physical and psychosocial status. Thus, a deterioration in the recipient's status can have strong negative psychological consequences for the donor, which can subsequently affect the relationship between donor and recipient. Accordingly, Gardner, August, and Githens (1977) recommend routine psychological evaluation of BMT donors because they found that some donors felt undue responsibility for the transplant outcome and subsequently developed inappropriate guilt feelings when graft-versus-host disease later occurred in the recipient. Therefore, bone marrow transplantation can adversely affect the QOL not only of the BMT recipient but also of the donor.

Other articles on BMT related primarily to physical and psychiatric symptoms in patients during the various stages of transplant. The articles did not focus on how these symptoms impacted on the patient's perceived QOL and ability to function, either physically or psychologically, posttransplant. Hence, the QOL of BMT patients is an area deserving of systematic and scientifically sound research. Furthermore, the issue of QOL following BMT takes on even greater significance because BMT patients tend to be younger and therefore potentially have a longer life ahead of them posttransplant (Kamani & August, 1984).

SIMILARITIES AND DIFFERENCES AMONG TRANSPLANT POPULATIONS

From this review of QOL after kidney, heart, liver, and bone marrow transplantation, one can derive certain conclusions. Generally, patients improve their QOL from before to after transplantation, although patients with psychiatric diagnoses may have less improvement in QOL after surgery. Problems with pain, energy, functional ability, emotional reactions, sleep, sexual function, and social isolation decrease after surgery. Furthermore, these improvements are sustained over time. However, worry, anxiety, and depression may still occur. Many transplant patients return to work; others choose to engage in volunteerism and recreational activities. Symptoms, depending upon the immunosuppressant drug regimen, are frequent and may cause distress. However, symptom frequency and distress may have little impact on perceived QOL and overall life satisfaction. Patients are thus apparently willing to make trade-offs between some distress after surgery in order to live longer, so they will view their QOL as good. These studies and personal reports contribute to the data base regarding QOL in transplantation and stimulate new questions for study in the future.

IMPLICATIONS FOR NURSING PRACTICE

Nurses must understand the impact of chronic illness upon patients' QOL while the patients are being evaluated, waiting for transplantation, and after receiving the transplant. Throughout the stages of transplantation, nursing diagnoses (Breu, Dracup, & Walden, 1987) are operative regarding QOL issues. Samples of these diagnoses are listed in Table 13.1. Understanding a patient's QOL and the changes that occur throughout the transplant process enables nurses to select appropriate nursing diagnoses and plan interventions to achieve specified patient outcomes.

CONCLUSION

Improved morbidity and mortality rates have encouraged researchers to study QOL in the transplant population. The measurement of QOL is still evolving; but in general, through the use of both objective and subjective measures of QOL in organ transplantation, researchers have found that patients experience improved QOL after this type of surgery. However, researchers realistically state that these patients still experience problems related to transplantation and have symptoms with which they must cope. Continued and more sophisticated study of QOL in this complex patient population will enlarge the body of knowledge from which we can gather information to provide better patient care.

TABLE 13.1 Nursing Diagnoses Related to Quality of Life Issues

Problem area	Sample nursing diagnoses
Activity/ability	Physical mobility: impaired
Attention	Attention, altered: distractibility
Communication	Communication: impaired verbal
Comfort/pain	Comfort patterns, altered: distress
Conduct/impulse process dysfunctional behaviors	Conduct/impulse processes, altered: dysfunctional behaviors, unpredictable behaviors
Coping: individual, family	Coping, ineffective individual
Diversional activity/recreation	Diversional activity deficit
Emotional integrity, feeling patterns, trauma response, violent behavior	Emotional integrity, alterations in: anxiety
Health maintenance	Self-care, altered: health maintenance
Home maintenance	Home maintenance management, impaired
Knowledge deficit	Knowledge, alterations in: deficit
Learning alterations	Learning, alterations in:
Memory	Memory altered: impaired short-term memory
Noncompliance	Participation, alterations in: individual noncompliance
Orientation	Orientation, altered: confusion
Participation: family, community	Participation, patterns, altered: ineffective individual participation
Role performance, parenting, family process	Role, alterations in: Parenting
Self-care	Self-care deficit
Self-concept, alterations in: disturbance in body image	Sexual dysfunction
	Sleep-pattern disturbance
Sexual dysfunction	Social interactions, impaired
Sleep/rest	Spiritual distress
Social interactions	Thought processes, alterations in
Spirituality	
Thought processes, judgment, decision processes	

Note. From "Integration of Nursing Diagnosis in the Critical Care Nursing Literature" by C. Breu, K. Dracup, & J. Walden, 1987, *Heart & Lung, 16*, p. 607. Copyright 1987 by C V Mosby. Reprinted by permission.

REFERENCES

Brennan, A. F., Davis, M. H., Buchholz, D. J., Kuhn, W. F., & Gray,L. A. (1987). Predictors of quality of life following cardiac transplantation. *Psychosomatics, 28,* 566–571.

Breu, C., Dracup, K., & Walden J. (1987) Integration of nursing diagnoses in the critical care nursing literature. *Heart & Lung, 16,* 605–616.

Christopherson, L. K., Griepp, R. B., & Stinson, E. B. (1976).Rehabilitation after cardiac transplantation. *Journal of the American Medical Association, 236,* 2082–2084.

Colonna,J. O., Brems,J. J., Hiatt,J. R., Millis,J. M., Ament,M. E., Baldrich-Quinones, W. J., Berquist, W. E., Besbris, D., Brill,J. E., Goldstein, L. I., Nuesse, B. N., Ramming, K. P., Salen, S.,Vargas, J. H., & Busuttil, R. W. (1988). The quality of survival after liver transplantation. *Transplantation Proceedings,20* (Suppl. 1), 594–597.

Croog, S. N., Levine, S., Testa, M. A., Brown, B., Bulpitt, C., Jenkins,D., Klerman, G., & Williams, G. H. (1986). The effects of antihypertensive therapy on the quality of life. *New England Journalof Medicine, 314,* 1657–1664.

Dean, H. (1985). Choosing multiple instruments to measure the quality of life. *Oncology Nursing Forum, 12,* 96–100.

Evans, R. W., Hart, L. G., & Manninen, D. L. (1984). A comparative assessment of the quality of life of successful kidney transplant patients according to source of graft. *Transplantation Proceedings, 16,* 1353–1358.

Evans, R. W., Manninen, D. L., Garrison, L. P., Hart, L. G., Blagg,C. R., Gutman, R. A., Hull, A. R., & Lowrie, E. G. (1985). The quality of life of patients with end-stage renal disease. *The New England Journal of Medicine, 312,* 553–559.

Evans, R. W., Manninen, D. L., Maier, A., Garrison, Jr., & Hart, L. G. (1985) The quality of life of kidney and heart transplant recipients. *Transplantation Proceedings, 17,* 1579–1582.

Ferrans, C. E., & Powers, M. J. (1985). Quality of life index: Development and psychometric properties. *Advances in Nursing Science, 8*(1), 15–24.

Gardner, C. G., August C. S., & Githens,J. (1977). Psychological issues in bone marrow transplantation. *Pediatrics, 60,* 625–631.

Hathaway, D. K., Winsett, R. P., & Peters, T. G. (1987). Psychosocial assessment of renal transplant recipients. *Dialysis & Transplantation, 16,* 442–444.

Hunt, S. M. (1985, September/October). Quality of life considerations in cardiac transplantation. *Quality of Life and Cardiovascular Care,* pp. 308–316.

Kamani, N., & August, C. S. (1984). Bone marrow transplantation. *Medical clinics of North America, 68,* 657–674.

Levine, S., & Croog, S. H. (1984). What constitutes quality of life?A conceptualization of the dimensions of life quality in healthy populations and patients with cardiovascular disease. In N. K. Wenger (Ed.), *Assessment of quality of life in clinical trials of cardiovascular therapies* (pp. 46–66). New York: LeJacq.

Lough, M. E., Lindsey, A. M., Shinn, J. A., & Stotts, N. A. (1985). Life satisfaction following heart transplantation. *Journal of Heart Transplantation, 4,* 446–449.

McDowell, I., & Newell, C. (1987). Quality of life and life satisfaction. In I. McDowell & C. Newell (Eds.), *Measuring health: A guide to rating scales and questionnaires* (pp. 204–228). New York: Oxford University Press.

Parfrey, P. S., Vavasour, H., Bullock, M., Henry, S., Harnett, J. D., & Gault, M. H. (1987). Symptoms in end-stage renal disease: Dialysis vs. transplantation. *Transplantation Proceedings, 19,* 3407–3409.

Schade, R. R. (1987). The changing indicators for liver transplantation. *Transplantation Proceedings, 19* (Suppl. 3), 2–6.

Sechrest, L., & Pitz, D. (1987). Commentary: Measuring the effectiveness of heart transplant programmes. *Journal of Chronic Disease, 40* (Suppl. 1), 155S–158S.

Simmons, R. G., Abress, L., & Anderson, C. R. (1988). Quality of life after kidney transplantation. *Transplantation, 45,* 415–421.

Simmons, R. G., Anderson, C., & Kamstra, L. (1984). Comparison of quality of life of patients on continuous ambulatory peritoneal dialysis, hemodialysis, and after transplantation. *American Journal of Kidney Disease, 4,* 253–255.

Starzl, T. E., Koep, L. J., Schröter, G. P., Hood, J., Halgrimson, C. G., Porter, K. A., & Weil, R. (1979). The quality of life after liver transplantation. *Transplantation Proceedings, 11,* 252–256.

Starzl, T. E., Van Thiel, D., Tzakis, A. G., Iwatsuki, S., Todo, S., Marsh, J. W., Koneru, B., Staschak, S., Stieber, A., & Gordon, R. (1988). Orthotopic liver transplantation for alcoholic cirrhosis. *Journal of the American Medical Association, 260,* 2542–2544.

Tarter, R. E., Van Thiel, D. H., Hegedus, A. M., Schade, R. R., Gavaler, J. S., & Starzl, T. E. (1984). Neuropsychiatric status after liver transplantation. *Journal of Laboratory Clinical Medicine, 103,* 776–782.

Wallwork, J., & Caine, N. (1985). A comparison of the quality of life of cardiac transplant patients and coronary artery bypass graft patients before and after surgery. *Quality of Life and Cardiovascular Care, 317–324,* 331.

Ware, J. (1984). Conceptualizing disease impact and treatment outcomes. *Cancer, 53,* suppliment 2316–2323.

Wenger, N. K., Mattson, M. E., Fursberg, C. D., & Elinson, J. (1984). Overview: Assessment of quality of life in clinical trials of cardiovascular therapies. In N. K. Wenger (Ed.), *Assessment of quality of life in clinical trials of cardiovascular therapies* (pp.1–22). New York: LeJacq.

Williams, J. W., Vera, S., & Evans, L. S. (1987). Socioeconomic aspects of hepatic transplantation. *American Journal of Gastroenterology, 82,* 1115–1119.

Wolcott, D. L., Fawzy, F. I., & Wellisch, D. K. (1987). Psychiatric aspects of bone marrow transplantation: A review and current issues. *Psychiatric Medicine, 4,* 299–319.

Wolcott, D. L., Wellisch, D. K., Fawzy, F. I., & Landsveux, J. (1986). Adaptation of adult bone marrow transplant recipient long-term survivors. *Transplantation, 41,* 478–484.

INDEX

A

ABO compatibility, 208, 277
Acute lymphoblastic anemia (ALL), 254–255
Acute tubular necrosis (ATN), 110, 111, 113, 114–115
  in heart transplant, 138
  in kidney rejection, 115
Acyclovir, 92, 110, 196, 214, 270
Adolescents, 271
  and compliance, 323
  self-image in, 269, 270, 321
Alcohol abuse, 188, 339
Allogeneic transplants, 206, 207, 215, 219, 225, 229
  in children, 252–253, 255
  graft-versus-host disease in, 221–224, 255
  and protected environment, 70
Allografts, 40–43
Allospecific antibodies, 42–43, 44
Amphotericin B, 63, 214
Anemia, 108, 114, 253–254
  aplastic, 204, 205, 253, 254
Anergy battery, 86
Angiography, 6, 8–9, 46, 152–153, 198
Antigen–antibody rejection, 42
Antigen-presenting cells (APC), 38–41

Antilymphocyte globulin (ALG), 108, 113, 178, 194, 197, 266
Antinuclear antibody (ANA) test, 92
Antiseptic bathing, 67
Antithymocyte globulin (ATG), 52–53, 148, 152, 223, 224
Anxiety
  assessment of, 319
  in children, 265
  concerning biopsy, 112
  concerning mechanical assist devices, 311
  dealing with, 54, 197
  in graft-versus-host disease, 224
Apnea testing, 7–8
Aspergillus organisms, 60, 62, 65, 68, 192
  and construction, 63, 68–69
  fumigatus, 61, 63, 68
Atelectasis, 193, 283
Autologous transplants, 50, 207, 219, 225, 226
  in children, 255
Autoperfusion, in heart–lung transplant, 25–26
Azathioprine, 111, 141, 148
  for children, 266
  in graft-versus-host disease, 223, 224
  infant dosages of, 285
  and leukopenia, 108

C

Protozoal infections, 60, 61, 62, 153,
215; *see also Pneumocystis carinii*
Psychological testing, 89, 97, 188,
322, 338
Psychosocial issues, 318–327
adjustment stages in, 324
assessment for, 318–319
in bone marrow transplant, 70,
224–226
in families of infants, 286
nursing care plan for, 325–327
in preoperative care of children,
255–256
Public Law 92–603, 4
Pulmonary embolus, 101
Pulmonary fibrosis, 166, 170
Pulmonary function tests, 88, 97,
152, 168
Pulmonary hygiene, 193
in children, 264–265
in neonates, 283
Purified protein derivative (PPD), 86
Pyelogram, intravenous, 98

Q

Quality of life, posttransplantation,
318, 329–342
components of, 330
importance of, 329
measurement of, 330–332
nursing diagnoses related to, 341,
342
and personality disorder, 337
studies of, 332–340 *see also specific
organ transplants*

R

Radiation, ionizing, 205
Rapid-flush technique, for liver
transplant, 28

Reimplantation response, 49, 138
Rejection process, 42–54
antibody-mediated, 42–43
in children, 266–268
classifications of, 43
diagnostic tests for, 48
and immunosuppressive
medications, 51–53
in neonates, 283–284
nursing care in, 53–54, 197, 284
patients' fears of, 54, 55, 197
signs/symptoms of, 48
of specific organs, 45–51,
112–116, 152, 178–179,
196–197
treatment of, 196–197
Renal scan, 111–112
Roller pump, 293, 297, 303
Rubella, screening for, 281, 285

S

Serologic markers, 66
Shumway, Norman E., 129, 130
Sibling donors, 206, 209, 253, 256,
259
Sickle cell anemia, 253–254
Sickness Impact Profile (SIP),
336–338
Skin
and corticosteroids, 151
hygiene, 72
involvement of in
graft-versus-host disease,
50–51, 222, 223, 269
maintaining integrity of, 193
Sodium nitroprusside, 135
Staphylococcus epidermidis,
213
Starzl, Thomas E., 186
Steroids; *see* Corticosteroids
Substance abuse, and kidney
transplantation, 83

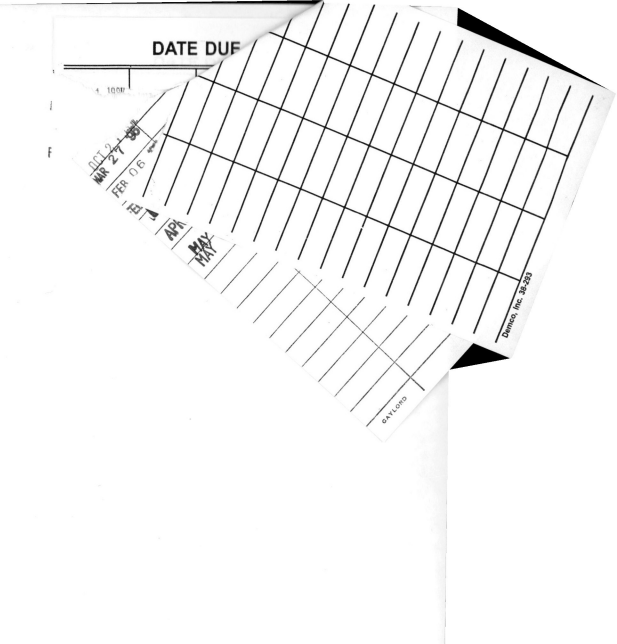